IAN Reviews in
Neurology 2023
Stroke and Headache

1695/-

IAN Reviews in
Neurology 2023
Stroke and Headache

Editor

PN Sylaja MD DM FRCP (Edinburgh) FESO FIAN
Professor and Head
In Charge, Comprehensive Stroke Care Program
Department of Neurology
Sree Chitra Tirunal Institute for Medical Sciences and Technology
Thiruvananthapuram, Kerala, India
Past President—Indian Stroke Association

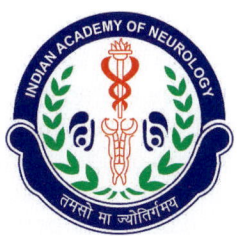

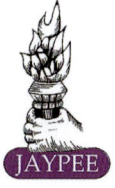

JAYPEE BROTHERS MEDICAL PUBLISHERS
The Health Sciences Publisher
New Delhi | London

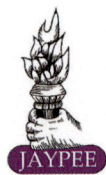
Jaypee Brothers Medical Publishers (P) Ltd

Headquarters
EMCA House
23/23-B, Ansari Road, Daryaganj
New Delhi 110 002, India
Landline: +91-11-23272143, +91-11-23272703
+91-11-23282021, +91-11-23245672
E-mail: jaypee@jaypeebrothers.com

Corporate Office
Jaypee Brothers Medical Publishers (P) Ltd.
4838/24, Ansari Road, Daryaganj
New Delhi 110 002, India
Phone: +91-11-43574357
Fax: +91-11-43574314
E-mail: jaypee@jaypeebrothers.com

Overseas Office
JP Medical Ltd.
83, Victoria Street, London
SW1H 0HW (UK)
Phone: +44-20 3170 8910
Fax: +44(0)20 3008 6180
E-mail: info@jpmedpub.com

Website: www.jaypeebrothers.com
Website: www.jaypeedigital.com

© 2024, Jaypee Brothers Medical Publishers

The views and opinions expressed in this book are solely those of the original contributor(s)/author(s) and do not necessarily represent those of editor(s) or publisher of the book.

All rights reserved. No part of this publication may be reproduced, stored or transmitted in any form or by any means, electronic, mechanical, photocopying, recording or otherwise, without the prior permission in writing of the publishers.

All brand names and product names used in this book are trade names, service marks, trademarks or registered trademarks of their respective owners. The publisher is not associated with any product or vendor mentioned in this book.

Medical knowledge and practice change constantly. This book is designed to provide accurate, authoritative information about the subject matter in question. However, readers are advised to check the most current information available on procedures included and check information from the manufacturer of each product to be administered, to verify the recommended dose, formula, method and duration of administration, adverse effects and contraindications. It is the responsibility of the practitioner to take all appropriate safety precautions. Neither the publisher nor the author(s)/editor(s) assume any liability for any injury and/or damage to persons or property arising from or related to use of material in this book.

This book is sold on the understanding that the publisher is not engaged in providing professional medical services. If such advice or services are required, the services of a competent medical professional should be sought.

Every effort has been made where necessary to contact holders of copyright to obtain permission to reproduce copyright material. If any have been inadvertently overlooked, the publisher will be pleased to make the necessary arrangements at the first opportunity.

Inquiries for bulk sales may be solicited at: jaypee@jaypeebrothers.com

IAN Reviews in Neurology 2023: Stroke and Headache / PN Sylaja

First Edition: **2024**

ISBN: 978-93-5696-309-2

Printed at: Samrat Offset Pvt. Ltd.

Contributors

EDITOR

PN Sylaja MD DM FRCP (Edinburgh) FESO FIAN
Professor and Head
In Charge, Comprehensive Stroke Care Program
Department of Neurology
Sree Chitra Tirunal Institute for Medical Sciences and Technology
Thiruvananthapuram, Kerala, India
Past President—Indian Stroke Association

CONTRIBUTING AUTHORS

Adreesh Mukherjee MBBS MD DM (Neurology)
Assistant Professor
Department of Neurology
Bangur Institute of Neurosciences
Institute of Post Graduate Medical Education and Research
Kolkata, West Bengal, India

Ajai Kumar Singh DM
Professor, Department of Neurology
Dr Ram Manohar Lohia Institute of Medical Sciences
Lucknow, Uttar Pradesh, India

Ajay Garg MD
Professor
Department of Neuroimaging and Interventional Neuroradiology
All India Institute of Medical Sciences
New Delhi, India

Ajay Hegde MCh DNB FRCS
Consultant Neurosurgeon
Department of Neurosurgery
Kasturba Medical College
Manipal Academy of Higher Education
Manipal, Karnataka, India

Akshaya Saravanan MD
Senior Resident
Department of Neuroimaging and Interventional Radiology
National Institute of Mental Health, and Neurosciences
Bengaluru, Karnataka, India

Alok Tyagi MD DNB OM FRCP
Honorary Clinical Senior Lecturer (Medicine)
Department of Neurology
Institute of Neurological Sciences
NHS Greater Glasgow and Clyde
Queen Elizabeth University Hospital
Govan, Glasgow, United Kingdom

Amit Kumar MD
Department of Laboratory Medicine
Rajendra Institute of Medical Sciences
Ranchi, Jharkhand, India

Angel Miraclin T MD
Assistant Professor
Department of Neurosciences
Christian Medical College Hospital
Vellore, Tamil Nadu, India

Aravinda HR MD DM
Professor and Deputy Medical Superintendent
Department of Neuroimaging and Interventional Radiology
National Institute of Mental Health, and Neurosciences
Bengaluru, Karnataka, India

Archana Sharma MD DM (Neurology)
Associate Consultant
AGRIM Institute of Neurosciences
Artemis Hospitals
Gurugram, Haryana, India

Ashish Kumar Duggal MD DM
Associate Professor
Department of Neurology
ABVIMS and Dr RML Hospital
New Delhi, India

Ayush Agarwal MD DM DNB MNAMS
Assistant Professor
Department of Neurology
All India Institute of Medical Sciences
New Delhi, India

Biswamohan Mishra MD DM
Assistant Professor
Department of Neurology
All India Institute of Medical Sciences
New Delhi, India

Chandrashekhar Deopujari MS MCh MSc
Professor and Head
Department of Neurosurgery
Bombay Hospital Institute of Medical Sciences
Mumbai, Maharashtra, India

Darshan Pandya MD
Senior Resident
Department of Neurology
Bombay Hospital Institute of Medical Sciences
Mumbai, Maharashtra, India

Debaleena Mukherjee MBBS MD DM (Neurology)
Senior Resident
Department of Neurology
Bangur Institute of Neurosciences
Institute of Post Graduate Medical Education and Research
Kolkata, West Bengal, India

Debashish Chowdhury DTCD MD (Medicine) DM (Neurology) FIAN FRCP (Edinburgh) Commonwealth Fellow in Stroke Medicine (Edinburgh)
Director Professor and Head
Department of Neurology
GB Pant Institute of Postgraduate Medical Education and Research
New Delhi, India

Deepti Vibha MD DM
Professor, Department of Neurology
All India Institute of Medical Sciences
New Delhi, India

Farsana MK MK MD
Senior Resident, Department of Neurology, National Institute of Mental Health, and Neurosciences
Bengaluru, Karnataka, India

George O Dickson MRCP
Honorary Clinical Lecturer (Medicine)
Department of Neurology
Institute of Neurological Sciences
NHS Greater Glasgow and Clyde
Queen Elizabeth University Hospital
Govan, Glasgow, United Kingdom

Girish Baburao Kulkarni MD DM MNAMS
Professor
Department of Neurology
National Institute of Mental Health, and Neurosciences
Bengaluru, Karnataka, India

Girish Menon MCh DNB FRCS
Professor and Head
Department of Neurosurgery
Kasturba Medical College
Manipal Academy of Higher Education
Manipal, Karnataka, India

Kamakshi Dhamija MBBS MD (Medicine) DM (Neurology)
Assistant Professor
Department of Neurology
Vardhman Mahavir Medical College and Safdarjung Hospital
New Delhi, India

Kamalesh Chakravarty MD DM
Associate Professor
Department of Neurology
Postgraduate Institute of Medical Education and Research (PGIMER)
Chandigarh, India

Kameshwar Prasad MD DM
Director and Head
Department of Neurology
Fortis Flt Lt Rajan Dhall Hospital
Vasant Kunj, New Delhi, India

Kanchana Pillai MD DM
Consultant Neurologist
Department of Neurology
Bombay Hospital Institute of Medical Sciences
Mumbai, Maharashtra, India

Meenakshisundaram U MBBS MD DM (Neurology)
Director of Neurology
SIMS Hospital, Chennai
Arunai Neuro Centre and Research Foundation
Chennai, Tamil Nadu, India

Mehul Desai MD DM
Consultant Neurologist
Department of Neurology
Bombay Hospital Institute of Medical Sciences
Mumbai, Maharashtra, India

Menka Jha MD DM
Associate Professor
Department of Neurology
All India Institute of Medical Sciences
Bhubaneswar, Odisha, India

MV Padma Srivastava MD DM FRCP (Edinburgh) FAMS FNASc FIAN FNA
Professor and Head
Department of Neurology
Chief – Neurosciences Centre
All India Institute of Medical Sciences
New Delhi, India

Padmasri Gorantla MD
Senior Resident
Department of Neuroimaging and Interventional Radiology
National Institute of Mental Health, and Neurosciences
Bengaluru, Karnataka, India

PN Sylaja MD DM FRCP (Edinburgh) FESO FIAN
Professor and Head
In Charge, Comprehensive Stroke Care Program
Department of Neurology
Sree Chitra Tirunal Institute for Medical Sciences and Technology
Thiruvananthapuram, Kerala, India

Ruby Chopra MD DM Fellowship
Headache Medicine
Consultant Neurologist
Department of Neurology
Delhi Heart and Multispeciality Hospital
Bathinda, Punjab, India

Samiran Chowdhury DNB
Department of Internal Medicine
Vivekananda Polyclinic and Institute of
Medical Sciences
Lucknow, Uttar Pradesh, India

Sanjay Prakash MBBS MD DM
Professor and Head
Department of Neurology
Smt BK Shah Medical Institute and
Research Centre
Sumandeep Vidyapeeth
Vadodara, Gujarat, India

Sanjay Rao Kordcal MD
Senior Resident
Department of Neurology
GB Pant Institute of Postgraduate
Medical Education and Research
New Delhi, India

Sanjeev Kumar Bhoi MD DM
Professor and Head
Department of Neurology
All India Institute of Medical Sciences
Bhubaneswar, Odisha, India

Sanjith Aaron MD DM Fellow
Cerebrovascular and Stroke
Professor and Head
Department of Neurosciences
Christian Medical College Hospital
Vellore, Tamil Nadu, India

Sapna Erat Sreedharan MD DM
Professor
Department of Neurology
Sree Chitra Tirunal Institute for Medical
Sciences and Technology
Thiruvananthapuram, Kerala, India

Sarah Miller MRCP (Neurology)
Consultant Neurologist
Department of Neurology
Institute of Neurological Sciences
NHS Greater Glasgow and Clyde
Govan, Glasgow, United Kingdom

Satish Khadilkar MD DM DNBE FIAN FICP FAMS FRCP
Dean and Head
Department of Neurology
Bombay Hospital Institute of Medical
Sciences
Mumbai, Maharashtra, India

Sonali Shah MD DMRD
Associate Professor
Department of Radiology
Bombay Hospital Institute of Medical
Sciences
Mumbai, Maharashtra, India

Soumya Sundaram MD DM
Additional Professor
Department of Neurology
Sree Chitra Tirunal Institute for Medical
Sciences and Technology
Thiruvananthapuram, Kerala, India

Sreenivas Meenakshisundaram
MBBS MD DM (Neurology)
Consultant Neurologist, Arunai Neuro
Centre and Research Foundation
Chennai, Tamil Nadu, India

Sucharita Ray MD DM PDF (Stroke and Cerebrovascular Disorders)
Associate Professor
Department of Neurology
Postgraduate Institute of Medical
Education and Research (PGIMER)
Chandigarh, India

Sumit Singh MD DM (Neurology)
Chief of Neurology and Co-Chief
Stroke Services, AGRIM Institute of
Neurosciences, Artemis Hospitals
Gurugram, Haryana, India

Surendra Kumar MD
Associate Professor
Department of Neurology
Rajendra Institute of Medical Sciences
Ranchi, Jharkhand, India

Tanushree Chawla MBBS MD (Medicine)
DM (Neurology)
Consultant Neurology
Department of Neurology
Institute of Neurosciences
Medanta – The Medicity
Gurugram, Haryana, India

Thomas Mathew MD DM
Professor and Head
Department of Neurology
St Johns Medical College
Bengaluru, Karnataka, India

Vimal Kumar Paliwal DM
Additional Professor
Department of Neurology
Sanjay Gandhi Postgraduate Institute
of Medical Sciences,
Lucknow, Uttar Pradesh, India

Vipul Gupta MD
Chief – Neurointerventional Surgery
and Co-Chief Stroke Unit
Neurointerventional Surgery
Artemis Hospital
Gurugram, Haryana, India

Vivek Nambiar MD DM
Associate Professor and Head of
Stroke Division
Department of Neurology
Amrita Institute of Medical Sciences
Kochi, Kerala, India

Preface

Historically, our engagement with headache dates back to 7000 BC when ancient civilizations considered it to be a sign of possession by evil spirits and demons, with a wide range of creative remedies to "release the demons" and relieve the symptoms. Early accounts of headache by Hippocrates are well known. *Ayurvedic* texts abound in descriptions of headache, and the doyens of Ayurveda, like *Charaka* and *Vagbhata*, grappled with the bane of headache. More recently, the scientific revolution began to unfold in the 16th century, and typically rejected the outlandish remedies of yore for headache and brought about rapid advances in our understanding of the affliction. Thomas Willis, considered to be the founder of clinical neuroscience, suggested that headache is caused by dilation of blood vessels. In the 20th century, Harold Wolffe studied headache in a modern laboratory setting and his experiments in the 1930s supported the theory that headache is due to vascular dilation. Today, as never before, we realize that the clinician should be abreast of recent advances in headache management that cannot be limited to pain relief measures. Not surprisingly, the causes of headache, and their management, continue to be an area of immense interest for researchers across the world. We are witness to an explosion of knowledge relating to the diagnosis and treatment of migraine and other headache disorders.

Of immense scientific interest and clinical relevance is the link between headache and underlying diseases that has lately attracted increasing attention. Notably, the focus on the relationship between headache and stroke has led to the recognition that the nature of headache may help predict and prevent a catastrophic event, and facilitate timely treatment.

This book is the inevitable outcome of our collective conviction that the time is ripe to put together ideas that explore the clinically relevant connection between headache and stroke. Apart from igniting interest in the subject, the compendium is expected to serve as a valuable addition to the repertoire of the practitioner, a tool that could potentially pave the way for more nuanced diagnosis, leading to treatment strategies that ensure better outcomes. Comprising 21 chapters, this compilation by eminent clinicians puts the spotlight on subjects ranging from diagnosis and management of migraine to complex headache disorders and headache associated with stroke.

It is pertinent to mention that this book, being thoughtfully brought out by the Indian Academy of Neurology, is an apt sequel to two earlier compilations, one on epilepsy and another on COVID-19 and Neurology. I consider myself singularly blessed to have been able to put together the trilogy.

PN Sylaja

Acknowledgments

As I come to the end of my term as Convener of the Continuing Medical Education Program of the Indian Academy of Neurology, I feel immensely happy that I too had an opportunity to contribute to the academic activities of the Academy. I am grateful to all my learned colleagues in the Academy for their unflinching support throughout my stint.

This collection, with its overriding focus on the link between headache and stroke, is a sequel to two earlier compilations, one on epilepsy and another on COVID-19 and Neurology. It has been an enormously satisfying endeavor to bring into a single volume a large body of clinically relevant insights on the subject. I thank the Indian Academy of Neurology for the opportunity to put together this magnificent compendium. In particular, I express my sincere gratitude to Dr Gagandeep Singh, President of the Academy, Dr Meenakshisundaram U, Secretary, and all the Executive Committee members for their support at all times.

I am beholden to all the authors whose steadfast commitment to this project, manifest in their firm adherence to tough timelines, has produced a piece of work of irrefutable clinical relevance. I am particularly obliged to Dr Debashish Chowdhury for being with me all the way, right from the start, providing timely guidance.

I thank the publication team at M/s Jaypee Brothers Medical Publishers, Ms Chetna Malhotra (Senior Director—Professional Publishing, Marketing and Business Development) and Ms Nedup Bhutia Pillai (Team Leader—Print Publishing), for their benevolent backing that has ensured the transformation of a fond dream into a coveted reality.

PN Sylaja

Contents

CHAPTER 1: **Reversible Cerebral Vasoconstriction Syndrome: Clinical Diagnosis and Management** 1
Vivek Nambiar, Sapna Erat Sreedharan

CHAPTER 2: **Pearls and Pitfalls in the Diagnosis and Management of Primary Angiitis of Central Nervous System** 9
PN Sylaja, Soumya Sundaram

CHAPTER 3: **Craniocervical Dissection: Diagnosis and Management** 16
Ayush Agarwal, MV Padma Srivastava

CHAPTER 4: **Approach to Thunderclap Headache** 21
Sucharita Ray, Kamalesh Chakravarty

CHAPTER 5: **Cerebral Sinus Venous Thrombosis—Management: An Update** 26
Sanjith Aaron, Angel Miraclin T

CHAPTER 6: **Cerebral Autosomal Dominant Arteriopathy with Subcortical Infarcts and Leukoencephalopathy: Recent Concepts** 34
Biswamohan Mishra, Deepti Vibha, Ajay Garg

CHAPTER 7: **Cerebral Vasospasm and Delayed Cerebral Ischemia Following Aneurysmal Subarachnoid Hemorrhage: Current Concepts** 46
Ajay Hegde, Girish Menon

CHAPTER 8: **Diagnosis and Management of Intracranial Dural Arteriovenous Fistulae** 54
Akshaya Saravanan, Aravinda HR, Padmasri Gorantla, Vipul Gupta

CHAPTER 9: **Headache in Stroke and Transient Ischemic Attacks** 65
Surendra Kumar, Amit Kumar, Kameshwar Prasad

CHAPTER 10: **Ditans and Gepants for Acute Migraine Treatment** 72
George O Dickson, Sarah Miller, Alok Tyagi

CHAPTER 11: **Non-headache Symptoms in Migraine: What do They Mean?** 81
Farsana MK, Thomas Mathew, Girish Baburao Kulkarni

CHAPTER 12: **Managing Chronic Migraine: An Update** 89
Kamakshi Dhamija, Tanushree Chawla

CHAPTER 13: Management of Cluster Headache: An Update — 103
Debashish Chowdhury, Sanjay Rao Kordcal, Samiran Chowdhury

CHAPTER 14: Uncommon Trigeminal Autonomic Cephalalgias: An Update — 116
Sanjay Prakash, Ajai Kumar Singh

CHAPTER 15: Tension-type Headache: Still an Enigma — 125
Menka Jha, Sanjeev Kumar Bhoi, Debashish Chowdhury

CHAPTER 16: Role of Greater Occipital Nerve Blocks in Headache Disorders — 133
Ashish Kumar Duggal, Ruby Chopra

CHAPTER 17: Hypnic Headache—Do We Know Enough — 147
Vimal Kumar Paliwal, Ajai Kumar Singh

CHAPTER 18: Diagnosis and Management of Idiopathic Intracranial Hypertension: An Update — 152
Debaleena Mukherjee, Adreesh Mukherjee

CHAPTER 19: Spontaneous Intracranial Hypotension — 162
Satish Khadilkar, Mehul Desai, Darshan Pandya, Kanchana Pillai, Sonali Shah, Chandrashekhar Deopujari

CHAPTER 20: Vestibular Migraine — 170
Meenakshisundaram U, Sreenivas Meenakshisundaram

CHAPTER 21: Neuromodulation in Headache Disorders — 174
Sumit Singh, Archana Sharma

Index — 183

CHAPTER 1

Reversible Cerebral Vasoconstriction Syndrome: Clinical Diagnosis and Management

Vivek Nambiar, Sapna Erat Sreedharan

ABSTRACT

Reversible cerebral vasoconstriction syndrome (RCVS), originally described by Call and Fleming, in peripartum subjects presents with recurrent thunderclap headaches with or without neurological deficits. It is a rare condition, mostly reported in adults with a female predilection; diagnostic hallmark is the angiographic demonstration of cerebral vasoconstriction, which reverses in 1–3 months. Though many have a severe presentation at onset, overall, they tend to have a good outcome with neurological sequelae rarely reported. Here, we present a brief review on this rare syndrome, its diagnostic markers, how to differentiate this condition from its clinical and radiological mimics, and the current evidence in management.

Keywords: Reversible cerebral vasoconstriction syndrome, Thunderclap headaches, Peripartum period, Hypertension, Angiography.

INTRODUCTION

Reversible cerebral vasoconstriction syndrome (RCVS) is a clinicoradiological syndrome characterized by severe headache with or without focal neurological symptoms with angiographic demonstration of cerebral vasoconstriction, which typically reverses in 1–3 months.[1] Termed postpartum angiopathy in the early 2000s due to its predilection in the peripartum period, subsequent reports suggest that the condition though chiefly affects young women, can occur even in 60s, and have many triggering factors.[2]

Though majority of patients have a uniphasic course of this condition, recurrent or ongoing symptoms necessitating hospitalization are not uncommon within first 3 months of the diagnosis[3] and on long-term follow-up.[4] Here, we give a brief overview of the clinical presentation, imaging findings, and how to differentiate from its close mimics followed by recent evidences in the treatment of this rare cerebrovascular syndrome.

EPIDEMIOLOGY

Though the actual incidence of RCVS remains unknown, there are many small and large case series reporting this condition since Calabrese proposed a diagnostic criteria in 2007 (**Box 1**).[5] Population-wide data from the US suggests that annual incidence of hospitalization for RCVS in adults is around 3 per million population per year.[6] The condition is reported across all ages from childhood to seventh decade of life, but the mean age of affected patients ranges between 42 and 50 years.[7,8] In adults, a definite female preponderance is noticed ranging from 1.8:1 to 8:1 depending on the study setting,[7,9] which may be secondary to hormonal or nonhormonal factors.[10] This condition is also reported in children, with a predilection for boys.[11]

A risk or precipitating factor is identified in 60–90% of patients presenting with RCVS, as shown in **Box 2**.

BOX 1: Diagnostic criteria of RCVS.

- Acute and severe headache (often thunderclap) with or without other neurological symptoms and signs
- Uniphasic course without new symptoms >1 month after clinical onset
- Segmental vasoconstriction of cerebral arteries shown by indirect (e.g., magnetic resonance or CT) or direct catheter angiography
- No evidence of aneurysmal SAH
- Normal or near-normal CSF (protein concentrations <100 mg/dL, <15 white blood cells/μL, and normal sugars)
- Complete or substantial normalization of arteries shown by follow-up indirect or direct angiography within 12 weeks of clinical onset or if patient dies in the acute phase, autopsy excludes alternate causes like CNS angiitis or aneurysmal SAH.

(CNS: central nervous system; CSF: cerebrospinal fluid; CT: computed tomography; SAH: subarachnoid hemorrhage; RCVS: reversible cerebral vasoconstriction syndrome)

Source: Adapted from Calabrese LH et al.[5]

BOX 2: Precipitating factors for RCVS.

- *Pregnancy and postpartum state*: With or without preeclampsia
- *Vasoactive medications*: Sympathomimetics, SSRIs, SNRIs, triptans, ergot preparations, and anti-inflammatory medications
- *Substance abuse/recreational drugs*: Alcohol, amphetamine, cocaine, ecstasy, and cannabis
- *Blood products*: Immunoglobulin, erythropoietin, and blood transfusions
- *Catecholamine secreting tumors*: Pheochromocytoma, bronchial carcinoid, and glomus tumors
- Miscellaneous trauma, migraine, head and neck surgery, carotid dissection, carotid endarterectomy, hypercalcemia, subdural spinal hematoma, and interferon alpha

(RCVS: reversible cerebral vasoconstriction syndrome; SNRIs: serotonin and norepinephrine reuptake inhibitors; SSRIs: selective serotonin reuptake inhibitors)

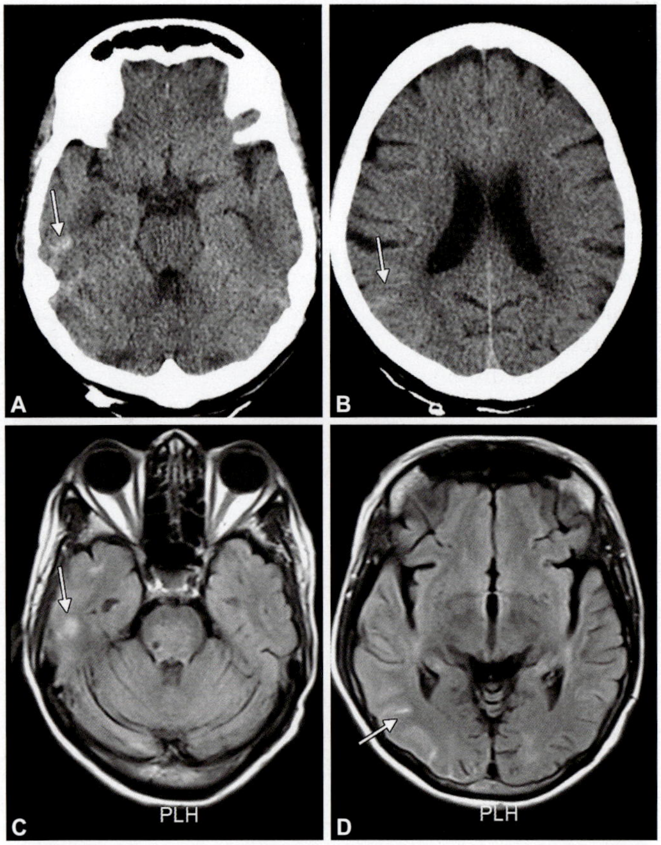

FIGS. 1A TO D: A 56-year-old lady with prior history of hypertension presented with acute onset left lower limb weakness, while she was watching TV without any headache, speech difficulty, visual symptoms or upper limb symptoms, or sensory disturbances, which completely resolved in 15 minutes. There were no preceding tonic–clonic movements also. She was found to have BP 160/90 mm Hg with no focal signs on examination. Noncontrast CT head done on the next day (A and B) showed cortical subarachnoid hemorrhage in the right temporal and right frontoparietal regions (arrows) with MRI brain FLAIR sequence (C and D) showing sulcal hyperintensity in the right parieto-occipital region with gyriform edema (arrow).

(BP: blood pressure; CT: computed tomography; FLAIR: fluid-attenuated inversion recovery; MRI: magnetic resonance imaging)

CLINICAL PRESENTATION

Clinical presentation of RCVS can range from uniphasic course of headache alone to rarely severe neurological deficits and death. Headache is the most common presentation of RCVS and is reported in 95–100% of series reporting this condition.[2] The classical headache in RCVS is thunderclap headache, which is usually recurrent, peaks in <1 minute, and can be associated with photophobia, nausea, vomiting, crying, and screaming in one-third to half of the affected patients. Though onset with recurrent thunderclap headaches is reported in 82–94% of RCVS[7-9] and can last for a week or so, recurrences up to 4 weeks are not uncommon. These attacks are triggered by bathing, stress, sexual intercourse, change in position, exertion, and coughing. In between the severe attacks, patients may report a moderate severity headache as well.

In around 5% of patients, only a single episode of thunderclap headache is reported, while a small fraction of patients can present without the classical thunderclap headache or even without headache also **(Figs. 1A to D)**.[9,12] The likely explanation given is that the headache may have been mild which could have been forgotten by the time the patient presented with a focal deficit, or subjects may be presenting with encephalopathy or seizures or aphasia where the history of headache cannot be elicited. Preceding history of migraine is reported in 20–40% of patients as well.

Other clinical presentations in RCVS include seizures, focal neurological deficits which may be transient or persistent, altered mentation, brain edema, and strokes secondary to complications of vasoconstriction. There is a wide range in the reported incidence of different symptoms across different clinical series of RCVS, reflecting mainly a recruitment bias.

Seizures are reported ranging from 1 to 17% in RCVS[1] and can be focal with or without generalization. They rarely persist beyond the acute phase and hence do not require long-term antiseizure medications. High blood pressure (BP) readings are noted in about one-third of patients with RCVS, especially during the acute attack, though history of hypertension is reported in <10% of patients.[7]

Focal neurological deficits can range from 8 to 43% and occur as a complication of vasoconstriction, which can outlast the resolution of headache. Deficits can be transient in around 16% of patients.[13] The most common clinical deficit reported in RCVS is visual disturbances followed by sensory, motor, or speech difficulties and ataxia. Deficits lasting for more than 24 hours are usually secondary to infarcts occurring in the watershed zones of cerebral hemispheres.

Neurological complications secondary to RCVS can be due to ischemia or hemorrhage or posterior reversible leukoencephalopathy syndrome (PRES). Hemorrhagic complications are the most common and occur early in the course of illness, within the first week of symptom onset. Vasoconstriction in the early course of illness along with high BP and cerebral autoregulatory failure can lead to rupture of pial vessels and cortical subarachnoid hemorrhage (SAH), which is reported in one-third of patients with RCVS. Parenchymal hemorrhage can also occur, ranging from 6 to 20% and is mostly single lobar, while some authors have reported subdural hemorrhage also in RCVS.[7,14]

In contrast, ischemic complications reported in 6–39% of patients with RCVS occur at least a week after hemorrhagic complications. Many patients may report resolution of headaches by the time they develop ischemic lesions **(Figs. 2C and D and Figs. 3F and G)** also, suggesting the persisting vasospasm as the underlying mechanism for the same.[7,9,15]

Reversible cerebral vasoconstriction syndrome and PRES are often encountered together and share many common clinical features and triggers.[16-19] PRES-like presentation in RCVS which is found in 9–38% of patients is characterized by headache and visual disturbances, ranging from hemianopia to cortical blindness and Balint syndrome, encephalopathy, and seizures. The incidence of seizures and focal neurological findings in this subgroup of RCVS is very high, as opposed to other presentations.

PATHOPHYSIOLOGY

The pathophysiology of RCVS is not fully understood. Two major hypotheses which are most accepted are disruption of cerebrovascular autoregulation and endothelial dysfunction.[20-24] Cerebral vessels are richly innervated by sympathetic nerve fibers. Sympathetic overactivity precipitated by vasoactive drugs, catecholamine secreting tumors, and hypertensive surges can disrupt the normal autoregulatory mechanism and lead to diffuse vasoconstriction and resultant complications. Once cerebral autoregulatory mechanisms are overwhelmed, there is endothelial dysfunction and increased blood–brain barrier (BBB) permeability. Vasospasm starts in the small distal arterioles initially in response to a precipitating factor and later progresses to involve medium and large arteries, which well explains the time course of symptoms and complications of this syndrome,[7] where neurological complications occur 1–2 weeks after the onset of headache. This hypothesis explains the phenomenon of vasoconstriction persisting beyond the resolution of headache in RCVS.

Endothelium plays a key role in perpetuating the syndrome by regulating vascular tone by secreting vasoactive substances. Endothelial dysfunction can result in altered permeability of BBB, which can be demonstrated by imaging also is the key to pathogenesis of RCVS. This mechanism explains the close association between RCVS and PRES, which occurs in over one-third of RCVS and has common precipitating causes.[9,21,25,26]

Peripartum period is one of the major risk factors of RCVS in young females, with factors secreted from placenta such as inflammatory cytokines and proangiogenic proteins such as placental growth factor and soluble endoglin having a major role in eliciting systemic immune response with endothelial dysfunction and vasoconstriction.[14,23]

Other factors which have been implicated in the development of RCVS are oxidative stress, humoral and biochemical factors, and genetic predisposition.[21,27] Estrogen modulates cerebral vascular tone and blood flow through genomic and nongenomic pathways, namely upregulating endothelial nitric oxide synthase (eNOS) expression, eNOS phosphorylation, shifting the prostanoid balance in favor of prostacyclin (PGI2), and reduction in vascular tone, ultimately leading to vasodilatation.[28,29] Estrogen has a significant role in modulating BBB permeability also, which explains why peripartum period with sharp drop in estrogen levels in maternal circulation is one of the major inciting factors for RCVS and PRES.[10,29]

Some authors have identified a genetic susceptibility in this syndrome as well, especially in subjects with no obvious precipitating causes. A genetic polymorphism of brain-derived neurotrophic factor gene (*Val66Met*) has been identified to increase the severity of vasoconstriction in RCVS.[27]

DIAGNOSIS

Diagnosis of RCVS is clinical and radiological. Cardinal clinical features include occipital or diffuse thunderclap headache recurring over days and weeks. These headaches may be associated with photophobia and phonophobia, focal neurological deficits, or focal seizures. An inciting event for the RCVS may be present in 60–90% of patients. Major precipitating factors include pregnancy and puerperium, drugs and toxins, pheochromocytoma, head trauma, neurosurgical procedures, etc. (**Box 2**). In the clinical context, neuroimaging including vascular imaging is required to confirm the diagnosis of RCVS and rule out close clinical differentials, which can present with similar clinical features acutely.

INVESTIGATIONS

Computed tomography (CT) with angiogram: Plain CT brain can identify intracerebral and SAH. In severe RCVS, there can be multiple territory ischemic infarcts. The SAH in RCVS is usually minimal in quantity and will be seen in the cerebral convexities (**Figs. 1A and B and Figs. 2A and B**). Large SAH at typical locations such as prepontine space, sylvian fissure, and anterior interhemispheric fissure are more favoring aneurysmal SAH rather than RCVS.

Even though CT angiogram can show the segmental narrowing and dilatation like beaded appearance of major intracerebral vessels in reconstructed images, vessel imaging can be normal in one-third of the cases in the initial week of illness.

Magnetic resonance imaging (MRI) and vessel wall MRI: Brain MRI helps to identify the sulcal SAH, especially after hyperacute stage when CT may miss the finding (**Figs. 1C and D**). In addition, it is highly sensitive in demonstrating parenchymal swelling, infarcts, or parenchymal bleed. (**Fig. 1D**). MR angiogram demonstrates the segmental narrowing of vessels and is a useful noninvasive tool for follow-up of patients as well. Vessel wall MRI with 3 Tesla MRI can be used to differentiate RCVS from its close clinical and imaging differential-intracranial atherosclerosis disease (ICAD) and central nervous system (CNS) vasculitis. In vessel wall imaging (VWI), RCVS shows no or mild (grade 1) concentric enhancement and no vessel thickening, while atherosclerotic stenosis shows eccentric wall thickening and enhancement and CNS angiitis shows thickening and circumferential uniform enhancement of medium vessels. Though in majority of patients with suspected RCVS, noninvasive imaging can help in arriving at a diagnosis and ruling out mimics, conventional angiography may be required in selected situations, especially when the possibility of aneurysmal SAH is high.

Digital subtraction angiogram (DSA): Angiographic demonstration of cerebral vasospasm (**Figs. 2 and 3**) and its reversibility still remains the gold standard confirmatory test in RCVS. It also rules out other clinical and imaging mimics such as aneurysms and cerebral venous thrombosis

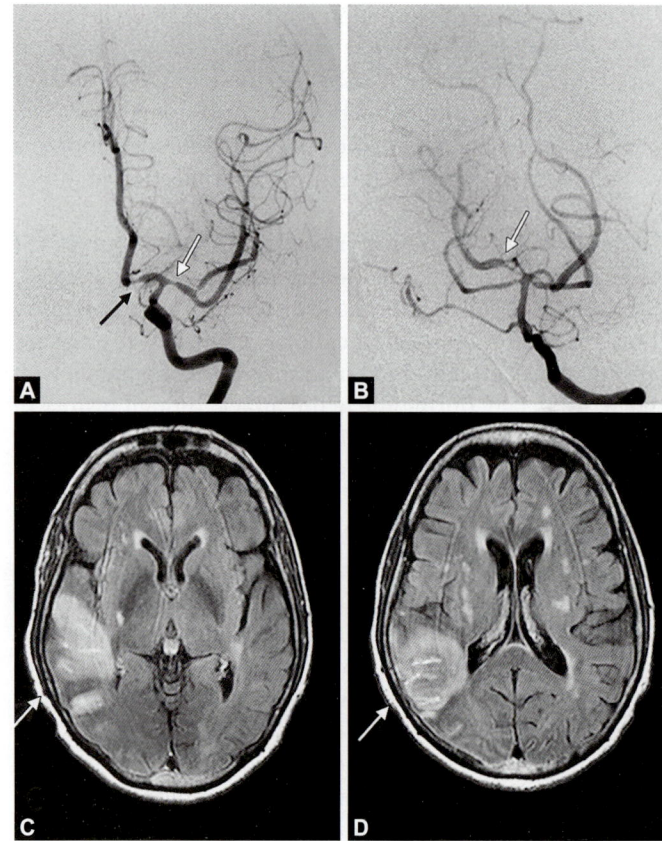

FIGS. 2A TO D: The DSA images of the same patient done on day 5 of symptom onset. (A) Left ICA injection with beading appearance (stenosis and dilatation), involving left MCA and ACA. (B) Left vertebral injection with classical beading in the right PCA origin suggestive of RCVS. She was initiated on nimodipine. The patient developed mild visual symptoms on day 8 of symptom onset and her repeat MRIs (C and D) show infarcts involving right MCA territory. She was continued on nimodipine and antihypertensives and on follow-up at 3 months, was completely asymptomatic except for left superior quadrantanopia.

(ACA: anterior cerebral artery; DSA: digital subtraction angiogram; ICA: internal carotid artery; MCA: middle cerebral artery; MRI: magnetic resonance imaging; PCA: posterior cerebral artery; RCVS: reversible cerebral vasoconstriction syndrome)

(CVT) and helps to differentiate from primary angiitis. Abrupt short segment stenosis is more likely seen in vasculitis, while response to vasodilator medications demonstrated in a repeat cerebral angiogram is helpful for confirmation of RCVS. The usual resolution of vessel spasm takes 1–3 months (**Fig. 3H**).

Transcranial Doppler (TCD): Arterial spasm causes significant increase in flow velocities and can be detected in bedside by TCD. The increase in velocity caused by RCVS does not meet the criteria for vasospasm after SAH, therefore can be used to follow-up imaging and therapeutic response. Noninvasive nature and bedside use make TCD a preferable tool for daily monitoring and can identify patients who are at high risk for delayed ischemia.[30,31]

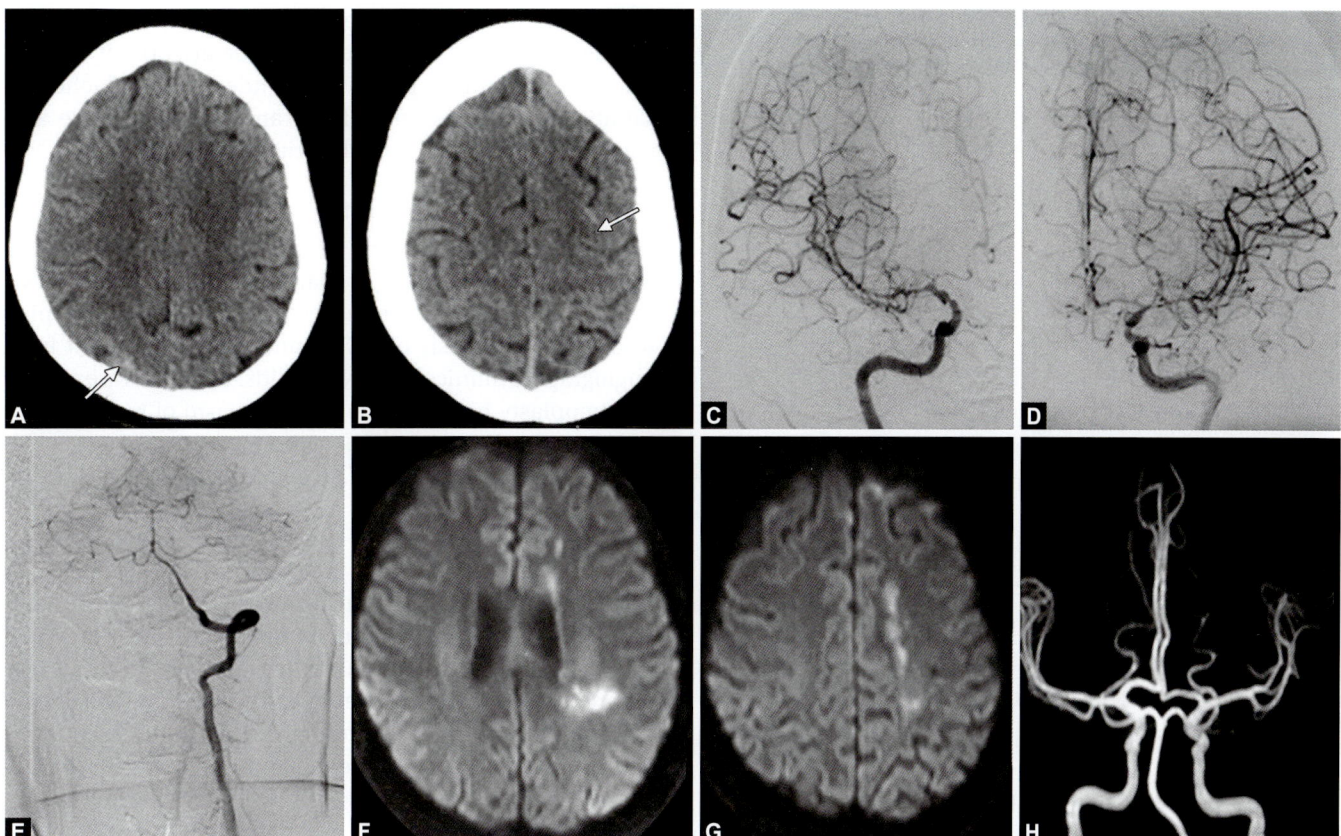

FIGS. 3A TO H: A 32-year-old lady, who underwent LSCS at term for poor progression of labor, without any significant antenatal history, developed acute-onset thunderclap headache on second day postpartum with dizziness. She was evaluated with CT head (A and B), which showed sulcal subarachnoid hemorrhage in left occipital (black arrow) and right high frontal region. CT venogram ruled out a cerebral venous thrombosis. She underwent DSA (C to E) on day 2 of symptom onset, which showed diffuse vasospasm involving right MCA M1 and ACA branches (C), left MCA (D), and left V4 segment of vertebral artery, basilar artery, and its branches (E). She was initiated on nimodipine. On day 6, she developed right hemiparesis with dysarthria. Her MRI DWI sequences showed acute infarcts left corona radiata and internal border zone (F and G). The patient was continued on nimodipine for 6 weeks along with physiotherapy and made a complete recovery. Her MRA repeated at 3 months (H) showed complete resolution of the diffuse vasospasm, confirming the diagnosis of RCVS.
(ACA: anterior cerebral artery; CT: computed tomography; DSA: digital subtraction angiogram; DWI: diffusion-weighted imaging; LSCS: lower segment cesarean section; MCA: middle cerebral artery; MRA: magnetic resonance angiography; MRI: magnetic resonance imaging; RCVS: reversible cerebral vasoconstriction syndrome)

DIFFERENTIAL DIAGNOSIS

Classical recurrent thunderclap headache and angiographic features, if present, make diagnosis of RCVS easy. In many situations, it may be difficult without classical features. Clinical differentials include other causes of isolated thunderclap headache, i.e., CVT, arterial dissection, SAH, spontaneous intracranial hypotension, and pituitary apoplexy. The most relevant differential is subarachnoid bleed in the first episode of thunderclap headache. Primary thunderclap headache is a rare headache disorder to be considered when a patient presents with recurrent thunderclap headache type and normal brain imaging.

The RCVS scoring system has been proposed by Rocha et al. with a high sensitivity and specificity in diagnosing RCVS and ruling out its mimics.[32] It is a clinicoradiological scoring utilizing clinical symptoms and imaging parameters and was able to differentiate RCVS from intracranial large and medium vessel vasculopathies **(Table 1)**.

Intracranial stenotic lesions with various MRI findings are a close differential for RCVS. Intracranial atherosclerosis and primary angiitis show more ischemic strokes. SAH and vasogenic edema predominate in RCVS. Multiple small, deep territory infarcts, extensive white matter changes, and contrast-enhancing lesions are more commonly seen with CNS angiitis.[33] Absence of brain MRI parenchymal lesions practically rules out CNS angiitis in this clinical scenario context.

TREATMENT

Treatment of RCVS is generally supportive along with management of complications. There is no evidence for a specific treatment improving the outcome.

TABLE 1: RCVS$_2$ scoring system.[32] A score of 2 or below practically excludes diagnosis of RCVS with 100% specificity.

Variable		Points
Gender:	Male	1
	Female	0
Precipitating factor for vasoconstriction:	Yes	1
	No	0
Thunderclap headache (single/multiple):	Yes	5
	No	0
Subarachnoid hemorrhage:	Yes	1
	No	0
Intracranial internal carotid artery affected:	Yes	2
	No	0

Total score of 2 or below: Negative for RCVS
3–4: Equivocal
5 or more: Positive diagnosis of RCVS
(RCVS: reversible cerebral vasoconstriction syndrome)

■ Supportive Measures

- *Pain management*: Adequate analgesia for the thunderclap headache and other types of headaches. Apart from nonsteroidal anti-inflammatory agents, opioids are also used for pain relief. Triptans and ergot alkaloids are avoided as they trigger vasospasm.
- *Blood pressure control*: Severe hypotension in a constricted artery can lead to infarcts, and uncontrolled BP can induce more vasospasm. Therefore, BP management is an act of balance, keeping systolic goal of 140-180 mm Hg, maintaining adequate cerebral perfusion, and avoiding rapid fluctuations in BP. Patients should be adequately hydrated with intravenous fluids—saline and intravenous antihypertensives such as labetalol and nicardipine are used for persistently high systolic BP values >180 mm Hg. Nimodipine, a cerebroselective calcium channel blocker, also reduces the BP and cerebral vasoconstriction.
- *Seizure control*: Appropriate antiepileptic medications are given for symptomatic seizures. There is no definite recommendation for prophylactic antiepileptic medications in RCVS.
- Empirical glucocorticoids are avoided as there is a chance of worse outcome.[9]
- No role for regular antiplatelets, statins, or anticoagulants even in case of infarcts, secondary to vasospasm

■ Specific Therapies

Treatment of Vasoconstriction

Vasoconstriction in RCVS generally reverses spontaneously over a period of 2–3 months. However, oral cerebroselective calcium channel blocker nimodipine has been tried in various studies but has been found to have no impact on angiographic resolution of the vasoconstriction. It reduces the intensity and frequency of thunderclap headaches.[7,30] Verapamil, magnesium sulfate, and dantrolene are also used in vasoconstriction with variable clinical effects.

Intra-arterial Therapies

Severe vasospasms are treated with intra-arterial nimodipine, milrinone, or papaverine and the reversal of vasospasm in the arterial territory of injection, helping to confirm diagnosis of RCVS, and differentiating it from angiographic mimics like CNS angiitis. There are rare reports of angioplasty being used in severe spasm of medium and larger cerebral arteries.[34,35]

COMPLICATIONS

Neurological complications are common with severe RCVS. These include seizures, posterior reversible encephalopathy syndrome, intraparenchymal bleed, and watershed infarctions. Anterior circulation watershed infarcts are common with RCVS in arterial dissection and neck vessel imaging is beneficial for ruling out carotid dissection.[36] A disabling neurological sequelae is seen with 5–10% of cases and usually are cases with severe peripartum angiopathy with eclampsia.

PROGNOSIS AND OUTCOME

Even though RCVS can have a turbulent course in acute phase, the prognosis is generally good in both adults and children. Long-term follow-up studies of RCVS showed an excellent outcome [modified Rankin Scale (mRS) = 0–1] in 90% of the patients.[37] Worse prognosis can be due to early infarcts and hemorrhagic transformation. Even with functional independence, a significant proportion of patients can have long-term moderate to severe headaches.[9] Recurrence of RCVS episodes are seen in 5% of cases and is usually clinically mild with isolated thunderclap headache.[4]

Avoiding exposure to known precipitating agents such as cocaine, selective serotonin reuptake inhibitor (SSRI), and other chemical agents will be helpful for prevention. Activities causing Valsalva maneuver, such as sexual activity, may be avoided for 4–6 weeks to avoid recurrent thunderclap headache.

CONCLUSION

Reversible cerebral vasoconstriction syndrome is a rare condition, which can present to stroke and headache specialists and needs to be differentiated from many clinical and radiological mimics, which vastly differ in their management strategies. With the availability of noninvasive imaging tools such as CT/MRI with angiogram and MR high-resolution VWI, diagnosis of RCVS can be made in majority of patients suspected with this clinical syndrome, though conventional angiogram remains the gold standard for confirmation of diagnosis. Management remains largely supportive, which includes identifying and avoiding exposure to the precipitating agents, maintaining euvolemia and cerebral perfusion to avoid complications, and cerebral vasodilators, though definite evidence regarding its efficacy is lacking. Overall, associated with a favorable outcome, rarely patients can develop delayed infarctions and neurological sequelae also.

REFERENCES

1. Ducros A. Reversible cerebral vasoconstriction syndrome. Lancet Neurol. 2012;11(10):906-17.
2. Erhart DK, Ludolph AC, Althaus K. RCVS: By clinicians for clinicians—a narrative review. J Neurol. 2023;270(2):673-88.
3. Garg A, Starr M, Rocha M, et al. Early Risk of Readmission Following Hospitalization for Reversible Cerebral Vasoconstriction Syndrome. Neurology. 2021;96(24):e2912-9.
4. Chen SP, Fuh JL, Lirng JF, et al. Recurrence of reversible cerebral vasoconstriction syndrome: A long-term follow-up study. Neurology. 2015;84(15):1552-8.
5. Calabrese LH, Dodick DW, Schwedt TJ, et al. Narrative review: Reversible cerebral vasoconstriction syndromes. Ann Intern Med. 2007;146(1):34-44.
6. Magid-Bernstein J, Omran SS, Parikh NS, et al. RCVS: Symptoms, Incidence, and Resource Utilization in a Population-Based US Cohort. Neurology. 2021;97(3):e248-53.
7. Ducros A, Boukobza M, Porcher R, et al. The clinical and radiological spectrum of reversible cerebral vasoconstriction syndrome. A prospective series of 67 patients. Brain. 2007;130(Pt 12):3091-101.
8. Choi HA, Lee MJ, Choi H, et al. Characteristics and demographics of reversible cerebral vasoconstriction syndrome: A large prospective series of Korean patients. Cephalalgia. 2018;38(4):765-75.
9. Singhal AB, Hajj-Ali RA, Topcuoglu MA, et al. Reversible cerebral vasoconstriction syndromes: Analysis of 139 cases. Arch Neurol. 2011;68(8):1005-12.
10. Topcuoglu MA, McKee KE, Singhal AB. Gender and hormonal influences in reversible cerebral vasoconstriction syndrome. Eur Stroke J. 2016;1(3):199-204.
11. Coffino SW, Fryer RH. Reversible Cerebral Vasoconstriction Syndrome in Pediatrics: A Case Series and Review. J Child Neurol. 2017;32(7):614-23.
12. Wolff V, Ducros A. Reversible Cerebral Vasoconstriction Syndrome Without Typical Thunderclap Headache. Headache. 2016;56(4):674-87.
13. Miller TR, Shivashankar R, Mossa-Basha M, et al. Reversible Cerebral Vasoconstriction Syndrome, Part 1: Epidemiology, Pathogenesis, and Clinical Course. AJNR Am J Neuroradiol. 2015;36(8):1392-9.
14. Stary JM, Wang BH, Moon SJ, et al. Dramatic intracerebral hemorrhagic presentations of reversible cerebral vasoconstriction syndrome: Three cases and a literature review. Case Rep Neurol Med. 2014;2014:782028.
15. Chen SP, Fuh JL, Wang SJ, et al. Magnetic resonance angiography in reversible cerebral vasoconstriction syndromes. Ann Neurol. 2010;67:648-56.
16. Singhal AB. Postpartum angiopathy with reversible posterior leukoencephalopathy. Arch Neurol. 2004;61:411-6.
17. Sadek AR, Waters RJ, Sparrow OC. Posterior reversible encephalopathy syndrome: A case following reversible cerebral vasoconstriction syndrome masquerading as subarachnoid haemorrhage. Acta Neurochir (Wien). 2012;154:413-6.
18. Soo Y, Singhal AB, Leung T, et al. Reversible cerebral vasoconstriction syndrome with posterior leucoencephalopathy after oral contraceptive pills. Cephalalgia. 2010;30:42-5.
19. Agarwal R, Davis C, Altinok D, et al. Posterior reversible encephalopathy and cerebral vasoconstriction in a patient with hemolytic uremic syndrome. Pediatr Neurol. 2014;50:518-21.
20. Chen SP, Yang AC, Fuh JL, et al. Autonomic dysfunction in reversible cerebral vasoconstriction syndromes. J Headache Pain. 2013;14(1):94.
21. Chen SP, Wang YF, Huang PH, et al. Reduced circulating endothelial progenitor cells in reversible cerebral vasoconstriction syndrome. J Headache Pain. 2014;15(1):82.
22. Lee MJ, Cha J, Choi HA, et al. Blood–brain barrier breakdown in reversible cerebral vasoconstriction syndrome: Implications for pathophysiology and diagnosis. Ann Neurol. 2017;81(3):454-66.
23. Pop A, Carbonnel M, Wang A, et al. Posterior reversible encephalopathy syndrome associated with reversible cerebral vasoconstriction syndrome in a patient presenting with postpartum eclampsia: A case report. J Gynecol Obstet Hum Reprod. 2019;48(6):431-4.
24. Chen SP, Fuh JL, Lirng JF, et al. Hyperintense vessels on flair imaging in reversible cerebral vasoconstriction syndrome. Cephalalgia. 2012;32(4):271-8.
25. Bartynski WS. Posterior reversible encephalopathy syndrome, part 2: Controversies surrounding pathophysiology of vasogenic edema. AJNR Am J Neuroradiol. 2008;29(6):1043-9.
26. Marra A, Vargas M, Striano P, et al. Posterior reversible encephalopathy syndrome: The endothelial hypotheses. Med Hypotheses. 2014;82(5):619-22.
27. Chen SP, Fuh JL, Wang SJ, et al. Brain-derived neurotrophic factor gene Val66Met polymorphism modulates reversible cerebral vasoconstriction syndromes. PLoS One. 2011;6(3):e18024.
28. Ospina JA, Duckles SP, Krause DN. 17beta-estradiol decreases vascular tone in cerebral arteries by shifting COX-dependent vasoconstriction to vasodilation. Am J Physiol Heart Circ Physiol. 2003;285(1):H241-50.
29. Bake S, Sohrabji F. 17beta-estradiol differentially regulates blood–brain barrier permeability in young and aging female rats. Endocrinology. 2004;145(12):5471-5.
30. Chen SP, Fuh JL, Chang FC, et al. Transcranial color doppler study for reversible cerebral vasoconstriction syndromes. Ann Neurol. 2008;63(6):751-7.
31. Merli N, Padroni M, Azzini C, et al. Reversible cerebral vasoconstriction syndrome: Strategies to early diagnosis and the role of transcranial color-coded doppler ultrasonography (TCCD). Neurol Sci. 2023;44(7):2541-5.
32. Rocha EA, Topcuoglu MA, Silva GS, et al. RCVS2 score and diagnostic approach for reversible cerebral vasoconstriction syndrome. Neurology. 2019;92(7):e639-47.

33. de Boysson H, Parienti JJ, Mawet J, et al. Primary angiitis of the CNS and reversible cerebral vasoconstriction syndrome: A comparative study. Neurology. 2018;91(16):e1468-78.
34. Song JK, Fisher S, Seifert TD, et al. Postpartum cerebral angiopathy: Atypical features and treatment with intracranial balloon angioplasty. Neuroradiology. 2004;46(12):1022-6.
35. Ringer AJ, Qureshi AI, Kim SH, et al. Angioplasty for cerebral vasospasm from eclampsia. Surg Neurol. 2001;56(6):373-8; discussion 378-9.
36. Cappelen-Smith C, Calic Z, Cordato D. Reversible Cerebral Vasoconstriction Syndrome: Recognition and Treatment. Curr Treat Options Neurol. 2017;19(6):21.
37. John S, Singhal AB, Calabrese L, et al. Long-term outcomes after reversible cerebral vasoconstriction syndrome. Cephalalgia. 2016;36:387-94.

CHAPTER 2

Pearls and Pitfalls in the Diagnosis and Management of Primary Angiitis of Central Nervous System

PN Sylaja, Soumya Sundaram

ABSTRACT

Primary angiitis of central nervous system (PACNS) is a rare inflammatory disorder, predominantly affecting the blood vessels of brain, leptomeninges, and spinal cord without any systemic involvement. Cerebral vasculitis due to systemic autoimmune and connective tissue disorders, drugs, infections, and malignancy is termed as secondary central nervous system vasculitis (CNSV). There are no objective clinical, imaging, or immunological markers, which can aid in the diagnosis of PACNS. A conglomeration of radiological findings of multiple infarcts of different ages, hemorrhages, and contrast enhancement in magnetic resonance imaging (MRI) of brain may suggest CNSV. The inflammation of vessels has to be demonstrated either in conventional digital subtraction angiogram (CA) or by biopsy. Since there are many conditions that mimic the similar imaging and angiographic findings, biopsy is required for a definitive diagnosis of vasculitis and to exclude alternate etiologies. High-resolution MR vessel wall imaging (HRVWI) has shown to be useful in differentiating various intracranial vasculopathies. Due to rarity of PACNS, randomized controlled trials for treatment are lacking. Induction therapy with combination of corticosteroids and cyclophosphamide (CYC) followed by maintenance therapy with azathioprine, mycophenolate mofetil (MMF), or methotrexate is the preferred line of management. Biological agents can be given in refractory cases. There are many uncertainties in the diagnosis and management of PACNS, which will be discussed in this chapter.

Keywords: Primary angiitis of central nervous system, CNSV, Diagnosis, Outcome, Treatment.

INTRODUCTION

Primary angiitis of central nervous system (PACNS) or primary central nervous system vasculitis (PCNSV) is a rare inflammatory disorder, predominantly affecting the blood vessels of brain and leptomeninges and rarely the spinal cord, but not secondary to any infective, neoplastic, or systemic causes.[1,2] Cerebral vasculitis due to systemic autoimmune and connective tissue disorders, drugs, viral, bacterial, fungal, and parasitic infections and malignancy is termed as secondary central nervous system vasculitis (CNSV). The neurological features are diverse and indistinguishable in primary and secondary CNSV. Stenosis, occlusion, necrosis, and destruction of cerebral vessels are the net effects of vasculitis leading to various clinical manifestations.[3]

PACNS is a difficult diagnosis for clinicians, since there are no objective clinical, imaging, or immunological markers, which can aid in the diagnosis.[4] The inflammation of vessels has to be demonstrated either in conventional digital subtraction angiogram (CA) or by biopsy. Since there are many conditions that can mimic the similar angiographic findings, biopsy is required for a definitive diagnosis of vasculitis and to exclude alternate etiologies.[5] To differentiate various intracranial vasculopathies, high-resolution MR vessel wall imaging (HRVWI) has shown to be a promising tool, especially in PACNS, intracranial atherosclerotic disease (ICAD), and moyamoya disease (MMD).[6,7]

The exact cause for PACNS is unknown and the immunological cascade triggered by infective organisms such as varicella zoster has been proposed, which needs further clarification. Therefore, immunosuppressive medications are the mainstay of treatment in PACNS.[8-10] Despite such aggressive treatment with corticosteroids and cyclophosphamide (CYC), a small proportion of patients progressively worsens with a fatal course. Rituximab and anti-tumor necrosis factor alpha (TNF-α) inhibitors are tried in refractory cases.[9-11] We still do not have clarity on the duration of treatment and when and how to de-escalate the treatment and how to manage refractory cases. In this chapter, we will be discussing the pitfalls in the diagnostic aspects of PACNS and its management.

CLINICAL FEATURES

There is no single clinical feature that is implicative of PACNS. The disease can affect individuals of any age group. The earlier reports have mentioned the median age of onset as 50 years with slight female preponderance.[4,12] However, the recent studies from India showed a median age of onset 34–36 years with male predilection.[13,14]

The clinical manifestations are manifold and depend on the type of vessels affected and the extend of the vasculitic process. The onset is variable ranging from days to months and comprises of headache, focal neurological deficits, dementia, and encephalopathy.[15] In the largest cohort of adult PACNS patients from Mayo Clinic, the most common clinical manifestations at presentation were headache (60%), cognitive dysfunction (54%), focal neurological deficits including stroke (41%) and seizures (20%).[12] Other frequent symptoms included hemiparesis, ataxia, dysarthria, aphasia, vertigo, impaired vigilance, visual impairment, and psychiatric features.[10] Headaches could precede by a few days or weeks or accompany other neurologic manifestations of PACNS.[8] Systemic manifestations of inflammation such as fever, fatigue, arthralgia, livedo reticularis, anorexia, and weight loss were seen in <10%.[12] If present, secondary causes need to be pursued. Patients with large- or medium-sized cerebral vasculitis more frequently present acutely with stroke. Small vessel cerebral vasculitis often present subacutely as rapidly progressive cognitive decline or encephalopathy and seizures.[10,15] Gamuts of other causes of rapidly progressive dementia encompassing autoimmune encephalitis, other inflammatory conditions, chronic CNS infections, and metabolic causes are important differentials in this scenario.[16] Stuttering course with stroke and cognitive decline can occur when there is diffuse involvement of cerebral vessels.

PACNS is an important diagnostic consideration along with other causes of vasculopathies, demyelinating disorders, and mitochondrial cytopathies in a patient with recurrent neurological events. Neurological deficits progressing over days with typical presentation of optic neuritis and myelopathy suggest CNS demyelination. Headache and seizures are unlikely in demyelinating

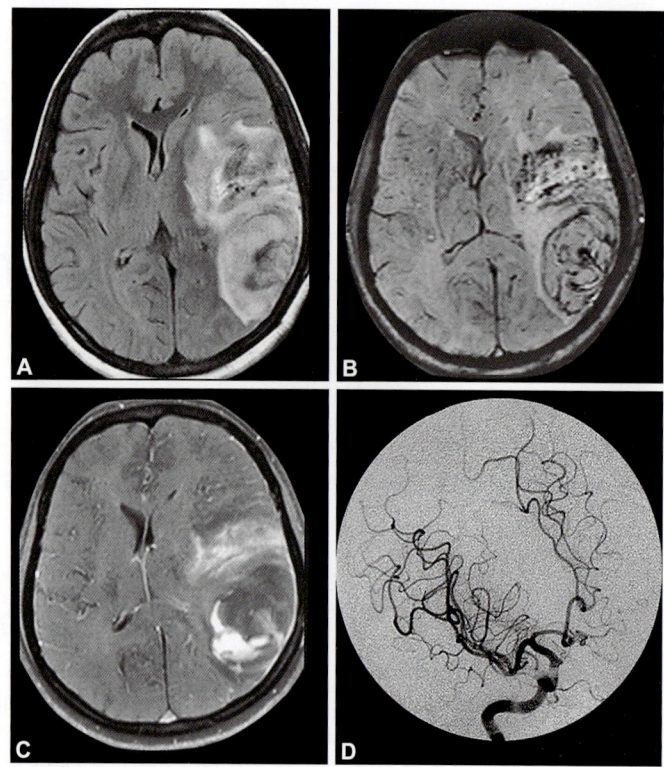

FIGS. 1A TO D: Neuroimaging of a 44-year-old female, who presented with subacute-onset progressive word-finding difficulty and right upper limb weakness. Magnetic resonance imaging of brain shows (A) tumor-like lesion with hyperintensity in the fluid-attenuated inversion recovery sequence, (B) blooming artifacts in the susceptibility-weighted sequence, (C) contrast enhancement after gadolinium administration in T1-weighted sequence, and (D) with normal angiogram in the right internal carotid artery injection. Meningocortical biopsy showed necrotizing pattern of cerebral vasculitis confirming the diagnosis of primary angiitis of central nervous system in this patient.

disorders.[17] However, encephalopathy, migraine, seizures, and stroke-like episodes are classical in mitochondrial encephalomyopathy, lactic acidosis, and stroke-like episodes (MELAS) syndrome.[18] The other rare presentations of PACNS are intracranial hemorrhage, tumor-like mass lesions **(Figs. 1A to D)**, and myelopathy.[8,13] Even if there are no pathognomonic clinical features in PACNS, this entity should be kept in the differential diagnosis and investigated in patients with strokes, encephalopathy, and cognitive decline.

INVESTIGATIONS

There are no blood based biomarkers identified till now for PACNS. Hematological, immunological, and serological tests are done to exclude alternate causes, rather than confirming the diagnosis of PACNS **(Table 1)**.[10] Sometimes elevated levels of C-reactive protein (CRP) in serum, low-titers of antinuclear antibodies (ANA) without anti-double-stranded

TABLE 1: Secondary causes of CNSV.	
Conditions causing CNSV	
Primary cerebral vasculitis	• Primary angiitis of CNS • Amyloid-β-related angiitis
Systemic vasculitis	• Behçet's disease • Churg–Strauss syndrome • Giant cell arteritis • Henoch–Schönlein purpura • Kawasaki disease • Polyarteritis nodosa • Takayasu arteritis
Connective tissue diseases	• Antiphospholipid antibody syndrome • Dermatomyositis • Mixed connective tissue disease • Rheumatoid arthritis • Sjögren's syndrome • Systemic lupus erythematosus • Systemic sclerosis
Other autoimmune disorders	• Cryoglobulinemia • Cogan's syndrome • Eales disease • Sarcoidosis
Infections	• Bacteria (tuberculosis, syphilis, *Mycoplasma*, rickettsia, *Listeria*, and Lyme disease) • Viral (varicella zoster, cytomegalovirus, Epstein–Barr virus, parvovirus B19, hepatitis C, hepatitis B, and HIV) • Fungi (aspergillosis, mucormycosis, histoplasma, and coccidioidomycosis) • Parasites (neurocysticercosis, toxoplasma, and malaria)
Neoplasms	• Atrial myxoma • Hodgkin and non-Hodgkin lymphomas • Intravascular lymphoma
Drugs	• Amphetamine • Cocaine • Epinephrine

(CNSV: central nervous system vasculitis; HIV: human immunodeficiency virus)

DNA positivity, and low titers of antineutrophil cytoplasmic antibodies (ANCAs) seen in PACNS can complicate the diagnosis. However, absence of constitutional symptoms and other organ system involvement argues against a systemic vasculitic or immune-mediated disorder.[8]

Magnetic resonance imaging (MRI) of brain with gadolinium contrast is the initial investigation of choice to delineate the underlying pathology behind the clinical presentation. If MRI is normal, then other causes should be explored. Multiple arterial territory infarcts, infarcts of different ages (acute, subacute, and chronic infarcts), hemorrhagic infarcts, microbleeds outside the infarct tissue and small vessel ischemic changes are seen in various combinations in patients with PACNS **(Figs. 2A to F)**. Hemorrhagic manifestations are very frequent and include parenchymal, subarachnoid hemorrhage (SAH), and rarely intraventricular hemorrhage.[19] Multiple microbleeds ≥5 were seen in one-third patients.[13] Intracranial hemorrhages are more frequent with necrotizing pattern of vasculitis, whereas parenchymal and leptomeningeal enhancement was more common with granulomatous pattern.[10] However ICAD, cardioembolism, cerebral amyloid angiopathy (CAA), amyloid beta-related angiiits (ABRA), cerebral autosomal dominant arteriopathy with subcortical infarcts and leukoencephalopathy (CADASIL), hematological disorders, and malignancies are a few conditions that can mimic the clinical and imaging features of PACNS.[20] In those presenting with stroke, a good number of older patients have vascular risk factors such as hypertension, hyperlipidemia, and diabetes mellitus, thereby mislabeling PACNS as ICAD.[2] Cardiac workup and luminal imaging can exclude the embolic and large artery atherosclerotic disease. In SAH presentations, reversible cerebral vasoconstriction syndrome (RCVS) is a possibility and a repeat CA after 3 months should be considered to demonstrate the disappearance of vasculitic features. Leptomeningeal enhancement is also unlikely in RCVS.[19] Myelopathy is rare and only 1 out of 12 patients showed longitudinally extensive transverse myelitis.[13]

Magnetic resonance angiography with contrast or time-of-flight (TOF-MRA) images can also detect features of vasculitis, but the sensitivity is low as compared to CA. In addition, TOF-MRA does not provide information on flow dynamics and collaterals and cortical branches are not reliably visible as compared to CA. In the French series of PACNS, multifocal narrowing in multiple vessels was demonstrated in one half of patients who underwent TOF-MRA.[19] In the Indian series also 10 out of 22 patients who underwent TOF-MRA showed vasculitic changes.[13] TOF-MRA can be utilized as the initial luminal imaging for suspected CNSV, and CA can be avoided if findings are certain. TOF-MRA could also be utilized for monitoring the disease activity, thereby avoiding repeated contrast injection with CA.[8] MMD, atherosclerotic plaque, dissection, and large vessel vasculitis such as Takayasu arteritis can also be detected with TOF-MRA.[21]

In order to demonstrate the features of vasculitis, luminal imaging technique preferably CA is favored over MRA/computed tomography angiogram (CTA). In suspected cases of CNSV, the diagnostic yield of CA can be up to 88%.[12] Steno-occlusive lesions in multiple vessels and beading pattern due to alternate dilations and stenosis is the most frequent finding.[3,8] Microaneurysms are rare. Isolated posterior circulation involvement is unusual. Small arteries are not visible in angiography and can be diagnosed

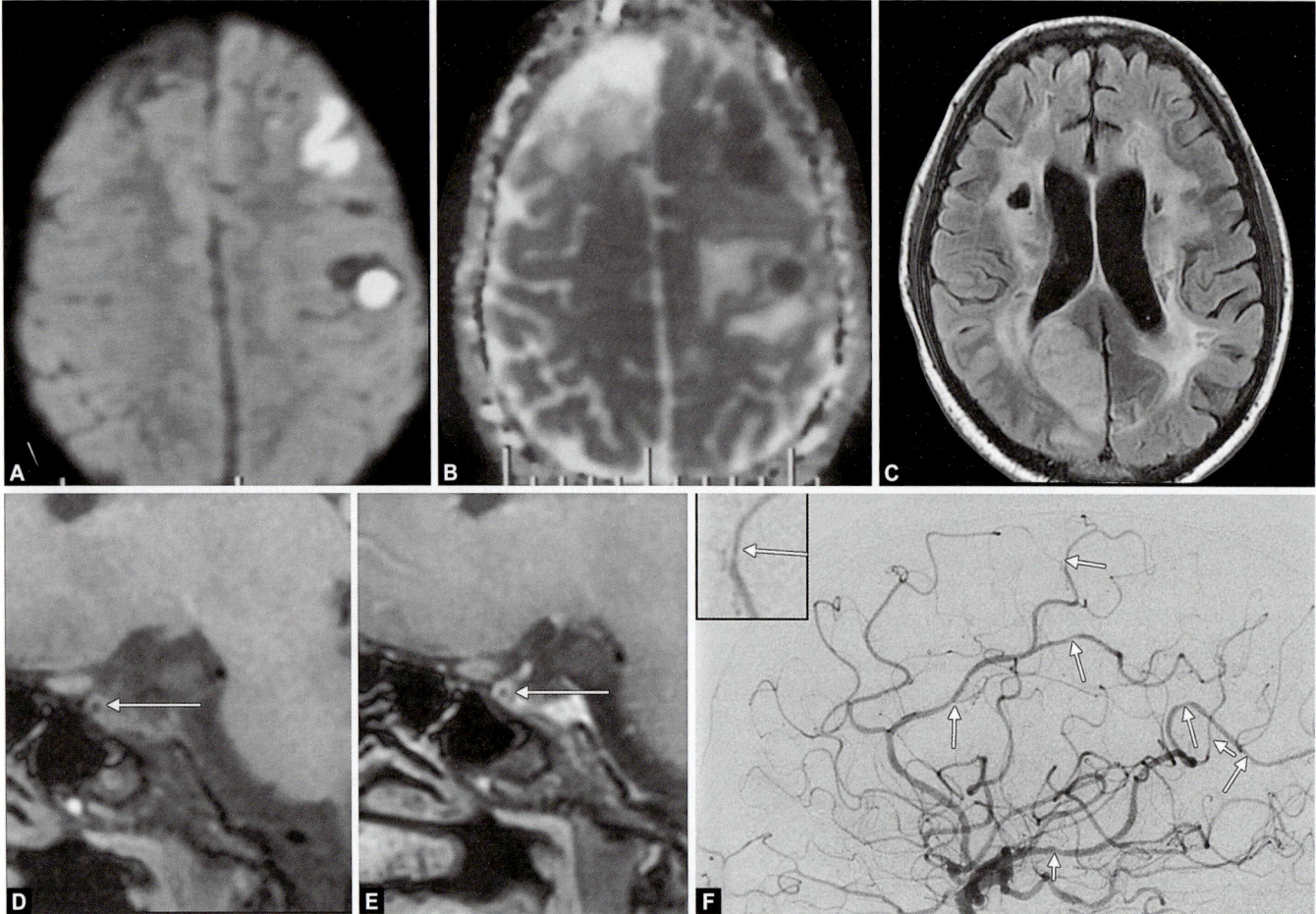

FIGS. 2A TO F: Neuroimaging in primary angiitis of central nervous system. (A) Diffusion-weighted and (B) apparent diffusion coefficient sequences show acute left middle cerebral artery territory infarcts. (C) Fluid-attenuated inversion recovery sequence shows small vessel ischemic changes. (D) High-resolution MR vessel wall imaging shows concentric vessel wall thickening in T1-weighted sagittal sequences and (E) concentric vessel wall enhancement in postgadolinium T1-weighted sagittal sequence and (F) conventional angiogram shows stenosis in multiple vessels.

only by biopsy.[4,8] Multiple stenosis in a single vessel is uncommon and may indicate a focal pathology. If middle cerebral artery (MCA) alone is involved, then varicella zoster vasculitis should be suspected, especially with antecedent history of varicella infection or by positive polymerase chain reaction (PCR)/antibody to the virus in cerebrospinal fluid (CSF). Vasculitic pattern in angiogram can be seen in other conditions also **(Box 1)**. Among them, ICAD and RCVS are important differentials.[3]

High-resolution MR vessel wall imaging is an encouraging novel investigative technique, which can be used to differentiate intracranial vasculopathies. Most of the ICAD lesions show eccentric wall thickening and enhancement. The specific feature of ICAD is the juxtaluminal T2 hyperintensity with adjacent T2 hypointense area indicating the fibrous cap and fatty core, respectively. In CNSV, concentric vessel wall thickening

BOX 1: Conditions mimicking vasculitis in angiography.

- Acute trauma
- Drugs
- Ehlers–Danlos syndrome
- Fibromuscular dysplasia
- Intracranial atherosclerosis
- Intravascular lymphoma
- Marfan syndrome
- Migraine
- Moyamoya disease and syndrome
- Radiation vasculopathy
- Reversible cerebral vasoconstriction syndrome
- Severe hypertension
- Sickle cell disease
- Subarachnoid hemorrhage

and concentric vessel wall enhancement are the classical features and the contrast enhancement of vessel walls may extend beyond the lumen to the periadventitial tissues or brain parenchyma.[6,7,22] Occasionally ICAD can also have circumferential vessel wall enhancement, but the T2 hyperintensity can point toward fibrous cap of ICAD rather than CNSV. MMD also needs exclusion in children and young adults and in them CTA/MRA itself can show stenosis/occlusion of terminal internal carotid artery (ICA), anterior cerebral artery (ACA), and MCA along with moyamoya vessels. Vessel wall imaging in MMD may also show concentric thickening with enhancement, but the outer wall diameter of the terminal ICA and proximal MCA are smaller in MMD patients.[7]

Computed tomography scan of chest, abdomen, and pelvis is done to rule out infective, inflammatory, or neoplastic causes.[3] CSF is abnormal in 90% of PACNS; however, the abnormalities are mild and nonspecific. Lymphocytic pleocytosis and mild elevation in protein without hypoglycorrhachia is commonly seen in PACNS.[4,12] Grossly abnormal CSF may indicate infective causes and PCR for viral and bacterial infections including tuberculosis and venereal disease research laboratory (VDRL) testing for syphilis has to be done. CSF immunoglobulin G (IgG) index and oligoclonal bands are elevated in inflammatory causes. Angiotensin-converting enzyme (ACE) level estimation in CSF for sarcoidosis is controversial due to low sensitivity and specificity.[23] CSF malignant cells cytology and flow cytometry can point toward neoplastic infiltration when abnormal. Whole body positron emission tomography (PET) may be required when underlying malignancy is a strong suspicion. Ophthalmological evaluation for features of retinal vasculitis and other ocular inflammation and choroid tubercles can give us a decisive diagnosis.[4]

■ Meningocortical Biopsy

A confirmation of cerebral vasculitis can be obtained only by brain biopsy and hence considered as the gold standard investigation in PACNS. Brain biopsy is a relatively safe option as the postprocedural mortality and permanent neurological deficits in patients who underwent biopsy for suspected CNSV are less. The adverse effects from immunosuppressive medications including flare up of the intracranial infections are more frequent, rather than the complications due to biopsy, thus arguing in favor of obtaining a tissue diagnosis.[3] In biopsies of suspected vasculitis or cryptogenic causes, infections are the alternative diagnosis that is often emerged.[24] The preferred biopsy site should be guided by the MRI brain with contrast and the areas should include contrast-enhanced parenchyma and meninges. The ideal sample should include dura, leptomeninges, cortex, and white matter.[4] The goal is to demonstrate the intramural inflammation of the blood vessels in the biopsied sample and exclude alternate causes like infections and malignancy.[3]

Targeted biopsy has better yield as compared to blind biopsy from nondominant temporal or frontal pole.[13,25]

In the Mayo Clinic cohort, 58 (72%) of the biopsied patients showed features of vasculitis. Granulomatous inflammatory pattern was observed in 34 (59%), lymphocytic pattern in 13 (22%), acute necrotizing pattern in 10 (17%), and mixed pattern in one patient. In this cohort, 20 patients with granulomatous pattern had accompanying vascular deposits of β-amyloid peptide. So, these patients had ABRA, an entity distinct from PACNS.[12] Lymphocytic vasculitis was the most frequent followed by necrotizing and granulomatous pattern in other studies.[8,13]

DIAGNOSIS

There are many factors that make the diagnosis of PACNS very demanding. There are no specific symptoms or findings for this condition. Even the neuroimaging features are mimicked by other vascular, infective, demyelinating, and neoplastic process. There are no laboratory, serological, or immunological markers, which can objectively diagnose this condition. The clinician's decision on pursuing meningocortical biopsy also determines the odds for the accurate diagnosis and exclusion of other causes. Lastly, very few centers have sufficient expertise in this field.[3]

Cravioto and Feigin first described the clinical and histopathological features of PACNS.[26] Later, Calabrese and Mallek in a series of eight patients described the clinical, angiographic, and histopathological features and proposed the first diagnostic criteria for PACNS: (1) Clinical features suggesting an acquired neurological deficit, which remains unexplained after the initial basic evaluation; (2) features of cerebral vasculitis in either angiography or histopathology, and (3) no evidence of systemic vasculitis or alternate condition to which the angiographical or pathological features could be secondary.[1] Many large observational studies have incorporated this criteria for inclusion of cases.[8,12,13] CA is often preferred over biopsy when CNSV is suspected since it is less invasive, easily available and safe, but the specificity is reported to be as low as 30%. Even the sensitivity of CA is only 30% when validated against histologically confirmed cases of PACNS.[27] Inflammation confined to small arteries, which are beyond the resolution of CA, can be missed and is detected only in biopsy. Angiography is often normal in patients with tumor-like lesions. So, a negative angiogram cannot preclude the diagnosis of PACNS.[19] Therefore, Birnbaum and Hellmann modified the diagnostic criteria and classified patients into two groups—definite and probable PACNS. Diagnosis confirmed by biopsy was labeled as definite PACNS and probable are cases when there is only angiographic evidence.[5] Biopsy is also not without any pitfalls. Not all PACNS can be diagnosed by biopsy because of low sensitivity. Vasculitic process can be patchy, which can account for negative biopsy. Large vessels are not biopsied; hence, vasculitis confined to large vessels can be missed.[4]

SUBTYPES OF PRIMARY ANGIITIS OF CENTRAL NERVOUS SYSTEM

Broadly, PACNS can be classified into two groups: biopsy-proven and angiography-proven (biopsy negative or not done).[8] Seizures, cognitive impairment, dyskinesia, and meningeal and parenchymal enhancement outside ischemic areas were more frequent in biopsy-proven PACNS, whereas focal neurological deficits and bilateral infarcts more common in CA proven PACNS.[19,28] Based on the size of the vessels, PACNS can be classified into large, medium, and small vessel vasculitis. Large and medium vessel involvement is determined by angiogram and small vessel vasculitis can be diagnosed only in biopsy. Therefore, this classification is similar to angiographically proven (large/medium vessel) and biopsy proven (small vessel). However, a strict subgrouping of patients into large, medium, and small vessel involvement may not be feasible, since patients can have inflammation of multiple vessels of different sizes.[13]

TREATMENT

The management of PACNS is challenging in many aspects. There are no direct evidence from randomized controlled trials for the treatment of PACNS and we are dependent on observational studies and case series for the treatment decisions. Majority of the studies had included angiographically diagnosed cases without biopsy confirmation, which casts uncertainty on the results.[8,9,12-14]

Cyclophosphamide and corticosteroids are the cornerstone of treatment in PACNS, and this treatment combination was first recommended by Cupp et al. in 1983 while describing a case series of four patients.[29] In the Mayo Clinic cohort, half of the patients were on corticosteroids alone as the initial treatment and of the 44 patients who relapsed, two-thirds were receiving only corticosteroids.[12] However, in the French cohort, majority received induction therapy with CYC and corticosteroids and only 14% received corticosteroids alone as initial treatment, which accounted for a reduced relapse rate.[8,9] Corticosteroids is given as pulse high-dose intravenous methyl prednisolone (1 g/day for 3–5 days) followed by oral prednisolone (1 mg/kg/day) for 6–8 weeks. Based on clinical response, oral prednisolone is slowly tapered and if needed a low dose can be maintained for 1–2 years.[9] The induction with CYC is by 750 mg/m^2 per month for six doses. Thereafter azathioprine, mycophenolate mofetil (MMF), or methotrexate is introduced as maintenance therapy. The total duration of therapy is decided based on clinical response and side effect profile.[9,15] If a patient worsens on this regimen, escalation of treatment with rituximab and anti-TNF-α inhibitors (infliximab and etanercept) can be considered. Biological agents could be an alternative to CYC if the complications, especially infertility, are unacceptable to the patient or if patients are intolerant.[10,12] However, sufficient literature is lacking for further immunotherapies, which can improve the outcome in refractory cases. We extrapolate the guidelines, that are available for systemic vasculitis to determine the treatment plan in these scenarios.

OUTCOME

To determine the outcome, the important parameters to assess are relapse, mortality, and modified Rankin scale (mRS). Relapse is defined as a recurrence or worsening of symptoms of PACNS or progression of existing deficits or appearance of new lesions on subsequent MRI irrespective of the treatment.[12] The relapse rate varied between 25 and 56%.[8,9,12,13] The interval from diagnosis to first relapse ranged between 2 and 63 months and the median is 19 months. Relapse was significantly higher in patients with meningeal enhancements and seizures.[8]

The most important factor determining the outcome is the initial treatment. Many studies have shown significant reduction in relapse and improved disability scores in patients treated with combination therapy rather than corticosteroids alone early in course of disease.[8,12] The reduced relapse rate and mortality observed in French cohort could also be related to the longer duration of corticosteroid usage and maintenance therapy.[8,9] Lymphocytic pattern had favorable outcome profile when compared to granulomatous or necrotizing pattern.[30] Delay in diagnosis was also related to poor outcome. In the recent study from India, the median delay in diagnosis from the first symptom was 39 months in patients with poor outcome as compared to 11 months in those with good outcome.[14]

The mortality reported in Mayo Clinic cohort was 15% and most of the death occurred in the first year and in those with severe disability. Increasing age, diagnosis by CA against biopsy, and large vessel involvement as compared to small vessel involvement were associated with increased mortality.[12] In the French cohort, the mortality was only 6%, which could be attributed to the aggressive initial combination therapy. The survivors were left with neurological deficits in 80%, but majority were ambulant independently.[8]

When short-term outcome was studied, at least one-third patients were discharged to another hospital for continued care and 5% patients died in the hospital. Only 6 out 10 patients were discharged directly to home. Older age, additional comorbid ischemic/hemorrhagic stroke, seizures, and medical complications were associated with discharge to another facility for continued care or in-hospital death.[2]

CONCLUSION

We have advanced our knowledge only very little in understanding the pathophysiological mechanism in PACNS. It is still challenging to clinicians to diagnose and treat as well as to monitor the outcome. Biopsy remains the confirmatory test. Advanced MRI protocol with vessel wall imaging, although promising, needs further validation with histopathological evidence. The combination therapy of CYC and corticosteroids followed by maintenance therapy has drastically improved the outcome in PACNS. The response to rituximab and anti-TNF-α inhibitors in refractory PACNS is encouraging, but needs to be proven in large studies.

REFERENCES

1. Calabrese LH, Mallek JA. Primary angiitis of the central nervous system. Report of 8 new cases, review of the literature, and proposal for diagnostic criteria. Medicine (Baltimore). 1988;67(1):20-39.
2. Patel SD, Oliver FO, Elmashad A, et al. Outcomes among patients with primary angiitis of the CNS: A Nationwide United States analysis. J Stroke Cerebrovasc Dis. 2022;31(11):106747.
3. Rice CM, Scolding NJ. The diagnosis of primary central nervous system vasculitis. Pract Neurol. 2020;20(2):109-14.
4. Salvarani C, Brown RD Jr, Hunder GG. Adult primary central nervous system vasculitis. Lancet. 2012;380(9843):767-77.
5. Birnbaum J, Hellmann DB. Primary angiitis of the central nervous system. Arch Neurol. 2009;66(6):704-9.
6. Mandell DM, Mossa-Basha M, Qiao Y, et al.; Vessel Wall Imaging Study Group of the American Society of Neuroradiology. Intracranial Vessel Wall MRI: Principles and Expert Consensus Recommendations of the American Society of Neuroradiology. AJNR Am J Neuroradiol. 2017;38(2):218-29.
7. Adhithyan R, Kesav P, Thomas B, et al. High-resolution magnetic resonance vessel wall imaging in cerebrovascular diseases. Neurol India. 2018;66(4):1124-32.
8. de Boysson H, Zuber M, Naggara O, et al.; French Vasculitis Study Group and the French NeuroVascular Society. Primary angiitis of the central nervous system: description of the first fifty-two adults enrolled in the French cohort of patients with primary vasculitis of the central nervous system. Arthritis Rheumatol. 2014;66(5):1315-26.
9. de Boysson H, Arquizan C, Touzé E, et al. Treatment and Long-Term Outcomes of Primary Central Nervous System Vasculitis. Stroke. 2018;49(8):1946-52.
10. Beuker C, Strunk D, Rawal R, et al. Primary Angiitis of the CNS: A Systematic Review and Meta-analysis. Neurol Neuroimmunol Neuroinflamm. 2021;8(6):e1093.
11. Paramasivan NK, Sundaram S, Sharma DP, et al. Rituximab for refractory primary angiitis of the central nervous system: Experience in two patients. Mult Scler Relat Disord. 2021;51:102907.
12. Salvarani C, Brown RD Jr, Christianson T, et al. An update of the Mayo Clinic cohort of patients with adult primary central nervous system vasculitis: description of 163 patients. Medicine (Baltimore). 2015;94(21):e738.
13. Sundaram S, Menon D, Khatri P, et al. Primary angiitis of the central nervous system: Clinical profiles and outcomes of 45 patients. Neurol India. 2019;67(1):105-12.
14. Agarwal A, Sharma J, Srivastava MVP, et al. Primary CNS vasculitis (PCNSV): a cohort study. Sci Rep. 2022;12(1):13494.
15. Sundaram S, Sylaja PN. Primary Angiitis of the Central Nervous System–Diagnosis and Management. Ann Indian Acad Neurol. 2022;25(6):1009-18.
16. Geschwind MD, Shu H, Haman A, et al. Rapidly progressive dementia. Ann Neurol. 2008;64(1):97-108.
17. Love S. Demyelinating diseases. J Clin Pathol. 2006;59(11):1151-9.
18. El-Hattab AW, Adesina AM, Jones J, et al. MELAS syndrome: Clinical manifestations, pathogenesis, and treatment options. Mol Genet Metab. 2015;116(1-2):4-12.
19. Boulouis G, de Boysson H, Zuber M, et al.; French Vasculitis Group. Primary Angiitis of the Central Nervous System: Magnetic Resonance Imaging Spectrum of Parenchymal, Meningeal, and Vascular Lesions at Baseline. Stroke. 2017;48(5):1248-55.
20. Akhtar T, Shahjouei S, Zand R. Etiologies of simultaneous cerebral infarcts in multiple arterial territories: A simple literature-based pooled analysis. Neurol India. 2019;67(3):692-5.
21. Garg A. Vascular brain pathologies. Neuroimaging Clin N Am. 2011;21(4):897-926, ix.
22. Sundaram S, Kumar PN, Sharma DP, et al. High-Resolution Vessel Wall Imaging in Primary Angiitis of Central Nervous System. Ann Indian Acad Neurol. 2021;24(4):524-30.
23. Stern BJ, Royal W 3rd, Gelfand JM, et al. Definition and Consensus Diagnostic Criteria for Neurosarcoidosis: From the Neurosarcoidosis Consortium Consensus Group. JAMA Neurol. 2018;75(12):1546-53.
24. Alrawi A, Trobe JD, Blaivas M, et al. Brain biopsy in primary angiitis of the central nervous system. Neurology. 1999;53:858-60.
25. Miller DV, Salvarani C, Hunder GG, et al. Biopsy findings in primary angiitis of the central nervous system. Am J Surg Pathol. 2009;33(1):35-43.
26. Cravioto H, Feigin I. Noninfectious granulomatous angiitis with a predilection for the nervous system. Neurology. 1959;9:599-609.
27. McVerry F, McCluskey G, McCarron P, et al. Diagnostic test results in primary CNS vasculitis: A systematic review of published cases. Neurol Clin Pract. 2017;7(3):256-65.
28. Salvarani C, Brown RD Jr, Calamia KT, et al. Primary central nervous system vasculitis: analysis of 101 patients. Ann Neurol. 2007;62(5):442-51.
29. Cupps TR, Moore PM, Fauci AS. Isolated angiitis of the central nervous system. Prospective diagnostic and therapeutic experience. Am J Med. 1983;74(1):97-105.
30. Salvarani C, Brown RD Jr, Christianson TJH, et al. Long-term remission, relapses and maintenance therapy in adult primary central nervous system vasculitis: A single-center 35-year experience. Autoimmun Rev. 2020;19(4):102497.

CHAPTER 3

Craniocervical Dissection: Diagnosis and Management

Ayush Agarwal, MV Padma Srivastava

ABSTRACT

Cervical artery dissection (CAD) is defined as blood collection in between the layers of the arterial wall of either the internal carotid or vertebral arteries. They result from an intimal tear, leading to the formation of a false lumen. This allows blood to enter, and form a mural hematoma. It is considered to be a multifactorial disease, with environmental factors being potential triggers in genetically predisposed individual. It accounts for 15–24% stroke cases in young. Internal carotid artery (ICA) dissections are more common than vertebral artery (VA) ones. The symptoms of CAD result either from intraluminal stenosis or occlusion, resulting in ischemia or compression of the adjacent nerves.

Neuroimaging is used to confirm the CAD diagnosis. The classical findings include the crescent sign, tapered arterial stenosis or occlusion, presence of a vascular flap or double lumen, and a dissecting aneurysm. Acute stroke care is the same as for patients without dissection and secondary prevention includes the use of antithrombotic therapy (antiplatelets or anticoagulants). The risk of recurrence is low, especially after a few weeks from symptom onset.

Keywords: Dissection, Cervical, CAD, Artery, Hematoma, Stroke.

INTRODUCTION

Arterial dissections result from separation of arterial wall layers, leading to a false lumen formation and are defined by the collection of blood and formation of intramural hematoma between these layers. Cervical artery dissection (CAD) entails dissection in either the internal carotid artery (ICA) or the vertebral artery (VA), and these occur either spontaneously or secondary to blunt or penetrating trauma.[1] Extracranial CADs are more common than intracranial ones, and ICA dissections are more common than VA dissections. Although the overall incidence of CAD is low (2.6–3 per 100,000 people/year), it is responsible for 15–24% cases of stroke in young.[2,3] The overall incidence of CAD is likely to be underestimated as asymptomatic patients or patients with local findings alone (Horner's syndrome, neck pain, and headache) are likely to be misdiagnosed.

ANATOMY

Dissections either result from an intimal tear resulting in the separation of arterial wall layers, which allows blood to enter and form an intramural hematoma or direct bleeding from ruptured vasa vasorum (**Fig. 1**). They usually occur at sites of high shear stress and the most common location is few centimeters above the carotid bifurcation for ICA dissection and in the V2–V3 segment for VA dissection.[4,5] Multiple dissections can occasionally occur in the same patient (13–22% of total cases).

The intramural hematomas can lead to dilatation of the vessel, leading to compression of adjacent nerves causing local symptoms such as headache, neck pain, Horner's syndrome, and cranial neuropathies.[6]

Intracranial dissections are more prone to pseudoaneurysm formation due to the absence of the external elastic lamina in intracranial vasculature. This leads to the

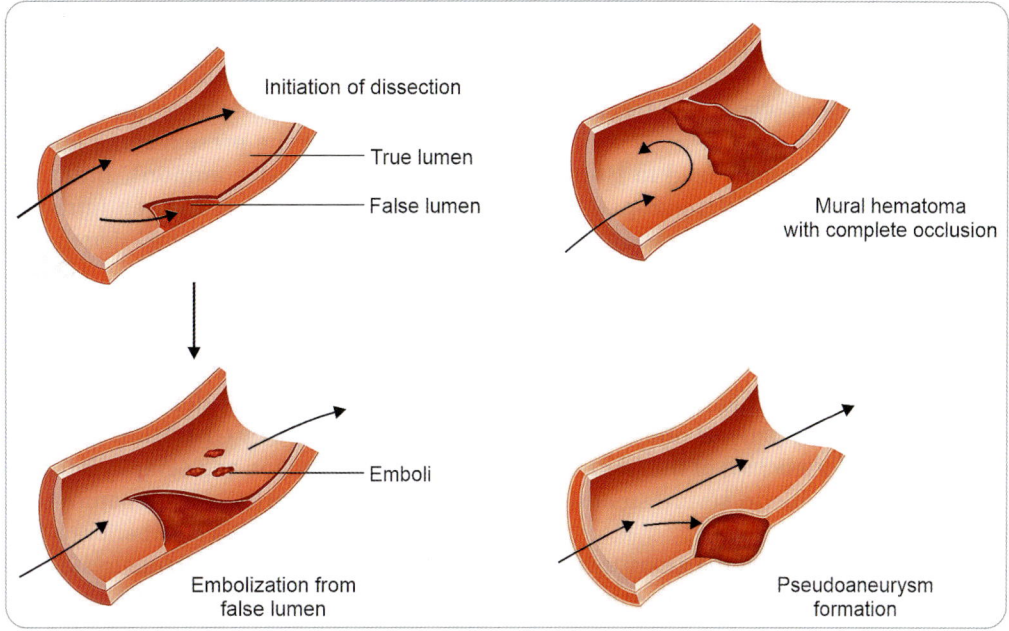

FIG. 1: Pathogenesis of cervical artery dissection.

formation of subadventitial hematoma growth, leading to the formation of dissecting aneurysms.

ETIOLOGY AND PREDISPOSING FACTORS

The exact pathophysiology of CAD is incompletely understood. The leading hypothesis considers CAD a multifactorial disease where environmental factors serve as second hits in patients who are genetically predisposed to dissections.[7]

Cervical artery dissection has been linked to some connective tissue and vascular disorders, of which fibromuscular dysplasia is the most common.[8] Approximately 2% CAD cases are related to monogenic connective tissue disorders such as type IV Ehlers–Danlos syndrome, Marfan syndrome, and osteogenesis imperfecta. However, since these disorders are rare per se, it remains to be ascertained whether their concomitant occurrence is higher than could occur by chance alone.[9]

Minor cervical trauma precedes approximately 50% CAD cases and can range from subtle neck hyperextensions to whiplash injuries. The common risk factors and triggers for CAD have been mentioned in **Table 1**.

CLINICAL PRESENTATION

Presentation from CAD can be broadly classified into local and ischemic/hemorrhagic events. Approximately 6% dissections are completely asymptomatic.
- *Local symptoms and signs*: Headache and neck pain are the most common occurring in approximately

TABLE 1: Common risk factors and triggers for cervical artery dissection.[1]

Minor trauma and other mechanical events	• Chiropractic manipulation • Severe coughing/sneezing • Sports-related injuries • Sudden neck movements (e.g., roller coaster rides) • Whiplash injury
Connective tissue and vascular diseases	• Alpha-1 antitrypsin deficiency • Aortic root dilation • Autosomal dominant polycystic kidney disease • Fibromuscular dysplasia • Cerebral aneurysms • Marfan syndrome • Osteogenesis imperfecta type 1 • Moyamoya disease • Reversible cerebral vasoconstriction syndrome • Turner syndrome • William syndrome • Vascular Ehlers–Danlos syndrome • Hyperhomocysteinemia • Hereditary hemochromatosis
Other risk factors	• Hypertension • Oral contraceptive intake (current) • Infection • Migraine • Pregnancy and postpartum period • Elongated styloid process • Winter/Autumn season

57–69% cases.[10] Patients with ICA dissection have headache, whereas VA dissection patients experience neck pain.[10] These are usually ipsilateral to the dissection and pain characteristics can vary but are usually migrainous.

ICA dissections can occasionally lead to Horner's syndrome (25% cases) and cranial neuropathies.[11] Horner's syndrome results from compression of the third order sympathetic nerve fibers by the enlarged ICA. The most common cranial neuropathies are hypoglossal, glossopharyngeal, and vagal.

- *Ischemic and hemorrhagic events*: These are the most feared complications of CAD. Ischemic injury occurs in approximately two-thirds of patients and can result from either artery-to-artery *embolism* of the intramural thrombus or *hypoperfusion* due to severe stenosis or occlusion at the dissection site.[1]

The stroke symptoms depend on the artery involved and are usually accompanied by local symptoms described above.

Subarachnoid hemorrhage is a rare complication (1% CAD cases) and results from rupture of dissecting aneurysms. These are more common in intracranial dissections or extracranial dissections with intracranial extension.[12]

EVALUATION AND DIAGNOSIS

A diagnosis of CAD should be suspected in any individual who develops acute-onset local symptoms (described earlier) or an ischemic stroke. These individuals should undergo neuroimaging to evaluate both the brain parenchyma and its vessels. The most commonly used modality is a computed tomography (CT) of the head with CT angiography (CTA) of the head and neck vessels because of its easier availability and low cost. However, it involves radiation exposure. An alternative is magnetic resonance imaging (MRI) of the brain with magnetic resonance angiography (MRA). The characteristic neuroimaging findings include the presence of a long-tapered stenosis or occlusion (most common), intimal flap, dissecting aneurysm, double lumen, or an intramural hematoma.[1] Crescent sign[13] is an additional sign that can be visualized only on MRA **(Figs. 2A and B)**.

Carotid Doppler and transcranial ultrasound are other imaging modalities that can be used.

Both of them are readily available and inexpensive, but are highly operator-dependent and lack the imaging resolution provided by CTA/MRA.

Digital subtraction angiography is the gold standard, but is rarely used due to its invasive nature and good diagnostic yield of CTA/MRA.[1] CTA is superior to MRA in identifying high-grade stenosis, pseudoaneurysms, and intimal flaps, and also better at visualizing VA dissections.[14] It has the same sensitivity and specificity for VA dissection diagnosis as digital subtraction angiography.[15] However, the same is not true for ICA dissections.

TREATMENT

Patients with CAD presenting with acute stroke should be managed under the same guidelines as all acute ischemic strokes. They should be assessed for eligibility for thrombolysis (alteplase or tenecteplase) and mechanical thrombectomy (MT).

- *Acute stroke treatment*: The landmark thrombolysis trials did not exclude dissection patients and subsequent studies have also demonstrated safety of alteplase and tenecteplase in acute ischemic stroke patients with dissection.[16] However, caution is warranted in individuals

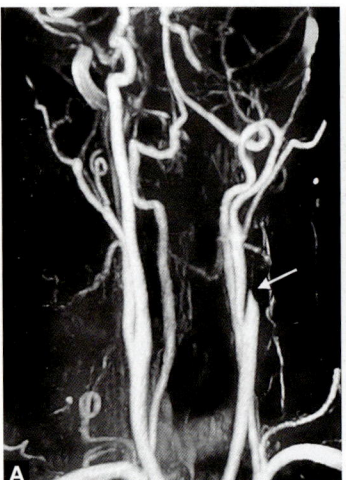 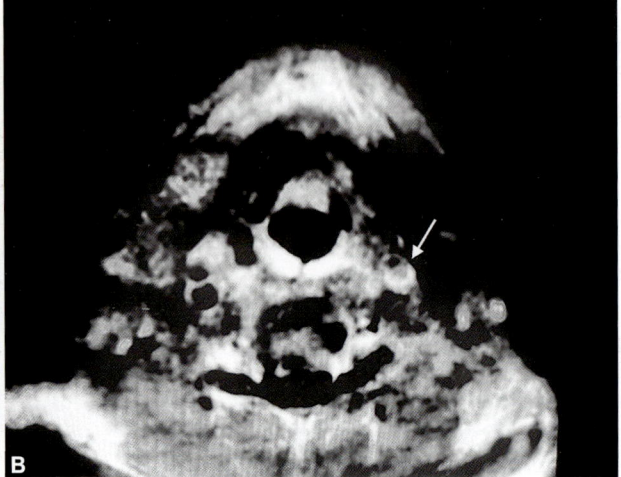

FIGS. 2A AND B: (A) MRA (MIP images) showing a long-tapered near complete occlusion of left ICA. (B) Axial T1-weighted MRA showing crescent sign of left ICA dissection (hyperintense crescent: mural hematoma; hypointense dot: flow void of left ICA).
(ICA: internal carotid artery; MIP: maximum intensity projection; MRA: magnetic resonance angiography)

with isolated intracranial dissection or extracranial dissection with intracranial extension.[17] This is due to an increased risk of intracerebral or subarachnoid hemorrhage in these patients. Also, patients with aortic dissections should avoid thrombolysis.

Patients with large vessel occlusions secondary to CADs should undergo MT, if they fulfill the criteria for MT.

Stenting can be considered for patients with persistent, high-grade stenosis even after achieving reperfusion. However, a multicenter, prospective study did not reveal any improvement in functional outcome in patients undergoing stenting when compared to those without, despite an improvement in successful reperfusion.[18]

- *Secondary prevention*: Antithrombotic therapy is prescribed to prevent stroke recurrence in patients with CAD. This can be as antiplatelets or anticoagulants. Current literature does not show any significant difference between the two and the treatment prescribed is usually based on the treating physician's discretion. Two randomized controlled trials [Cervical Artery Dissection In Stroke Study (CADISS) and aspirin vs. anticoagulation in CAD (TREAT-CAD)] had compared antiplatelets with anticoagulants in this patient population and have been summarized in **Table 2**.

Due to this inconclusive evidence, the recent secondary stroke prevention guidelines by American Heart Association (AHA)/American Stroke Association (ASA) recommend the use of either vitamin K antagonists or aspirin in patients with ischemic stroke or transient ischemic attack (TIA) secondary to CAD.[19] The physician's decision is usually based on multiple factors including infarct size, presence or absence of intraluminal thrombus, occlusion, and presence of dissecting aneurysm. There is no consensus on the dose of aspirin (TREAT-CAD used 300 mg/day whereas CADISS left it to the physician's discretion) and a dose between 81–325 mg/day is considered reasonable.[1] Treatment with dual antiplatelets (aspirin and clopidogrel) for 21 days following a minor stroke [the National Institutes of Health Stroke Scale (NIHSS) <4] or high-risk TIA (ABCD2 score ≥2) can be considered. The use of antiplatelets should be delayed by 24 hours in patients who get thrombolyzed. In patients being considered for anticoagulant therapy, the infarct size determines when it is started. Although vitamin K antagonists were used in CADISS and TREAT-CAD, observational data has suggested that direct oral anticoagulants are both safe and effective.[20]

No randomized controlled trials (RCTs) have assessed the management of intracranial dissection. However, antiplatelets are preferred to anticoagulants due to the increased risk of subarachnoid hemorrhage.

The rate of stroke recurrence is 0–13% at 1 year.[21] Most cases have recurrence within the first 2 weeks. However, the optimal duration of secondary prevention therapy is unclear and the AHA recommends antithrombotic therapy for at least 3 months. In practice, physicians usually prescribe antithrombotic therapy for at least 6 months. Patients receiving anticoagulants are usually switched from them to antiplatelets after 2–3 months.

OUTCOME

The functional outcome after CAD is largely dependent on the severity of the ischemic insult. Grossly, the outcomes appear favorable with 75–82% individuals achieving a modified Rankin Scale (mRS) 0–1 and the mortality rate is <5%.[21] Dissection of ICA and complete occlusion of the vessel are the indices associated with poorer outcome.[22]

The stroke recurrence and functional outcome is independent of vessel recanalization status.[1] Repeat vascular imaging is usually performed between 3 and

Study name	Aim	Study design	Patient no.	Primary outcome	Follow-up	Results
CADISS	Compare antiplatelets to anticoagulants for stroke prevention in CAD	Multicenter, open label RCT	250	Ipsilateral stroke or death at 90 days	3 months; 1 year	@3 months: OR 0.335; 95% CI 0.006–4.233 @1 year: OR 0.56, 95% CI 0.10–3.21
TREAT-CAD	Test the noninferiority of aspirin to vitamin K antagonist treatment in CAD patients	Multicenter, open-label, randomized noninferiority trial	194	Composite of clinical (stroke, major hemorrhage, or death) or MRI outcomes (new ischemic or hemorrhagic brain lesions) at 14 days and clinical outcomes only at 90 days	3 months	21 (23%) in aspirin group; 12 (15%) in vitamin K antagonist group. Absolute difference: 8% (95% CI −4 to 21). Noninferiority not shown

(CAD: cervical artery dissection; CADISS: Cervical Artery Dissection In Stroke Study; CI: confidence interval; OR: odds ratio; MRI: magnetic resonance imaging; TREAT-CAD: aspirin vs. anticoagulation in CAD)

6 months poststroke. Most recanalization occur within the first few months poststroke (1 month—16%, 3 months—50%, 6-12 months—60%).[23] The presence of complete occlusion decreases the likelihood of complete recanalization.

CONCLUSION

Cervical artery dissection is a multifactorial disease and an important cause of stroke in young and should be ruled out in all young individuals with stroke. Early diagnosis and treatment lead to better functional outcomes and prevention of stroke recurrence. CAD patients are the candidates for thrombolysis or MT and AHA/ASA guidelines recommend treatment with either antiplatelets or anticoagulants for secondary prevention. The risk of recurrence is highest in the first 2 weeks poststroke, highlighting the need for early aggressive management. Future studies should aim to further elucidate the interplay and influence of genetic and environmental factors in arterial dissection to further enhance our understanding of this multifactorial disorder.

REFERENCES

1. Omran SS. Cervical artery dissection. Continuum (Minneap Minn). 2023;29(2, Cerebrovascular Disease):540-65.
2. Lee VH, Brown RD, Mandrekar JN, et al. Incidence and outcome of cervical artery dissection: a population-based study. Neurology. 2006;67(10):1809-12.
3. Putaala J, Metso AJ, Metso TM, et al. Analysis of 1008 consecutive patients aged 15 to 49 with first-ever ischemic stroke: the Helsinki young stroke registry. Stroke. 2009;40(4):1195-203.
4. Lleva P, Ahluwalia BS, Marks S, et al. Traumatic and spontaneous carotid and vertebral artery dissection in a level 1 trauma center. J Clin Neurosci Off J Neurosurg Soc Australas. 2012;19(8):1112-4.
5. Arnold M, Bousser MG, Fahrni G, et al. Vertebral artery dissection: presenting findings and predictors of outcome. Stroke. 2006;37(10):2499-503.
6. Arnold MJ, Jonas CE, Carter RE, et al. Pain as the only symptom of cervical artery dissection. J Neurol Neurosurg Psychiatry. 2006;77(9):1021-4.
7. Raser JM, Mullen MT, Kasner SE, et al. Cervical carotid artery dissection is associated with styloid process length. Neurology. 2011;77(23):2061-6.
8. Talarowska P, Dobrowolski P, Klisiewicz A, et al. High incidence and clinical characteristics of fibromuscular dysplasia in patients with spontaneous cervical artery dissection: the ARCADIA-POL study. Vasc Med Lond Engl. 2019;24(2):112-9.
9. Debette S, Goeggel Simonetti B, et al. Familial occurrence and heritable connective tissue disorders in cervical artery dissection. Neurology. 2014;83(22):2023-31.
10. Silbert PL, Mokri B, Schievink WI. Headache and neck pain in spontaneous internal carotid and vertebral artery dissections. Neurology. 1995;45(8):1517-22.
11. Lyrer PA, Brandt T, Metso TM, et al. Clinical import of Horner syndrome in internal carotid and vertebral artery dissection. Neurology. 2014;82(18):1653-9.
12. Krings T, Mandell DM, Kiehl TR, et al. Intracranial aneurysms: from vessel wall pathology to therapeutic approach. Nat Rev Neurol. 2011;7(10):547-59.
13. Hakimi R, Sivakumar S. Imaging of carotid dissection. Curr Pain Headache Rep. 2019;23(1):2.
14. Vertinsky AT, Schwartz NE, Fischbein NJ, et al. Comparison of multidetector CT angiography and MR imaging of cervical artery dissection. Am J Neuroradiol. 2008;29(9):1753-60.
15. Chen CJ, Tseng YC, Lee TH, et al. Multisection CT angiography compared with catheter angiography in diagnosing vertebral artery dissection. Am J Neuroradiol. 2004;25(5):769-74.
16. Zinkstok SM, Vergouwen MDI, Engelter ST, et al. Safety and functional outcome of thrombolysis in dissection-related ischemic stroke: a meta-analysis of individual patient data. Stroke. 2011;42(9):2515-20.
17. Bernardo F, Nannoni S, Strambo D, et al. Intravenous thrombolysis in acute ischemic stroke due to intracranial artery dissection: a single-center case series and a review of literature. J Thromb Thrombolysis. 2019;48(4):679-84.
18. Marnat G, Lapergue B, Sibon I, et al. Safety and outcome of carotid dissection stenting during the treatment of tandem occlusions: a pooled analysis of TITAN and ETIS. Stroke. 2020;51(12):3713-8.
19. Kleindorfer DO, Towfighi A, Chaturvedi S, et al. 2021 guideline for the prevention of stroke in patients with stroke and transient ischemic attack: a guideline from the American Heart Association/American Stroke Association. Stroke. 2021;52(7):e364-e467.
20. Debette S, Mazighi M, Bijlenga P, et al. ESO guideline for the management of extracranial and intracranial artery dissection. Eur Stroke J. 2021;6(3):XXXIX-LXXXVIII.
21. Debette S, Leys D. Cervical-artery dissections: predisposing factors, diagnosis, and outcome. Lancet Neurol. 2009;8(7):668-78.
22. Traenka C, Grond-Ginsbach C, Goeggel Simonetti B, et al. Artery occlusion independently predicts unfavorable outcome in cervical artery dissection. Neurology. 2020;94(2):e170-80
23. Nedeltchev K, Bickel S, Arnold M, et al. R2-recanalization of spontaneous carotid artery dissection. Stroke. 2009;40(2):499-504.

CHAPTER 4

Approach to Thunderclap Headache

Sucharita Ray, Kamalesh Chakravarty

ABSTRACT

Thunderclap headache (TCH) is a medical emergency that heralds a number of conditions that demand urgent medical or surgical attention. Even though it has been canonically used to signify the sentinel headache of an unruptured aneurysm, there have been many other conditions that have since been found to present with this intensity. It is crucial for students of neurology to develop an approach to first learn about the various differentials that can present as a TCH and then subsequently to manage it. This chapter will aid students in doing just that.

Keywords: Thunderclap, Headache, Emergency, Aneurysm, CVST, RCVS.

INTRODUCTION

Thunderclap headache (TCH) is described as an acute and very severe headache that reaches maximal intensity less than a minute from the onset and stays for at least 5 minutes.[1] Historically, the term was first used by Day and Raskin to describe an intense sentinel headache of an unruptured aneurysm.[2] However, over the years, many other causes have been attributed to this dramatic presentation.[3] It becomes extremely important not just to learn to identify this medical emergency but also approach in a way toward managing it.

ETIOLOGY

Thunderclap headache is usually a symptom with varied etiology affecting the vasculature as well as the brain parenchyma. Subarachnoid hemorrhage (SAH) and rupture of intracranial aneurysms are some of the most common causes. Reversible cerebral vasoconstriction syndrome (RCVS) is often considered to be the second most common cause.[4] However, there may be many other causes as listed in **Table 1**. Headache that seems to rise to peak within seconds to peak within 1 minute of onset and lasts hours to

TABLE 1: Causes of thunderclap headache.	
Ruptured intracranial aneurysm	Third ventricle colloid cyst
Subarachnoid hemorrhage	Pituitary apoplexy
RCVS	Aqueductal stenosis
Cerebral venous sinus thrombosis	Retroclival hematoma
Cervical artery dissection	Brain tumor
Subdural hematoma	Miscellaneous causes
Giant cell arteritis	Hypertensive crisis
Stroke, both ischemic and intracerebral hemorrhage	Spontaneous intracranial hypotension
Primary vasculitis of CNS	Pheochromocytoma
Infective causes	Illicit drugs
Complicated sinusitis	Cannabis
Meningitis	Cocaine
Medications	Amphetamine
Triptans	Methamphetamine
Oral contraceptives	Khat
Nasal decongestants	Ecstasy

Continued

Continued

Intravenous immunoglobulin	LSD
Antidepressants-serotonergic	Heroin
Ergot alkaloids	Remote causes
Surgical manipulation	Cardiac cephalgia
Strenuous physical or sexual activity	Aortic arch dissection

(CNS: central nervous system; LSD: lysergic acid diethylamide; RCVS: reversible cerebral vasoconstriction syndrome)

days if untreated is considered to be the definition of TCH.[5] In every case, an exhaustive workup should be considered to rule out all possible causes.

SPECTRUM OF CLINICAL PRESENTATION

The excruciating headache of acute onset reaching a peak before 1 minute is the hallmark in all cases. Nausea and vomiting, photo and phonophobia, transient or prolonged visual obscurations, diplopia and even seizures, and alterations in sensorium can occur in many patients.[6] TCH can sometimes be lateralized to the side of the SAH or the unruptured aneurysm.[7] Vision loss and diplopia arising from cranial nerve palsies, especially third cranial nerve palsy with pupillary involvement, may be seen in pituitary apoplexy.[8] Elderly patients can present with severe headache and vision loss with pulselessness indicating giant cell arteritis (GCA) or strokes. A meticulous and detailed history taking is necessary in all cases of TCH. History taking should be meticulous even if the first episode of TCH presents to the emergency.

HOW TO APPROACH THUNDERCLAP HEADACHE?

It is important to know that TCH does not always arise de novo from before. It may occur in many against a background of longstanding headaches.[5] It is traditionally attributable to causes other than the usual migraine, and it is very important to determine that TCH is not merely an exacerbation of previous headaches, like migraine.[3] The next step of diagnosis of TCH is to be aware of the wide variety of clinical presentations accompanying a TCH. Often the associated findings are neurological, but many a times, even non-neurological symptoms and signs may be seen, and these findings are very helpful in narrowing down the possibilities in TCH. However, there is a big chance of these associated findings to be obscured under the severe headache. As a clinician, it is more important to pay attention to these findings as they hold a clue to the diagnosis of the etiology of TCH.

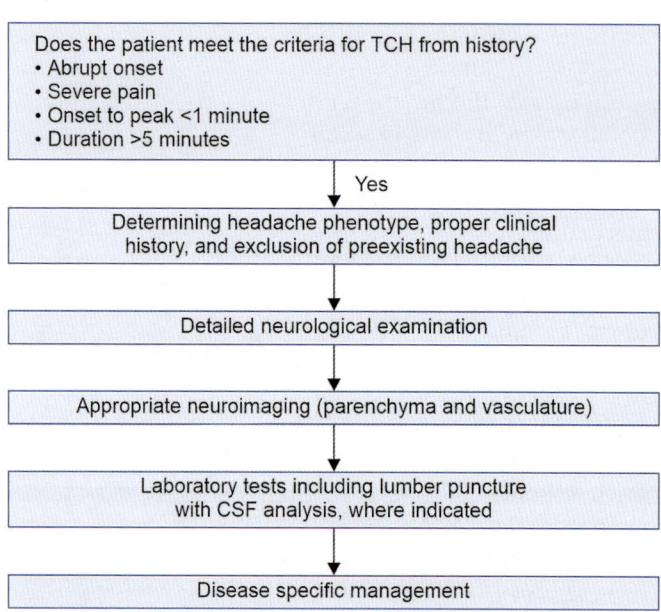

FLOWCHART 1: Algorithm for approach to a patient with TCH.
(CSF: cerebrospinal fluid; TCH: thunderclap headache)

Once the clinical history has sufficiently ruled out a mere exacerbation of a preexisting headache disorder and established the possibility of a TCH, the next step in approaching the case relies on a meticulous history taking and a thorough clinical examination. Neurological examination confirms and verifies the clinical history, and the signs help in narrowing down the possibilities. This is complemented by judiciously decided imaging protocols and relevant laboratory examinations. It is more important to know that a normal neurological examination and initial imaging do not exclude a serious cause of TCH **(Flowchart 1)**.[9]

COMPONENTS OF HISTORY TAKING

Headache Phenotypes

Approach to TCH must begin with a meticulous history taking. Headache history should include inquiry into location, severity, lateralization, and radiation of headache. Associated features such as nausea, vomiting, photophobia and phonophobia, transient visual obscurations, neck rigidity, or neck pain should be enquired after. It is more important to ask about a change in the phenotype of headache, which can hold a clue toward the etiology. The site and location of headache may not give a clue toward the etiology, but usually the concept of the "worst headache of life" or an acute-onset severe headache lasting several hours is a clue toward something serious. Physical exertion or sexual activity may precede an SAH as well as other kinds of headache, but headache requiring an emergency visit has a chance to be an SAH due to aneurysm rupture.

Thunderclap headache was incorporated as a component of the Ottawa Subarachnoid Hemorrhage (OSAH) clinical decision rule. The other components are age older than 40 years, pain in the neck, limited flexion or neck stiffness, loss of consciousness, and onset during exertion. It had 100% sensitivity but only 7.6% specificity in predicting SAH, thus limiting its use in emergency department.[10] A sentinel headache predating the rupture of an aneurysm may accompany it in 10–43% of the cases. This headache is often severe, abrupt, and can continue for days, and is usually caused due to the leakage from a tiny berry aneurysm.[11] On the other hand, the headache in GCA is throbbing and localized to both temples, and is often associated with jaw claudication due to ischemia of the maxillary artery, which supplies the muscles of mastication. Many visual symptoms may accompany GCA such as amaurosis, visual loss, or diplopia. TCH is associated but not universal for GCA, whereas new-onset headache is considered to be a cardinal symptom.[12] Additionally, headache in intracerebral hemorrhage, venous sinus thrombosis, and even cervical artery dissection can also occur in a thunderclap manner but do not follow any special characteristics.[3]

Drug History in Thunderclap Headache

History of intake of drugs and other interactions should be asked in detail. There should be a detailed history of drug intake. Cocaine, cannabis, amphetamine, and methamphetamines are some of the commonly implicated substances implicated in causing TCH.[13] History of triptan use for preexisting headaches should always be inquired as they can cause TCH by causing reversible cerebral constriction syndrome.[14] Use of nasal decongestants, ergot alkaloids, oral contraceptives, cyclophosphamide or erythropoietin, or intravenous immunoglobulin injections are some of the other common medications, which can precipitate TCH **(Table 1)**.[13,15] It is also important to ask a history of medications for a preexisting headache disorder as many cases of chronic unrelenting headache result from medication overuse and can confuse the diagnosis.[16]

Conducting a Complete Neurological Examination

A detailed neurological examination should complement a meticulous history of headaches. An assessment of blood pressure and fundus evaluation for papilledema and cranial nerves should be evaluated. Focal neurological deficits can hold an important clue to diagnosis. For example, unilateral dilated pupil with headache around the periorbital area without meningeal irritation usually points to an aneurysm of posterior communicating artery. Pituitary apoplexy can present with many systemic as well as neurologic symptoms. Nausea, vomiting, impaired consciousness, and signs of meningeal irritation accompany many cranial nerve palsies

and ophthalmoplegia in this condition.[17] Usually, it requires imaging and hormonal studies for confirmation. Patients may also be very reluctant to sit up as the same exacerbates headaches in spontaneous intracranial hypotension. Patients with ischemic and hemorrhagic stroke are usually seen with upper motor neuron facial palsy and hemiparesis or hemisensory symptoms or crossed deficits with various cranial nerve palsies. Seizures are commonly seen in patients of venous sinus thrombosis. Patients with SAH present with signs of meningeal irritation and neck rigidity in addition to TCH. The history of a sentinel headache may be seen in up to 30% of cases up to 2 weeks before the presentation. But its absence does not rule out a SAH.[11]

Laboratory Tests

Laboratory parameters for evaluation of pituitary hormones, especially prolactin, cortisol, and growth hormone, should be considered when indicated. Additionally, total leukocyte count, thyroid profile, and serum glucose levels should be considered. Cerebrospinal fluid (CSF) examination is of vital importance in elucidating the causes of TCH. It can rule out an infection of leptomeninges. Xanthochromia in CSF is 100% sensitive for indicating the presence of blood in the subarachnoid layer as occurs in SAH.[18] However, it should be carried out a minimum of 12 hours after a suspected SAH for blood breakdown products to appear. Opening pressure of the CSF can be useful in monitoring the intracranial pressure and also help in relieving the same in cases of cerebral venous sinus thrombosis (CVST) obstructing vision. Histopathological examination is required in cases of suspected intracranial space-occupying lesions and also when suspecting primary central nervous system (CNS) vasculitis. A toxicological and drug level should accompany all cases of suspected substance abuse. A hormonal profile is very useful in diagnosis of pituitary apoplexy and serum and urine osmolality, and sodium levels can help in diagnosing it in cases of accompanying syndrome of inappropriate antidiuretic hormone (SIADH). Imaging protocols are very important in etiological diagnosis of TCH and should be ordered in all cases and as early as feasible.

Deciding Imaging Protocols in Thunderclap Headache

Imaging protocols are decided based on suspected etiology of TCH and are crucial to establish the diagnosis in many unclear cases. Noncontrast computed tomography (NCCT) head is the most sensitive imaging modality to detect the acute blood of SAH with sensitivity and specificity reaching up to 98%. Magnetic resonance imaging (MRI) employing T2 fluid-attenuated inversion recovery (FLAIR) sequences may prove to be more helpful in the subacute stage once the hemoglobin begins to degrade.[19] Angiograms are best used for the visualization of aneurysms. Sensitivity for detection of aneurysms 4-10 mm in size using a 64 slice CT scan approaches 100%. NCCT as well as MRI are useful to detect ischemic as well as hemorrhagic strokes and venous infarcts. Cord sign on NCCT scan is indicative of venous thrombosis. MRI demonstrates the absence of a flow void and the presence of altered signal intensity. To confirm the involved vessel, venography can be used both using CT and MRI to find the involved vein.[20]

Magnetic resonance imaging is very useful in detection of spontaneous intracranial hypotension showing diffuse enhancement of dura with the subdural fluid collection, compensatory engorgement of venous structures, pituitary hyperemia, and sagging of the brain.[21] The classical imaging pattern associated with RCVS is a beaded appearance in the angiogram of medium to large caliber vessels, both intracranially as well as extracranially. The imaging may be confusing, with evidence of bilateral disease, which often waxes and wanes on sequential studies. One-third of the cases can be imaging negative at presentation. The final diagnosis is based on the reversibility of the previously identified areas of vasoconstriction, usually by 12 weeks, as per the diagnostic criteria.[15] For patients presenting with TCH due to pituitary apoplexy, sequences involving the pituitary to see the overall size, areas of hyperdensity on CT scan, and hyperintensity on MRI are utilized. Susceptibility weighted imaging (SWI) and gradient echo (GRE) sequences of MRI can also reveal blooming in brain parenchyma, which can be used to demonstrate the presence of hemorrhages. The presence of microhemorrhages is strongly suggestive of vasculitis and needs to be corroborated with clinical presentation and other laboratory markers. Cervical and vertebral artery dissection can also be associated with SAH and can be easily diagnosed using CT scan and CT and MR angiography. Vessel wall imaging is an emerging modality of investigation that can be used to supplement and aid in the diagnosis of complicated cases of differentials of TCH such as RCVS, SAH, vasculitis, or aneurysmal SAH. Some patterns on vessel wall imaging such as extent of thickening [pattern of thickening (focal vs. diffuse)], the region of thickening (concentric vs. eccentric), presence and pattern of enhancement if any, and resolution of previous enhancement can all give important clues to the diagnosis of the condition.[22] Conventional angiography is used to detect a cervical artery dissection but cannot detect a mural hematoma. The latter is best visualized by MRI. Some of the signs encountered are a candle flame appearance of the internal carotid sparing the bifurcation, or a long and irregular stenosis that spares the bulb. Occasionally, a dissecting aneurysm, an intimal flap, or a false channel is also seen that can suggest dissection, although it is important to bear in mind that a normal appearance does not exclude the diagnosis.[23]

How to Manage Thunderclap Headaches?

Management of TCH revolves around symptomatic relief and treatment of underlying cause. Because it is a rare entity in emergencies, there is no established guideline or management algorithm for its management. Here, we outline the empirical management of the common conditions causing a TCH.[9] Whenever medical drugs such as triptans, ergot alkaloids, prostaglandins or oral contraceptive pills, illicit drugs, or erythropoietin are found to be given in the patient, the same must be withdrawn immediately even if the association is unclear.[14] Headache can be treated with nonsteroidal analgesics such as naproxen, ibuprofen, piroxicam, paracetamol, and diclofenac. Doses can be repeated up to their maximum tolerable doses. In cases of severe pain, injectable analgesics or opioids may be required. The patient needs to be stabilized with intravenous fluids, proton pump inhibitors, sedatives, and antianxiety medications. Steroids have no proven benefit in all cases of TCH and must be given on a case-to-case basis only when indicated. Management of RCVS involves the withdrawal of offending agents if any. Symptomatic management requires analgesics to manage headaches, monitoring of blood pressure, and control of hypertension. Calcium channel blocking agents such as nimodipine are used to reverse vasospasm in the same doses as in cases of aneurysmal SAH (30-60 mg every 4-8 hours orally or 0.5-2 mg/kg/h). Glucocorticoids should be summarily avoided because they are ineffective in preventing clinical worsening and may further worsen the sympathetic hyperactivity. Refractory cases may require intra-arterial administration of calcium blockers, prostacyclin, and even balloon angioplasty has been tried. Adequate patient stabilization is required until the condition reverses by itself.[24]

Pituitary apoplexy with TCH is a vision-threatening emergency that usually requires high-dose steroids for symptoms control or surgical decompression in refractory cases.[8] SAH needs management of aneurysms on an emergent basis by neurosurgical clipping or coiling of the aneurysm. Postoperative period needs to be monitored for symptomatic vasospasm, which requires high-dose calcium channel blockers. There are established protocols for strokes, both ischemic or hemorrhagic strokes in emergencies and subsequent follow-up. Cervical dissection is another common cause, which may require management with dual antiplatelets, anticoagulants, or intracranial or extracranial stenting in selected cases. Intracranial hemorrhage requires management of blood pressure and evacuation of hematoma where appropriate. Venous thrombosis requires anticoagulation and thrombus retrieval by endovascular means in the early stages. Patients presenting with venous thrombosis with extensive areas of venous ischemic strokes may benefit with decompression. Space-occupying lesions need to be stabilized first for intracranial pressure and surgical treatment as appropriate. Symptomatic treatment may require antiepileptics to control seizures. Primary CNS vasculitis requires high-dose steroids and immunosuppression. Cases of raised intracranial pressure frequently require drainage of CSF in large volumes as well as acetazolamide to reduce CSF production in select cases.

CONCLUSION

A TCH is a neurological emergency with many differentials with severe consequences on morbidity and mortality. Localizations involve several sites involving cerebral vasculature, parenchyma, or even systemic causes. Judicious approach involves delineating it from severe forms of preexisting headache, a proper and thorough clinical examination and appropriate imaging and laboratory tests to narrow down the possibilities.

REFERENCES

1. Gobel H. 4.4 Primary thunderclap headache. The International Classification of Headache Disorders, 3rd edition. [online] Available from https://ichd-3.org/other-primary-headache-disorders/4-4-primary-thunderclap-headache/ [Last accessed June, 2023].
2. Day JW, Raskin NH. Thunderclap headache: Symptom of unruptured cerebral aneurysm. Lancet Lond Engl. 1986;2(8518):1247-8.
3. Dodick D. Thunderclap headache. J Neurol Neurosurg Psychiatry. 2002;72(1):6-11.
4. Chen CY, Fuh JL. Evaluating thunderclap headache. Curr Opin Neurol. 2021;34(3):356-62.
5. Matharu MS, Schwedt TJ, Dodick DW. Thunderclap headache: An approach to a neurologic emergency. Curr Neurol Neurosci Rep. 2007;7(2):101-9.
6. Dilli E. Thunderclap headache. Curr Neurol Neurosci Rep. 2014;14(4):437.
7. Yang CW, Fuh JL. Thunderclap headache: An update. Expert Rev Neurother. 2018;18(12):915-24.
8. Equiza J, Rodríguez-Antigüedad J, Campo-Caballero D, et al. Pituitary apoplexy causing thunderclap headache: Easy to miss. Pract Neurol. 2020:002625.
9. Long TR, Hein BD, Brown MJ, et al. Posterior reversible encephalopathy syndrome during pregnancy: Seizures in a previously healthy parturient. J Clin Anesth. 2007;19(2):145-8.
10. Bellolio MF, Hess EP, Gilani WI, et al. External validation of the Ottawa subarachnoid hemorrhage clinical decision rule in patients with acute headache. Am J Emerg Med. 2015;33(2):244-9.
11. de Falco FA. Sentinel headache. Neurol Sci. 2004;25 Suppl 3:S215-7.
12. Mollan SP, Paemeleire K, Versijpt J, et al. European Headache Federation recommendations for neurologists managing giant cell arteritis. J Headache Pain. 2020;21(1):28.
13. Short K, Emsley HCA. Illicit Drugs and Reversible Cerebral Vasoconstriction Syndrome. The Neurohospitalist. 2021;11(1):40-4.
14. Kato Y, Hayashi T, Mizuno S, et al. Triptan-induced Reversible Cerebral Vasoconstriction Syndrome: Two Case Reports with a Literature Review. Intern Med. 2016;55(23):3525-8.
15. Arrigan MT, Heran MKS, Shewchuk JR. Reversible cerebral vasoconstriction syndrome: An important and common cause of thunderclap and recurrent headaches. Clin Radiol. 2018;73(5):417-27.
16. Tepper SJ. Medication-overuse headache. Contin Minneap Minn. 2012;18(4):807-22.
17. Pyrgelis ES, Mavridis I, Meliou M. Presenting Symptoms of Pituitary Apoplexy. J Neurol Surg A Cent Eur Neurosurg. 2018;79(1):52-9.
18. Arora S, Swadron SP, Dissanayake V. Evaluating the sensitivity of visual xanthochromia in patients with subarachnoid hemorrhage. J Emerg Med. 2010;39(1):13-6.
19. Mortimer AM, Bradley MD, Stoodley NG, et al. Thunderclap headache: Diagnostic considerations and neuroimaging features. Clin Radiol. 2013;68(3):e101-13.
20. Leach JL, Fortuna RB, Jones BV, et al. Imaging of cerebral venous thrombosis: Current techniques, spectrum of findings, and diagnostic pitfalls. Radiographics. 2006;26 suppl 1:S19-41.
21. Spelle L, Boulin A, Pierot L, et al. Spontaneous intracranial hypotension: MRI and radionuclide cisternography findings. J Neurol Neurosurg Psychiatry. 1997;62(3):291-2.
22. Rustici A, Merli E, Cevoli S, et al. Vessel-wall MRI in thunderclap headache: A useful tool to answer the riddle? Interv Neuroradiol. 2021;27(2):219-24.
23. Hassen WB, Machet A, Edjlali-Goujon M, et al. Imaging of cervical artery dissection. Diagn Interv Imaging. 2014;95(12):1151-61.
24. Ducros A, Wolff V. The Typical Thunderclap Headache of Reversible Cerebral Vasoconstriction Syndrome and its Various Triggers. Headache. 2016;56(4):657-73.

Cerebral Sinus Venous Thrombosis—Management: An Update

Sanjith Aaron, Angel Miraclin T

ABSTRACT

Cerebral venous thrombosis (CVT), a condition once considered rare, is now being increasingly diagnosed due to increased awareness and better access and availability of imaging facilities. The rapid advances being made in the management of ischemic strokes are also being reflected in CVT, especially in the areas of endovascular therapies and surgical interventions. However, there are certain subsets of CVT that need different management strategies, and in some of them, there are still many grey areas in the treatment. There is also equipoise in the ideal duration of anticoagulants and anticonvulsants in the follow-up phase of CVT.

The coronavirus disease 2019 (COVID-19) pandemic has thrown up fresh challenges as both the COVID-19 infection and the adenoviral vector-based COVID vaccines are known to trigger CVT.

In this chapter, we have described the importance of targeting and treating various steps in the pathophysiology of CVT simultaneously and the need for different treatment approaches for some of the subtypes of CVT.

Keywords: Cerebral venous thrombosis, Management update, COVID, CVT, Cortical vein thrombosis, BIH presentation of CVT, Deep cerebral venous thrombosis.

INTRODUCTION

Cerebral vein and dural sinus thrombosis can be caused either by the occlusion of the dural venous sinuses, the superficial cortical veins, or a combination of both. There are many acquired and hereditary causes of cerebral venous thrombosis (CVT). Being a relatively rare condition that presents in a myriad of ways, CVT can often get missed or misdiagnosed. However, in the last two decades, with increased awareness of this condition and the wide availability of imaging modalities, especially magnetic resonance imaging (MRI), CVT has been increasingly recognized and treatment initiated early. This is reflected in the mortality rates of CVT cases, which, compared to earlier cohorts, have come down to 5.6% in the acute phase and 9.4% at follow-up.[1] Earlier registries had uniformly indicated a female predilection; however, some recent studies indicate this gender predilection is narrowing.[2] In recent years, we have gained a better understanding of the pathophysiology of CVT. However, there are still many grey areas in the management of CVT. In this chapter, we have attempted to review the latest evidence and delineate the practical guidelines in management of patients with CVT.

PATHOGENESIS OF CEREBRAL VEIN AND DURAL SINUS THROMBOSIS

When there is occlusion of a dural venous sinus **(Fig. 1A)**, the cortical veins draining into that sinus will get congested, causing an increase in the postcapillary venous pressure and intracranial pressure (ICP) **(Fig. 1B)**. The brain will try to compensate for this by creating collateral pathways of venous drainage and also by increasing cerebrospinal fluid (CSF) absorption. However, if the superior sagittal and lateral dural sinuses (the principal sites for CSF absorption where the arachnoid granulation are located) are thrombosed, then this absorption can be impaired,

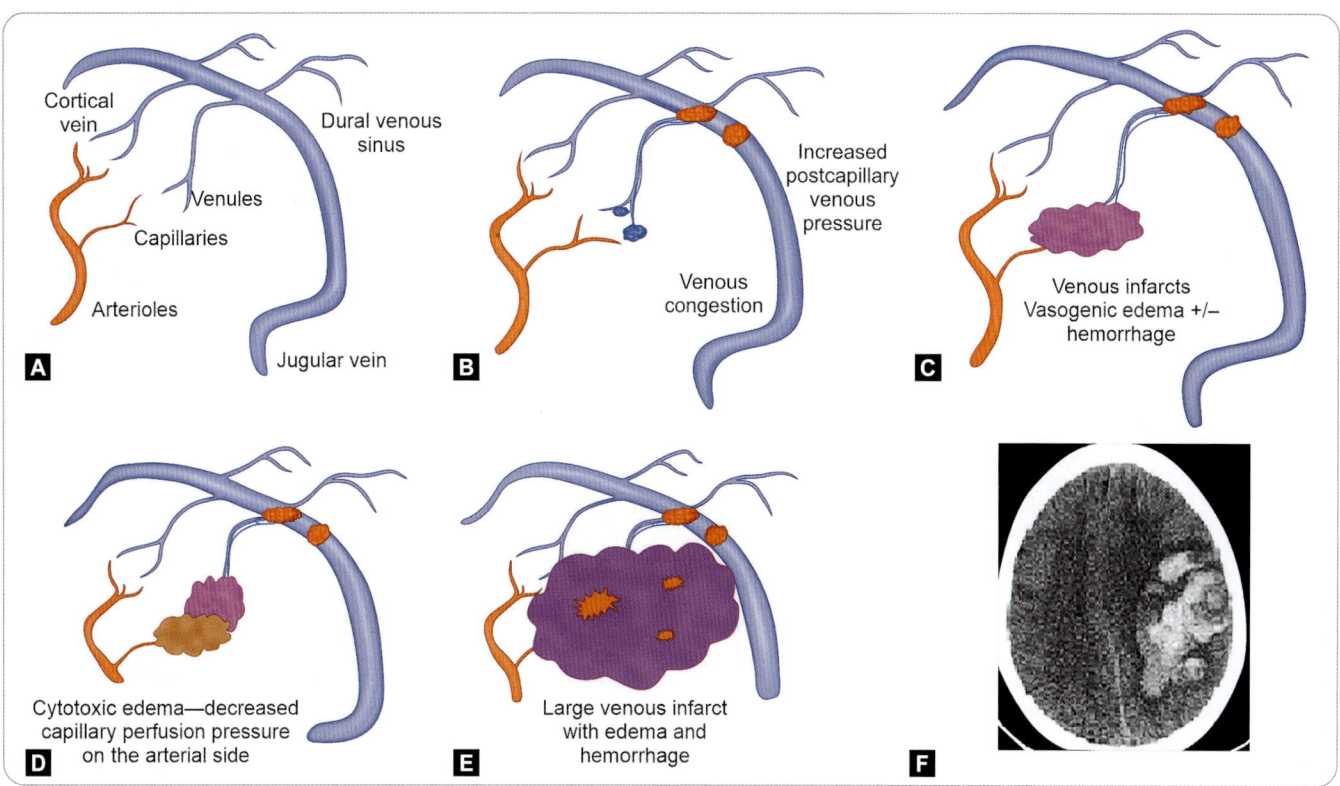

FIGS. 1A TO F: Pathogenesis of large venous infarcts. (A) Normal anatomy showing the cortical veins, venules, and dural sinuses (blue) and the arteries, arterioles, and capillaries (red). (B) Thrombus in the superior sagittal sinus causing congestion and back pressure changes in the draining vein. (C) Further increase in venous pressures resulting in venous infarcts and vasogenic edema, which can be accompanied by venous hemorrhages. (D) Any further increase in pressures can reflect on the arterial side through a drop in capillary perfusion pressure resulting in cytotoxic edema. (E) If not intervened the final result can be large venous infarcts with edema (both cytotoxic and vasogenic) and hemorrhage. (F) Plain computed tomography (CT) scan showing a large venous infarct on the left side with edema, hemorrhage, and mass effect causing a midline shift.

resulting in the failure of this CSF buffer, causing a further increase in the ICP and, in some cases, leading to the development of a communicating hydrocephalus. As the postcapillary venous pressure can increase further, there can be blood–brain barrier disruption and leakage of blood plasma into the interstitial space, resulting in vasogenic edema and venous infarcts with or without hemorrhage **(Fig. 1C)**. If this continues, decreased capillary perfusion pressure will start developing on the arterial side, resulting in cytotoxic edema **(Fig. 1D)**, culminating in the formation of large venous infarcts with both vasogenic and cytotoxic edema with or without hemorrhage, and resulting in a mass effect and potential herniation **(Figs. 1E and F)**. The clinical presentation and severity of CVT will depend on the venous territory involved, the extent of thrombosis, the robustness of the venous collaterals, the variation in the venous anatomy, and the chronicity of the thrombus.

TREATMENT

Treatment should target multiple pathophysiological mechanisms simultaneously **(Fig. 2)**, and some subsets of CVT cases may warrant different treatment strategies. Also, close monitoring of patients is required, especially in the acute phase, and in those cases where patients are not responding, different treatment strategies may be needed to prevent them.

■ Restoration of Venous Flow

Preventing the propagation of the thrombus any further and restoring the venous flow are the cornerstones of the treatment of CVT. Recanalization was found to cause regression of the venous infarcts, especially if hemorrhage has not yet set in, resulting in a good functional recovery. Immediate systemic anticoagulation should be initiated with either partial thromboplastin time (PTT)-adjusted intravenous (IV) unfractionated heparin (UFH) or body-weight-adjusted low-molecular-weight heparin (LMWH).[3] Since studies have shown superiority for LMWH over UFH,[4] unless there are contraindications for the use of LMWH like renal insufficiency or situations where a reversal of the anticoagulation is anticipated (surgical intervention), LMWH is recommended over UFH. Full therapeutic anticoagulation should be initiated even in CVT patients

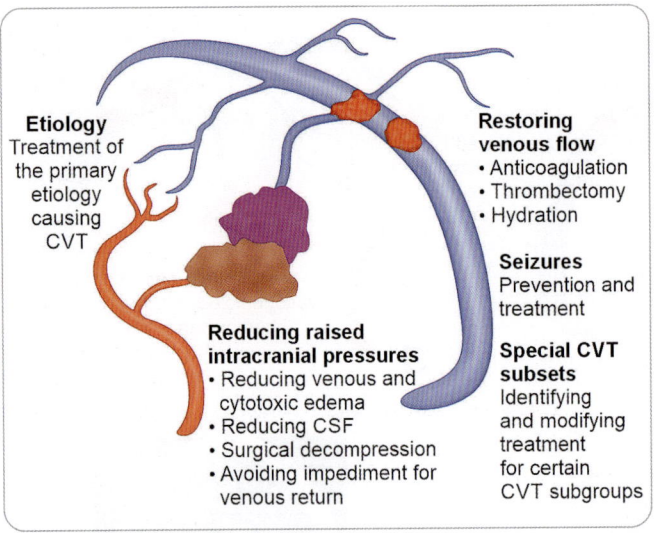

FIG. 2: Potential targets for therapy in cerebral vein and dural sinus thrombosis.
(CSF: cerebrospinal fluid; CVT: cerebral venous thrombosis)

with venous hemorrhage and/or subarachnoid hemorrhage since the underlying venous outflow occlusion is the cause of these bleeds.[5]

In cases where patients develop progressive neurologic worsening despite adequate anticoagulation without other causes for the worsening, repeat imaging should be done. If the repeat imaging shows progression or no recanalization, endovascular thrombolysis or mechanical thrombectomy may be considered. A randomized controlled trial [Thrombolysis or Anticoagulation for Cerebral Venous Thrombosis (TO-ACT)] failed to show benefit with thrombectomy with or without chemical thrombolysis over anticoagulation. However, this study was underpowered, and the endovascular strategies used were heterogeneous.[6] In a recent study, balloon-assisted mechanical thrombectomy was found to be effective in a subset of younger patients with severe CVT without hemorrhagic infarction and noninvolvement of the frontoparietal lobes who had failed medical therapy.[7]

Reducing the Raised Intracranial Pressures

Factors which impede the venous return should be avoided. Nursing should be done by elevating the head of the bed without neck rotation or flexion, avoiding tight-fitting collars and mask or bands. Jugular catheters should be avoided. Hyperosmolar therapy with 3% saline should be initiated, and in severe cases while contemplating surgery or endovascular options, mannitol can be given. If ventilator care is needed, it should be done with full sedation, avoiding high positive end expiratory pressures (PEEP) and frequent suctioning. Carbonic anhydrase inhibitors like acetazolamide, which can reduce CSF production, can also be used to complement other therapies targeting raised ICP. Steroids can potentially promote thrombosis and have failed to show benefit in CVT patients with parenchymal lesions.[8] In CVT, steroids use should be limited to those cases of CVT caused by systemic lupus erythematosus (SLE), Behçet's disease, and other autoimmune conditions. Therapeutic lumbar puncture is another option to reduce ICP in cases where there are no contraindications caused by parenchymal lesions. In patients where medical treatment has failed with the parenchymal lesions causing a life-threatening impending herniation, decompressive surgery (hemicraniectomy or hematoma evacuation) should be carried out. Giving space for the swollen brain to bulge and reducing the ICP can be a lifesaving measure. A good functional outcome can be expected even in patients with pupillary asymmetry, especially if done early and in those below 40 years.[9,10] The DECOMPRESS-2 trial, a large prospective international multicentric study looking at outcomes of decompressive surgery for patients with severe cerebral venous thrombosis, showed two-thirds of CVT patients were alive and more than one-third were independent 1 year after decompressive surgery. Decompressive neurosurgery was judged worthwhile by 4 out of 5 patients who survived and their care givers.[11]

Treatment and Prevention of Seizures

Seizures are a common complication of CVT, occurring in 34–50% of patients, either in the early phase of the disease or as a late symptom. In the acute setting, antiepileptic drugs should be initiated in patients presenting with seizures. Levetiracetam or sodium valproate is preferred since they have fewer drug interactions with vitamin K antagonist (VKA) used for anticoagulation. The role of prophylactic antiepileptic medications and the optimal duration to continue the antiepileptic agents are not clear. Late seizures (seizures occurring after 7 days) can occur in 10% of patients. Status epilepticus at presentation, hemorrhagic supratentorial lesions, and those who had undergone decompression are more prone to this and may constitute a subgroup of CVT cases where prophylactic antiepileptic agents may be needed and also consider long-term antiepileptic treatment.[12,13]

Postacute Stage

There is an overall risk of recurrence of 5.8% for both CVT and thrombosis in other venous beds after the acute phase of CVT. Most of these events were found to occur in the first year after CVT.[14] Hence follow-up oral anticoagulants is recommended. Oral VKA with an international normalized ratio (INR) target of 2.5 (acceptable range: 2–3) can be given. The RE-SPECT CVT trial showed that dabigatran 150 mg twice a day is equally safe and effective for preventing recurrent venous thromboembolisms (VTEs) in patients with CVT.[15] In the retrospective ACTION-CVT (Direct Oral Anticoagulants Versus Warfarin in the Treatment of Cerebral Venous Thrombosis) study, similar risks of recurrent venous thrombosis and death, as well as similar rates of recanalization on follow-up imaging, were observed.[16] However, in these trials, CVT patients with underlying malignancy, antiphospholipid antibody (APLA) syndrome, renal failure, and pregnancy were excluded. Hence for these groups of CVT, VKA should be preferred over direct oral anticoagulants (DOACs). However, there are no clear guidelines on the optimum duration of oral anticoagulants after the acute phase. European Academy of Neurology guidelines[3] recommend giving oral anticoagulants for 3-6 months in CVT caused by transient risk factors like pregnancy and infection, 6-12 months for those with CVT associated with "mild" thrombophilia, and continuing the anticoagulants lifelong in those with an underlying malignancy or combined or "severe" thrombophilia [e.g., two or more prothrombotic abnormalities; antithrombin III (AT III), protein C or S deficiencies, APLA, and malignancy]. There is an ongoing study comparing the efficacy and safety of short-term (3-6 months) versus long-term (12 months) anticoagulation after cerebral vein thrombosis for the prevention of such venous thromboembolic events.[17] Women should be advised not to take oral contraceptive preparations and other hormonal therapies post-CVT.

SPECIAL SUBSETS OF CEREBRAL VEIN AND DURAL SINUS THROMBOSIS PATIENTS

There are some special subsets of CVT patients where the clinical presentations and imaging findings can differ from the usual CVT cases. For some of these subgroups, different treatment strategies may need to be employed. It is important to have a high index of suspicion to identify these subgroups of CVT cases early to prevent serious morbidities and mortality.

■ Benign Intracranial Hypertension-like Presentation of Cerebral Vein and Dural Sinus Thrombosis

Visual impairment can complicate CVT through multiple mechanisms:
- Venous infarcts involving the occipital cortex
- Raised ICP following the development of a secondary dural arteriovenous (AV) fistula
- Arterial occipital infarcts occurring as a late complication due to posterior cerebral artery compression secondary to herniation

However, one of the causes that can get misdiagnosed is case of CVT without any parenchymal involvement with optic nerve dysfunction secondary to raised ICP, which can mimic benign intracranial hypertension (BIH) **(Figs. 3A to D)**. The presentation can be a young patient with chronic headache with subsequent visual impairment and papilledema on examination. The CT brain can appear normal, and the CSF can be cellular with high opening pressures.[18] In a series evaluating BIH, 10% had CVT on MRI/magnetic resonance venography (MRV).[19] It is very important to identify these patients early to avoid the progression of visual deterioration and loss. Before starting treatment, a primary or secondary dural arteriovenous fistula (DAVF) should be ruled out. Anticoagulants and acetazolamide should be started early with close monitoring of the vision using optical coherence tomography (OCT) or serial ultrasounds to measure the optic nerve head diameter or visual fields in chronic cases. Serial therapeutic lumbar punctures can be carried out if there are no contraindications in cases of deterioration while on medical treatment. Optic nerve sheath fenestration[20] and endovascular procedures to open up the blocked venous channels should also be attempted to prevent blindness in refractive cases. CSF diversion procedures like thecoperitoneal (TP) shunts can be attempted in cases that worsen despite these measures, especially in patients with sustained intracranial hypertension and no parenchymal lesions.[21]

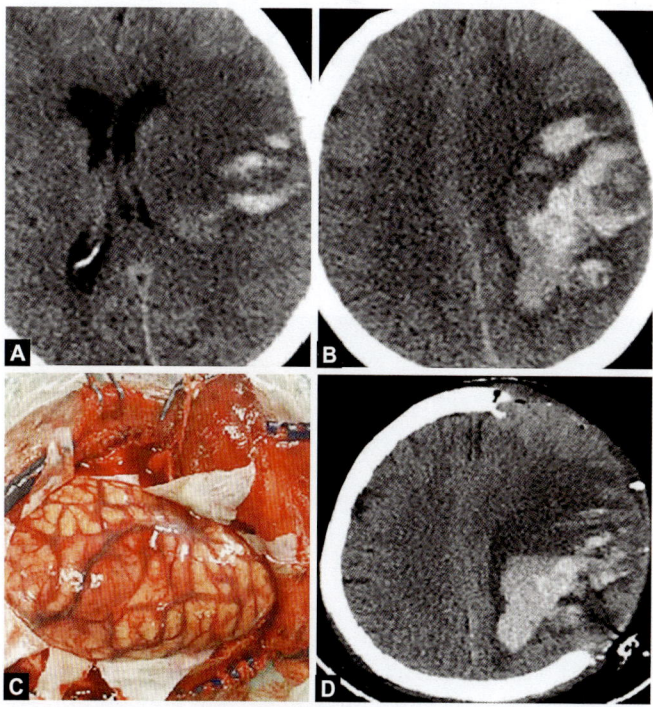

FIGS. 3A TO D: Decompressive hemicraniectomy in cerebral vein and dural sinus thrombosis. (A and B) Plain computed tomography (CT) scan showing a large venous infarct with hemorrhage with mass effect causing midline shift. (C) Decompressive hemicraniectomy. (D) Postoperative CT scan showing a reduction in the midline shift.

Isolated Cortical Vein Thrombosis

Isolated cortical vein thrombosis (ICoVT) without involvement of the dural sinuses is rare. These patients can present with focal sensorimotor seizures. Headache is seen less frequently, and papilledema is usually absent. Signs of increased ICP are less common in ICoVT compared with cerebral venous sinus thrombosis (CVST), whereas localized cerebral edema or hemorrhagic lesions are more frequent in ICVT.[22,23] ICoVT can get missed on CT and MRI, with a T2*-gradient echo sequence may be required to demonstrate the thrombus in the occluded cortical vein **(Figs. 4A to C)**.[24] Susceptibility weighted imaging (SWI) showing cord sign was observed in 100% of the cases. The treatment is the same as for CVT, and a longer duration of antiepileptic drugs should be considered.

Isolated Deep Cerebral Venous Thrombosis

Involvement of the deep cerebral veins can occur occasionally with superficial venous thrombosis. However, it is associated with a poor prognosis with mortality of 30% in the ISCVT Study.[25] Isolated thrombosis of the deep cerebral venous system is very rare. Thrombosis of the internal cerebral vein (formed from the choroidal, septal, and thalamostriate veins), basal vein of Rosenthal, Vein of Galen, or straight sinus can lead to the involvement of the deep structures, including bilateral thalami, and can result in diencephalic dysfunction **(Figs. 5A to C)**. Hydrocephalus may occur as a consequence of edema and swelling of both thalami. In these patients, there may be a delay in

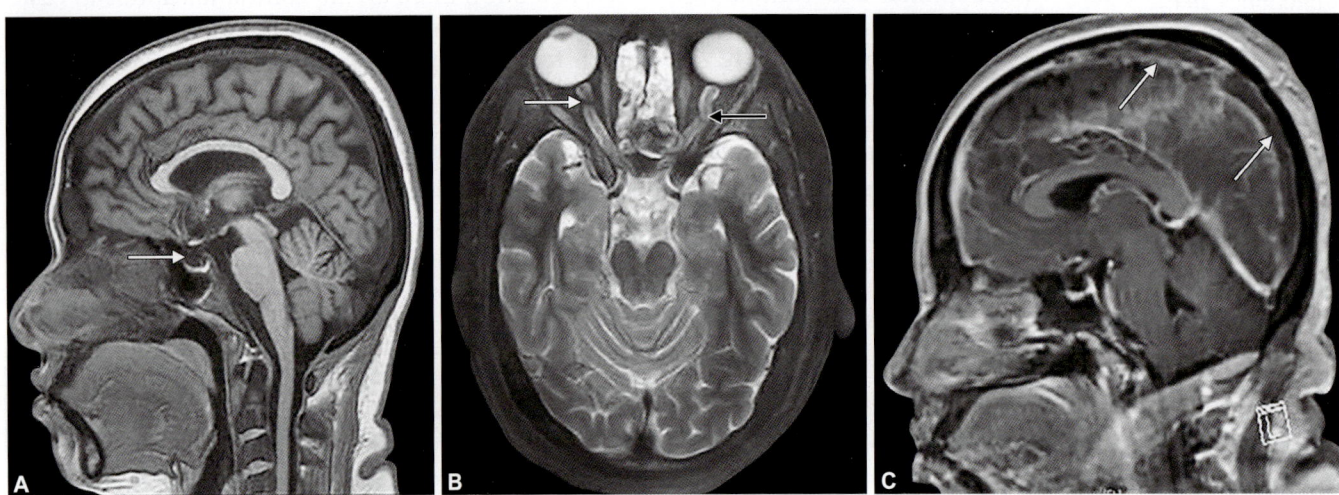

FIGS. 4A TO C: Benign intracranial hypertension presentation of chronic cerebral vein and dural sinus thrombosis. (A) Magnetic resonance imaging (MRI) of brain—sagittal view showing empty sella. (B) Tortuous optic nerves with periorbital cerebrospinal fluid (CSF) flare and flattening of posterior sclera. (C) Chronic cerebral venous thrombosis (CVT) with partial recanalization in the anterior two-thirds of the superior sagittal sinus.

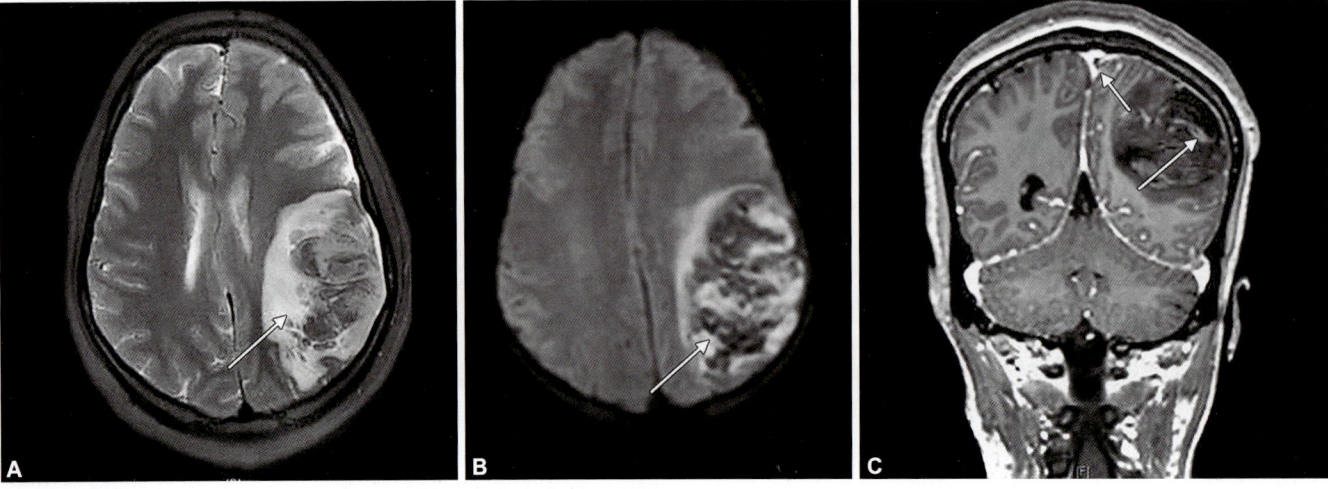

FIGS. 5A TO C: Isolated cortical vein thrombosis. (A and B) Magnetic resonance imaging (MRI) of brain—left parietal hemorrhagic venous infarct. (C) Postcontrast images showing multiple thrombosed cortical veins.

the diagnosis as the presenting symptoms can only be a diencephalic dysfunction, altered sensorium, or coma without any focal neurological deficit or seizures. A high index of suspicion based on the appropriate clinical setting and early imaging findings is warranted.[26] Plain CT is usually the first examination performed in an emergency setting and may pick up isolated DVCT only in 25% of cases.[7,27] Thrombus appearing hyperdense can be seen in the internal cerebral veins, and the bilateral venous edema involving the basal ganglia and thalamus can be seen as a butterfly-shaped hypodense area. A contrast MRI with MRV should be done in suspected cases if the CT findings are inconclusive. Early initiation of appropriate treatment, including endovascular therapies **(Figs. 6A to F)**, can lower mortality.

Septic Cerebral Venous Sinus Thrombosis

Infections can cause CVT due to multiple mechanisms.
- *Spread of infection from adjacent structures*: The cerebral veins, emissary veins, and dural venous sinuses have no valves, allowing blood to flow in either direction depending on the pressure gradients. This can potentially cause the spread of infection from adjacent structures and result in septic thrombophlebitis.[28] Infections in the sphenoid and ethmoid sinuses, the dangerous triangle of the face, and mastoiditis (which can cause lateral sinus thrombophlebitis) are all potential causes.
- *Systemic infection*: It can precipitate thrombosis due to the release of proinflammatory cytokines, leading to the activation of the coagulation system, activation of tissue factor (TF), which can covert factor X to factor Xa, intravascular fibrin deposition, and impaired fibrin degradation.
- Septic sinus thrombosis can complicate meningitis, especially pneumococcal meningitis.[29] In patients having sudden raised ICP features or developing new focal deficits after a period of excellent initial recovery, a delayed cerebral thrombosis should be suspected. Some infections, like HIV infection and invasive fungal infections, can cause CVT through multiple mechanisms. Treatment should include early surgical drainage of the primary site of infection if possible, appropriate intravenous antibiotics, and systemic anticoagulation. Corticosteroids are of uncertain benefit; some reports have shown a favorable response.

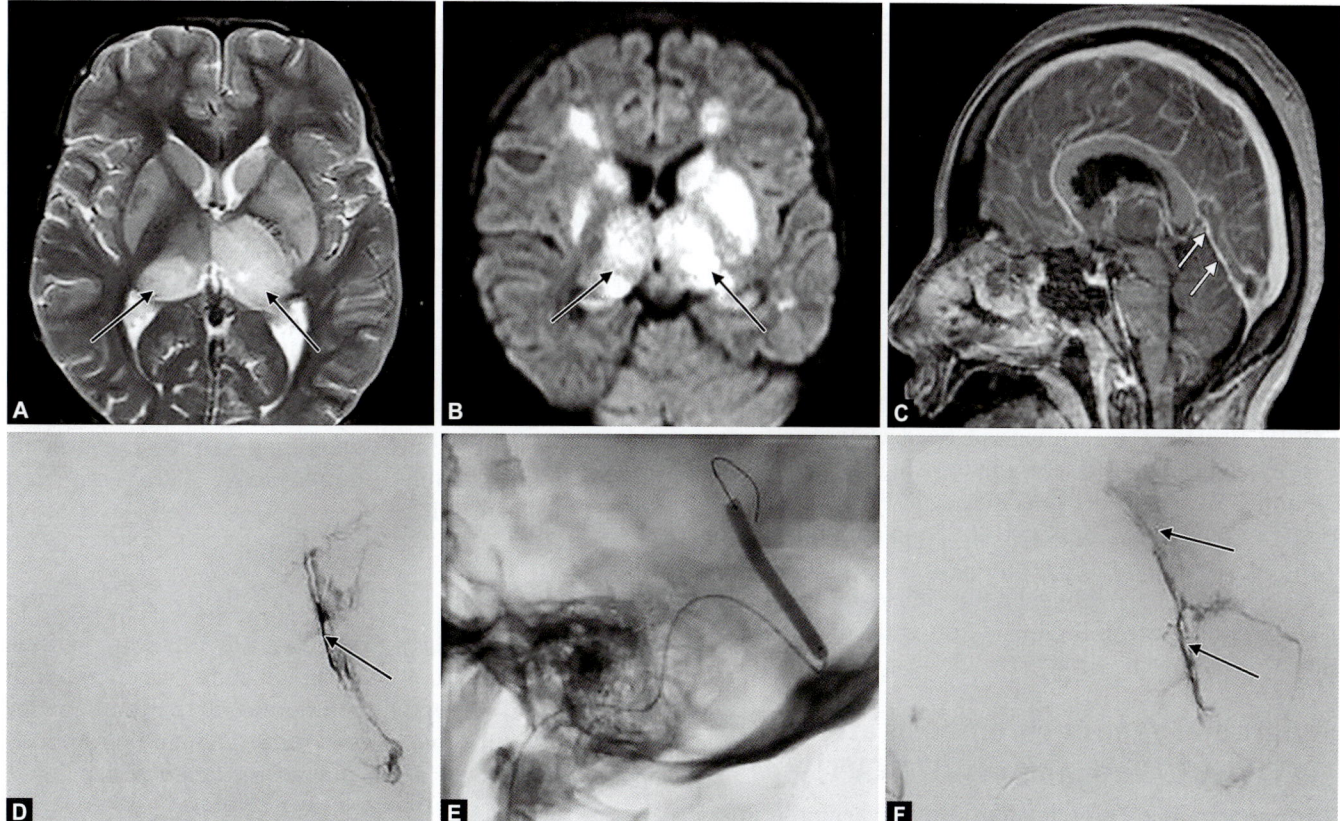

FIGS. 6A TO F: Deep cerebral venous sinus thrombosis treated with balloon thromboplasty. (A and B) Magnetic resonance imaging (MRI) of brain—vasogenic edema and venous infarction of bilateral basal ganglia and thalamus. (C) MRI of brain with contrast showing thrombosis of the straight sinus. (D) Digital subtraction angiogram (DSA) showing filling defect in the straight sinus. (E) Modified Fogarty Balloon thromboplasty of the straight sinus. (F) Postprocedure DSA showing partial recanalization of the straight sinus.

Women with a Previous History of Cerebral Vein and Dural Sinus Thrombosis Planning Pregnancy

There are no contraindications for future pregnancies in women with a previous history of CVT. However, they should be informed regarding a slightly higher risk of both recurrent CVT (9 per 1,000 pregnancies) as well as noncerebral VTE (27 per 1,000 pregnancies).[30] Studies and meta-analyses have shown the safety and efficacy of antithrombotic prophylaxis (LMWH) without an increase in hemorrhagic complications in such patients. Miscarriage did not differ significantly in women undergoing antithrombotic therapy or not (11.3% vs. 18.8%; $p = 0.34$).[31] Prophylactic anticoagulation with subcutaneous LMWH throughout pregnancy and continuing up to 8 weeks postpartum is warranted for these patients at high risk of CVT. Coumarins can cross the placenta and can potentially cause coumarin embryopathy, especially if exposed between 6 and 12 weeks of gestation. Hence, if a pregnancy is planned while on coumarins, it should be substituted with LMWH ahead of conceiving. There is no data on the safety of non-vitamin K antagonist oral anticoagulants (NOACs) in pregnancy, and hence it should not be used.

COVID-19 Infection-related Cerebral Vein and Dural Sinus Thrombosis

Coronavirus disease 2019 (COVID-19) infection can induce a procoagulant milieu by increasing the concentrations of coagulation factors and APLAs and decreasing the concentrations of endogenous anticoagulant factors. This can induce thrombosis in various venous and arterial beds, including the cerebral veins and sinuses. It is important to note that CVT could be the only presentation of the COVID-19 infection. The systemic and pulmonary symptoms and signs may or may not manifest. Hence, COVID-19 testing should be done as a standard workup for all CVT cases and in those COVID-19 patients presenting with headaches or seizures.[32] COVID-associated CVT cases can have high D-dimer levels, inflammatory markers like erythrocyte sedimentation rate (ESR) and C-reactive protein (CRP), and antiphospholipid antibodies (anti-beta-2-glycoprotein). The platelet count will be normal. The treatment is the same as for non-COVID CVT and the outcome depends on early diagnosis and initiation of therapy.

Cerebral Venous Thrombosis after COVID-19 Vaccination (VITT-CVT)

Thromboembolic complication termed vaccine-induced immune thrombotic thrombocytopenia (VITT). It can occur following COVID-19 vaccination using adenoviral vector-based vaccines ChAdOx1 nCov-19 (Oxford-AstraZeneca) and Covishield (Oxford-AstraZeneca). This VIIT can also cause CVT (VITT-CVT). An evolving model suggests a two-hit process in which the vaccine stimulates neoantigen formation (the first hit) along with a systemic inflammatory response (the second hit), which together lead to the production of anti-PF4 antibodies.[33] Young female patients are at increased risk for this complication, and the onset of symptoms occurs 5–10 days postvaccination. It is important to note that headaches occur in around 50% of patients within the first 72 hours postvaccination, and this will usually be associated with systemic symptoms such as fatigue, fever, myalgia, and arthralgia.[34] Usually, this headache settles within the first few days. In individuals with headaches or those who develop delayed-onset headaches (within 30 days) postvaccination, CVT should be suspected and investigated. Also, one should suspect VIIT-CVT in patients with CVT who are worsening without any obvious reason while on heparin and in those developing extracranial venous thrombosis. The laboratory tests will show (1) thrombocytopenia 1.5 lakhs, or a falling platelet count; (2) high D-dimer levels >4,000 FEU (fibrinogen equivalent units), and (3) positive antibody against PF4 [enzyme-linked immunosorbent assay (ELISA)]. It is important to suspect and diagnose VIIT-CVT since these patients should not be given heparins (UFH or LMWH) since PF4, being a positively charged protein, may combine with heparin to form neoantigens, and the action of antibodies against PF4 can increase in the presence of heparin. VIIT-CVT should be treated with heparinoids (fondaparinux and danaparoid) and followed up with a factor Xa inhibitor or direct thrombin inhibitor. Anticoagulants should be continued for 3 months after normalization of the platelet count. In the acute state, high-dose intravenous immunoglobulin (IVIG) should be initiated to counter the antibody to PF4, and in refractory cases. Therapeutic plasma exchange (TPE) or immunosuppression with rituximab (RTX) should be tried. Platelet transfusions can cause a potential worsening of thrombosis and should be reserved for patients with life-threatening bleeding or the need for emergency surgery. Overall mortality is higher than non-VIIT-CVT, especially in those with platelet counts below 30,000/mm^3 and intracranial hemorrhage.

PROGNOSIS

We can use risk scores like the IN-REvASC score[35] or the ISCVT-RS score[36] to predict the outcome of patients with CVT. In CVT cases with underling active malignancy presenting with coma, altered sensorium, and thrombosis of the deep venous system, prognosis is guarded.

CONCLUSION

Even though the prognosis of CVT has improved in the last few decades, it is still an important cause of stroke in the young causing mortality and morbidity. It is important to identify certain subsets of CVT patients where a different treatment strategy may need to be employed. There are still many areas of diagnostic and therapeutic equipoise, where we do not have robust evidence-based guidelines. There are many unanswered questions as to who benefits with endovascular therapy, optimal duration of anticoagulation as well as antiepileptic therapy. All these answers require further research. In the future, we can expect newer treatment modalities such as factor XI and factor XIa inhibitors for treatment and biomarkers that can aid in diagnosis and prognosticating patients with CVT.

REFERENCES

1. Coutinho JM, Zuurbier SM, Stam J. Declining mortality in cerebral venous thrombosis: A systematic review. Stroke. 2014;45(5):1338-41.
2. Ruuskanen JO, Kytö V, Posti JP, et al. Cerebral Venous Thrombosis: Finnish Nationwide Trends. Stroke. 2021;52(1):335-8.
3. Ferro JM, Bousser MG, Canhão P, et al. European Stroke Organization guideline for the diagnosis and treatment of cerebral venous thrombosis - endorsed by the European Academy of Neurology. Eur J Neurol. 2017;24(10):1203-13.
4. Misra UK, Kalita J, Chandra S, et al. Low molecular weight heparin versus unfractionated heparin in cerebral venous sinus thrombosis: a randomized controlled trial. Eur J Neurol. 2012;19(7):1030-6.
5. Wingerchuk DM, Wijdicks EF, Fulgham JR. Cerebral venous thrombosis complicated by hemorrhagic infarction: factors affecting the initiation and safety of anticoagulation. Cerebrovasc Dis Basel Switz. 1998;8(1):25-30.
6. Coutinho JM, Zuurbier SM, Bousser MG, et al. Effect of Endovascular Treatment With Medical Management vs Standard Care on Severe Cerebral Venous Thrombosis: The TO-ACT Randomized Clinical Trial. JAMA Neurol. 2020;77(8):966-73.
7. Alwan A, Miraclin AT, Bal D, et al. Management of Severe Cerebral Venous Sinus Thrombosis Using Mechanical Balloon Assisted Thrombectomy. Stroke Vasc Interv Neurol. 2023;3(1):e000574.
8. Canhão P, Cortesão A, Cabral M, et al. Are steroids useful to treat cerebral venous thrombosis? Stroke. 2008;39(1):105-10.
9. Ferro JM, Crassard I, Coutinho JM, et al. Decompressive surgery in cerebrovenous thrombosis: a multicenter registry and a systematic review of individual patient data. Stroke. 2011;42(10):2825-31.
10. Aaron S, Alexander M, Moorthy RK, et al. Decompressive craniectomy in cerebral venous thrombosis: a single centre experience. J Neurol Neurosurg Psychiatry. 2013;84(9):995-1000.
11. ESOC. (2021). Conference Abstracts. [online] Available from https://2021.eso-conference.org/conference-abstracts/ [Last accessed June, 2023].
12. Ferro JM, Canhão P, Bousser MG, et al.; ISCVT Investigators. Early seizures in cerebral vein and dural sinus thrombosis: risk factors and role of antiepileptics. Stroke. 2008;39(4):1152-8.
13. Sánchez van Kammen M, Lindgren E, et al. Late seizures in cerebral venous thrombosis. Neurology. 2020;95(12):e1716-23.
14. Miranda B, Ferro JM, Canhão P, et al. Venous thromboembolic events after cerebral vein thrombosis. Stroke. 2010;41(9):1901-6.
15. Ferro JM, Coutinho JM, Dentali F, et al. Safety and Efficacy of Dabigatran Etexilate vs Dose-Adjusted Warfarin in Patients With Cerebral Venous Thrombosis: A Randomized Clinical Trial. JAMA Neurol. 2019;76(12):1457-65.
16. Yaghi S, Shu L, Bakradze E, et al. Direct Oral Anticoagulants Versus Warfarin in the Treatment of Cerebral Venous Thrombosis (ACTION-CVT): A Multicenter International Study. Stroke. 2022;53(3):728-38.
17. Miranda B, Aaron S, Arauz A, et al. The benefit of EXtending oral antiCOAgulation treatment (EXCOA) after acute cerebral vein thrombosis (CVT): EXCOA-CVT cluster randomized trial protocol. Int J Stroke Off J Int Stroke Soc. 2018;13(7):771-4.
18. Biousse V, Ameri A, Bousser MG. Isolated intracranial hypertension as the only sign of cerebral venous thrombosis. Neurology. 1999;53(7):1537-42.
19. Lin A, Foroozan R, Danesh-Meyer HV, et al. Occurrence of cerebral venous sinus thrombosis in patients with presumed idiopathic intracranial hypertension. Ophthalmology. 2006;113(12):2281-4.
20. Xue X, Zhou C, Gao Y, et al. Optic nerve sheath fenestration for visual impairment in cerebral venous diseases. Front Neurol. 2023;14:1065315.
21. Lobo S, Ferro JM, Barinagarrementeria F, et al. Shunting in acute cerebral venous thrombosis: a systematic review. Cerebrovasc Dis Basel Switz. 2014;37(1):38-42.
22. Urban PP, Müller-Forell W. Clinical and neuroradiological spectrum of isolated cortical vein thrombosis. J Neurol. 2005;252(12):1476-81.
23. Coutinho JM, Gerritsma JJ, Zuurbier SM, et al. Isolated cortical vein thrombosis: systematic review of case reports and case series. Stroke. 2014;45(6):1836-8.
24. Boukobza M, Crassard I, Bousser MG, et al. MR imaging features of isolated cortical vein thrombosis: diagnosis and follow-up. Am J Neuroradiol. 2009;30(2):344-8.
25. Ferro JM, Canhão P, Stam J, et al.; ISCVT Investigators. Prognosis of cerebral vein and dural sinus thrombosis: results of the International Study on Cerebral Vein and Dural Sinus Thrombosis (ISCVT). Stroke. 2004;35(3):664-70.
26. Provenzale JM, Kranz PG. Dural Sinus Thrombosis: Sources of Error in Image Interpretation. Am J Roentgenol. 2011;196(1):23-31.
27. Kalita J, Sachan A, Dubey AK, et al. A clinico-radiological study of deep cerebral venous thrombosis. Neuroradiology. 2022;64(10):1951-60.
28. Jacob MS, Gunasekaran K, Miraclin AT, et al. Clinical Profile and Outcome of Patients with Cerebral Venous Thrombosis Secondary to Bacterial Infections. Ann Indian Acad Neurol. 2020;23(4):477-81.
29. Lucas MJ, Brouwer MC, van de Beek D. Delayed cerebral thrombosis in bacterial meningitis: a prospective cohort study. Intensive Care Med. 2013;39(5):866-71.
30. Aguiar de Sousa D, Lucas Neto L, Arauz A, et al. Early Recanalization in Patients With Cerebral Venous Thrombosis Treated With Anticoagulation. Stroke. 2020;51(4):1174-81.
31. Bain E, Wilson A, Tooher R, et al. Prophylaxis for venous thromboembolic disease in pregnancy and the early postnatal period. Cochrane Database Syst Rev. 2014;(2):CD001689.
32. Miraclin TA, Aaron S, Sivadasan A, et al. Management and Outcomes of COVID-19 Associated Cerebral Venous Sinus Thrombosis. J Stroke Cerebrovasc Dis. 2022;31(4):106306.
33. Greinacher A, Selleng K, Palankar R, et al. Insights in ChAdOx1 nCoV-19 vaccine-induced immune thrombotic thrombocytopenia. Blood. 2021;138(22):2256-68.
34. Pavord S, Scully M, Hunt BJ, et al. Clinical Features of Vaccine-Induced Immune Thrombocytopenia and Thrombosis. N Engl J Med. 2021;1680-9.
35. Klein P, Shu L, Nguyen TN, et al. Outcome Prediction in Cerebral Venous Thrombosis: The IN-REvASC Score. J Stroke. 2022;24(3):404-16.
36. Ferro JM, Bacelar-Nicolau H, Rodrigues T, et al. Risk score to predict the outcome of patients with cerebral vein and dural sinus thrombosis. Cerebrovasc Dis Basel Switz. 2009;28(1):39-44.

CHAPTER 6

Cerebral Autosomal Dominant Arteriopathy with Subcortical Infarcts and Leukoencephalopathy: Recent Concepts

Biswamohan Mishra, Deepti Vibha, Ajay Garg

ABSTRACT

Cerebral autosomal dominant arteriopathy with subcortical infarcts and leukoencephalopathy (CADASIL) is an autosomal dominant inherited nonamyloid angiopathy predominantly involving the central nervous system (CNS). CADASIL is phenotypically diverse and affects multiple molecular systems in the small blood vessels of the brain. A key characteristic of CADASIL is cerebral white matter changes visible in magnetic resonance imaging (MRI) of young adult patients, often preceding the onset of severe symptoms, which triggers genetic testing. The location of neurogenic locus notch homolog protein 3 *(NOTCH3)* mutations is highly variable and correlates with disease severity. These mutations consistently disrupt the balance of cysteine residues in extracellular NOTCH3. Based on advances in genetic evaluation, numerous variants in the *NOTCH3* gene that cause CADASIL have been identified. However, the mechanism underlying the disease remains poorly understood and is an area of active research. Another unique feature of CADASIL is the presence of granular osmiophilic material (GOM) deposits around blood vessels, which appear to play a role in sequestering proteins essential for blood vessel homeostasis. There is currently no treatment for CADASIL. As our understanding of CADASIL continues to increase, translational research that bridges basic science and clinical findings will be essential for the discovery of biomarkers and therapeutic targets.

Keywords: Cerebral autosomal dominant arteriopathy with subcortical infarcts and leukoencephalopathy (CADASIL), Stroke in young, Familial stroke syndromes, Stroke with migraine, Genetic stroke syndrome, Headache with stroke.

INTRODUCTION

Cerebral autosomal dominant arteriopathy with subcortical infarcts and leukoencephalopathy (CADASIL) is a monogenic hereditary small vessel disease (SVD).[1] It is currently recognized as the most common genetic cause of stroke and dementia in adults.[2] It is caused by mutations in the neurogenic locus notch homolog protein 3 (*NOTCH3*) gene on chromosome 19p13.2-p13.1 that are inherited in an autosomal dominant pattern, with missense mutations being the most common type (95%). The disease has an insidious onset and usually begins to manifest in the third or fourth decade of life. Clinical manifestations of CADASIL include migraine with aura, recurrent ischemic strokes, transient ischemic attacks (TIAs), progressive white matter degeneration, memory loss, major cognitive impairment, as well as various psychiatric symptoms. This chapter aims to summarize the current understanding, identification, and management of CADASIL.

EPIDEMIOLOGY

Cerebral autosomal dominant arteriopathy with subcortical infarcts and leukoencephalopathy is considered a rare disease, with a prevalence of mutation carriers between 0.8 and 5 per 100,000.[3] Recent data suggest a higher prevalence of *NOTCH3* pathogenic variants in the general population worldwide, particularly in Asiatic descendants, suggesting that CADASIL may manifest with milder clinical variants.[4-6] Further studies have indicated that the frequency of pathogenic variants in the *NOTCH3* gene that affect cysteine residues may be much higher, possibly affecting as many as 1 in 300 people globally. These variants have been linked to an increased risk of stroke and vascular dementia, as well as increased white matter hyperintensity volume, especially in the anterior temporal lobes.[4] The clinical presentations of pathogenic variants in the *NOTCH3* gene can be quite diverse depending upon the level of penetrance.[7] Despite the variability in clinical manifestations, all CADASIL patients inevitably progress to dementia and disability, with more than half of patients older than 58 years unable to walk, and close to 65% unable to attend their own bodily needs or requiring constant nursing care by the age of 65 years.[8] Moreover, CADASIL reduces life expectancy, with a mean age at death of 64.4 years in men and 70.7 years in women.[9]

PATHOPHYSIOLOGY (FLOWCHART 1)

The *NOTCH3* gene on chromosome 19p13 encodes a transmembrane receptor that is mainly expressed on vascular smooth muscle cells (VSMCs) and pericytes. The receptor has three domains: One extracellular domain (ECD) for ligand binding, one transmembrane domain, and one intracellular domain for intracellular signaling. The ligand binding induces a proteolytic cleavage of the ECD, which releases it into the interstitial space between cells. The intracellular domain then translocates to the nucleus and regulates the expression of specific target genes involved in VSMCs differentiation, vascular development during embryogenesis, and vascular response to injury.

The ECD is composed of three Notch/LIN repeats and 34 epidermal growth factor-like repeats (EGFRs) rich in cysteine residues, which form disulfide bonds that are responsible for the protein's tertiary structure.[10,11] CADASIL mutations typically involve EGFR-encoding sequences, leading to changes in cysteine residues, and causing receptor misfolding. Misfolded proteins are sequestered by the endoplasmic reticulum (ER) for refolding and trafficking, but mutant NOTCH3 proteins are highly resistant to degradation, leading to their retention in the ER for a long time. This retention causes ER stress, reactive oxygen species formation, and impaired cell growth and

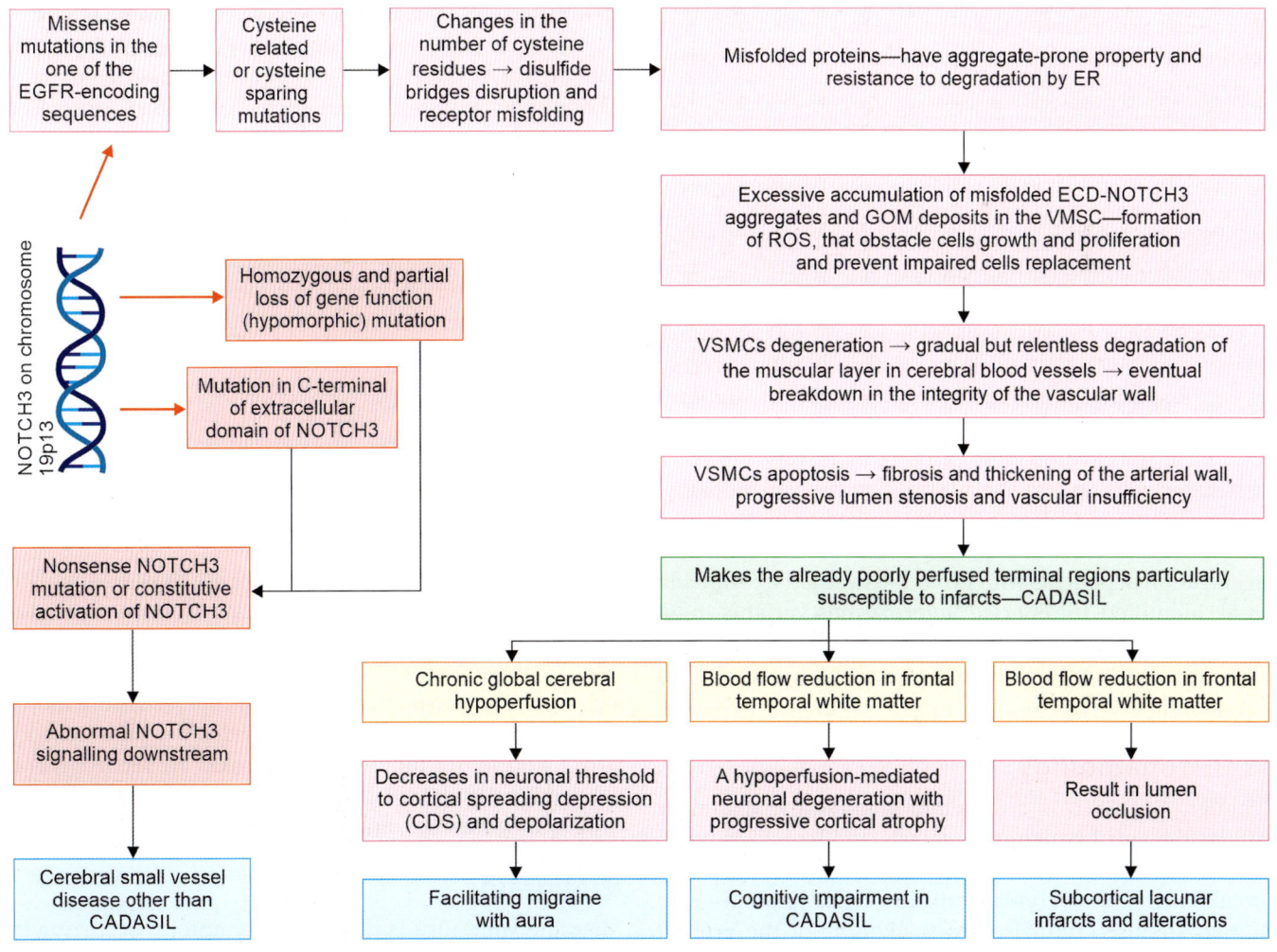

FLOWCHART 1: Current understanding of pathogenesis of CADASIL.
(CADASIL: cerebral autosomal dominant arteriopathy with subcortical infarcts and leukoencephalopathy; ECD: extracellular domain; EGFR: epidermal growth factor-like repeat; ER: endoplasmic reticulum; GOM: granular osmiophilic material; VSMCs: vascular smooth muscle cells; ROS: reactive oxygen species)

proliferation. Misfolded proteins may not interact properly with chaperones and proteases that normally mediate protein degradation, and abnormal prolonged association between NOTCH3 aggregates and calnexin could facilitate retention of the aggregates in the ER.[12,13] Mutant VSMCs have lower proliferation rates and impaired mitochondrial function with abnormal mitochondria, which may play a role in CADASIL pathology **(Flowchart 1)**.

Recent studies have shown that endothelial cells and astrocytes are also affected in CADASIL, suggesting a more widespread impairment of the gliovascular unit. This highlights the complexity of CADASIL pathogenesis and the need for a better understanding of the underlying mechanisms.[14,15]

■ Molecular Pathology

Cerebral autosomal dominant arteriopathy with subcortical infarcts and leukoencephalopathy mutations are mainly found in exons 2-23 of *NOTCH3* gene, which encode the 34 EGFR on the ECD. Over 40% of mutations involve exons 3 and 4, with the majority of mutations involving exon 4.[16,17] Mutations are mainly missense variants (95%) and less frequently small in-frame deletions, duplications, or splice-site mutations.[18,19]

More than 300 pathogenic variants have been described in CADASIL patients worldwide, all of them involving cysteine residues. Genetic variants not involving cysteine have also been described, but their pathogenic role in disease occurrence remains uncertain. Recent studies have examined the correlation between *NOTCH3* variant position and clinical features and molecular markers of CADASIL. In a cohort of 38 probands, Hu et al. found 23 different *NOTCH3* variants, with patients carrying cysteine-sparing pathogenic variants experiencing later symptom onset and milder temporal lobe involvement.[20] Cho et al. discovered that variants in EGFRs 1–6 were associated with earlier onset of stroke and encephalopathy, while variants in EGFRs 7–34 were linked to lower stroke risk.[21] Gravesteijn et al. reported lower levels of NOTCH3 aggregation in patients with EGFR 7–34 variants.[22] Almeida et al. identified 15 different heterozygous variants in 24 Portuguese families with suspected CADASIL, suggesting that genetic testing should focus on exons 4, 8, and 11 in this population.[23]

■ Histopathology

Though CADASIL is a systemic angiopathy, it mainly affects the small penetrating vessels and leptomeningeal arteries in the brain, causing VSMCs degeneration and breakdown in the vascular wall. This leads to progressive lumen stenosis, fibrosis, and thickening of the arterial wall, making the already poorly perfused regions more susceptible to infarcts **(Flowchart 1)**.[24,25]

Cerebral autosomal dominant arteriopathy with subcortical infarcts and leukoencephalopathy patients often exhibit cerebral microbleeds throughout the brain, which occur independently from ischemic lesions and suggest that CADASIL microangiopathy is the cause of both ischemic lesions and petechial hemorrhages. The presence of microbleeds is associated with a higher risk of hemorrhagic stroke, dementia, and urge incontinence, and predicts a higher risk of ischemic stroke. Nonamyloid granular osmiophilic material (GOM) in the media of affected vessels is a hallmark of CADASIL.[26]

CLINICAL FEATURES

The usual clinical presentation in patients with CADASIL usually consists of one or more of the following: TIAs, cognitive decline, migraine with aura, acute reversible encephalopathy disturbance, and psychiatric disturbances. The disease progression and age at onset differ between families and individuals. The clinical symptomatology, age of onset, and temporal course of disease progression can be highly variable, even among members of the same family.

Cerebral autosomal dominant arteriopathy with subcortical infarcts and leukoencephalopathy usually develops in adulthood, but there have been rare cases of children and adolescents with genetically confirmed CADASIL.[27,28] The earliest onset reported was in a 3-year-old boy with global developmental delay, whose brain magnetic resonance imaging (MRI) revealed multiple foci of increased T2 signal, and genetic sequencing identified a *NOTCH3* pathogenic variant.[29] Considering the clinical heterogeneity of CADASIL, various other neurological conditions can mimic the disorder, which need to be thoroughly excluded. **Flowchart 2** shows a step-by-step approach in patient with suspected CADASIL. Differentials include multiple sclerosis and primary angiitis of central nervous system (CNS), which if diagnosed can be managed with definitive treatment.

■ Transient Ischemic Attacks and Stroke

Transient ischemic attacks and stroke are most frequent, in about 85% of symptomatic individuals. Ischemic episodes typically occur at a mean age of 47 years (range: 20–70 years).[30,31] Ischemic episodes in CADASIL often manifest as a classic lacunar syndrome (ataxic hemiparesis, pure motor stroke, dysarthria-clumsy hand syndrome, pure sensory stroke, and sensorimotor stroke). Strokes are recurrent and can lead to motor and cognitive decline, gait disturbance, urinary incontinence, and pseudobulbar palsy.

■ Migraine

Migraine with aura is a common symptom, occurring in almost half of symptomatic cases, and may be the first manifestation of the disease. It can also be the only symptom

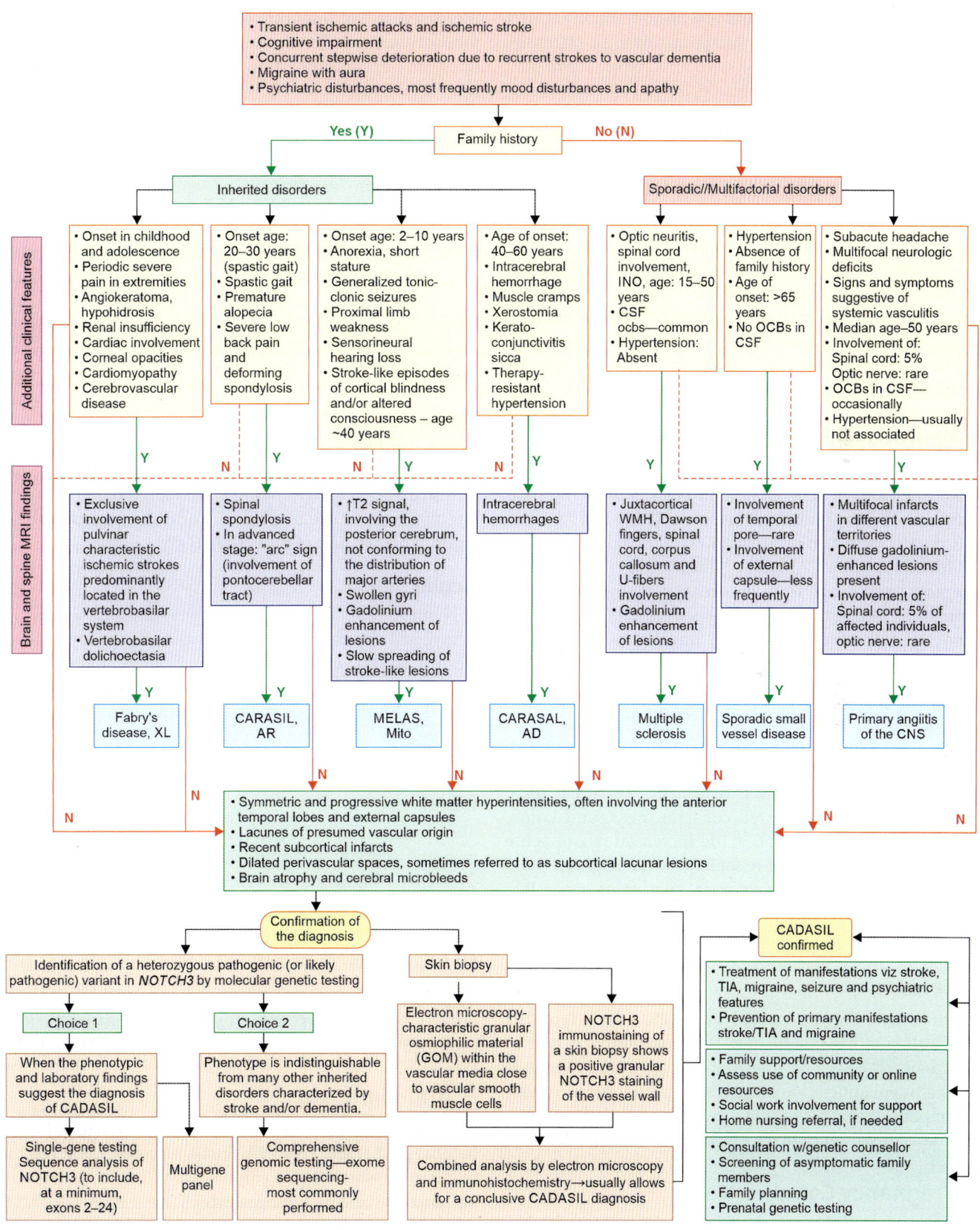

FLOWCHART 2: Approach to a patient with suspected CADASIL.

(AD: autosomal dominant; AR: autosomal recessive; CADASIL: cerebral autosomal dominant arteriopathy with subcortical infarcts and leukoencephalopathy; CARASAL: cathepsin A-related arteriopathy with strokes and leukoencephalopathy; CARASIL: cerebral autosomal recessive arteriopathy with subcortical infarcts and leukoencephalopathy; CNS: central nervous system; CSF: cerebrospinal fluid; MELAS: mitochondrial encephalomyopathy, lactic acidosis and stroke-like episodes; Mito: mitochondrial inheritance; OCB: oligoclonal bands; TIA: transient ischemic attack; XL: X-linked recessive) in some patients. Onset of migraine with aura usually occurs around the age of 30 years. Symptoms of aura primarily affect the visual and sensory system, but atypical aura may include motor symptoms, confusion, altered consciousness, hallucinations, or basilar symptoms, which can be challenging to distinguish from ischemic episodes.[32,33]

Cognitive Impairment and Dementia

Cognitive decline is a common feature of CADASIL, with up to 75% of affected individuals developing dementia, often accompanied by apathy. The pattern of cognitive dysfunction is initially characterized by deficits in executive function, verbal fluency, and memory, with some preservation of recognition and semantic memory. Cognitive decline may start as early as age 35 years and becomes more apparent with aging and disease progression.

Neuropsychiatric Symptoms

Psychiatric disturbances are common in CADASIL, with about one-third of affected individuals experiencing such symptoms.[34] The prevalence is variable: 7–74%. Apathy is a particularly common manifestation, affecting 40% of individuals with CADASIL.[35] The nature of psychiatric symptoms can range from personality changes to severe depression. While the pathogenesis of these disturbances is not yet fully understood, they have been reported as presenting symptoms of CADASIL in some cases.[11,36]

Acute Reversible Encephalopathy

About 10% of individuals with CADASIL may experience acute encephalopathy, which is characterized by symptoms such as pyrexia, confusion, headache, seizures, focal neurological deficits, altered consciousness, and coma, and can sometimes be fatal.[34] The increased risk of acute encephalopathy has been associated with migraine with aura, particularly confusional aura, suggesting a possible shared pathophysiologic mechanism between the two conditions.[37]

Seizures

Seizures have been reported in 5–10% cases, typically manifesting in the middle age. The most common type of seizure observed is a focal seizure, but generalized seizures and status epilepticus have also been reported. Seizures may accompany episodes of acute reversible encephalopathy or may be a consequence of structural brain damage.[38,39]

Pregnancy Complications

Complications, such as transient ischemic episodes, migraine, and preeclampsia-like symptoms, may arise in women with CADASIL during pregnancy. Pregnancy, particularly during puerperium, has been linked to an increased risk of migraine with aura. Despite limited and inconsistent data on the subject, it seems that CADASIL does not necessarily lead to unfavorable outcomes for the mother or fetus.[40]

Other Clinical Features

Cardiac

The association between CADASIL and cardiac involvement is controversial. One study found that nearly 25% of individuals with CADASIL had a history of acute myocardial infarction or pathologic Q-waves on electrocardiogram, a percentage significantly higher than controls without a heterozygous *NOTCH3* pathogenic variant.[41] However, another study found no signs of previous myocardial infarction in CADASIL patients.[42]

Nerve

Nerve biopsies of individuals with CADASIL may demonstrate signs of axonal damage, demyelination, and ultrastructural changes of the endoneurial blood vessels,[43] but there is no clear clinical evidence that peripheral neuropathy is a part of the CADASIL.[44]

Ocular

Subclinical retinal lesions have been reported. Fundoscopy may reveal clinically silent retinal vascular abnormalities.[45] Optical coherence tomography may show abnormalities such as reduced subfoveal choroidal thickness, retinal arterial luminal narrowing, retinal venous luminal enlargement, and reduced vessel density of the deep retinal plexus.[46,47]

Renal

Accumulation of NOTCH3 and GOM has been detected in renal arteries, and stenosis of renal arteries has been described. There is currently no evidence that kidney function is affected.[48,49]

DIAGNOSIS

At present, there are no widely agreed-upon diagnostic criteria for CADASIL. However, some researchers have proposed a CADASIL diagnostic screening tool **(Table 1)**.[50-52]

Brain Imaging

On MRI of the brain, two major types of abnormalities can be observed **(Figs. 1A to F)**: Small, circumscribed regions that appear isointense to cerebrospinal fluid (CSF) on both T1- and T2-weighted images, which are usually consistent with lacunar infarctions in terms of their size, shape, and location, and less well-demarcated T2 hyperintensities of variable size that may have different degrees of hypointensity on T1-weighted images, but are clearly different from

TABLE 1: Diagnostic criteria proposed for CADASIL.		
Study	Criteria or scale	Salient features of the study
Pescini et al., 2012[50]	*CADASIL scale*: • Migraine: 1 point • Migraine with aura: 3 points • TIA or stroke: 1 point • TIA/stroke onset ≤50 year: 2 points • Psychiatric disturbances: 1 point • Cognitive decline/dementia: 3 points • Leukoencephalopathy: 3 points • Leukoencephalopathy extended to temporal pole: 1 point • Leukoencephalopathy extended to external capsule: 5 points • Subcortical infarcts: 2 points • Family history* in at least 1 generation: 1 point • Family history* in at least 2 generations: 2 points The total score (ranging from 0 to 25) is obtained by the sum of the score attributed to each variable. A total score ≥15 is predictive of CADASIL diagnosis. CADASIL indicates cerebral autosomal-dominant arteriopathy with subcortical infarcts and leukoencephalopathy. *For at least 1 of the typical disturbances (headache, TIA/stroke, cognitive decline, and psychiatric disturbances)	• In this study, researchers developed a preliminary scale to assess the likelihood of CADASIL based on common disease features • The scale was tested for accuracy by applying it to CADASIL patients and NOTCH3-negative patients (those without a pathogenic mutation in the *NOTCH3* gene) • An optimization algorithm was then used to refine the scale, and a third group of patients with sporadic small-vessel disease was included to evaluate its stability • The final CADASIL scale had a sensitivity of 96.7% and a specificity of 74.2% • It proved to be a reliable screening tool for identifying patients with a high probability of having CADASIL and determining who should undergo genetic testing

Mizuta et al., 2017[51]	*Clinical criteria*:
	1. Age at onset (clinical symptom 2 or white matter lesions) ≤55 years old
	2. At least two of the following clinical findings:
	  a. Either of subcortical dementia, long tract signs, or pseudobulbar palsy
	  b. Stroke-like episode with a focal neurological deficit
	  c. Mood disorder
	  d. Migraine
	3. Autosomal dominant inheritance
	4. White matter lesions involving the anterior temporal pole by MRI or CT
	5. Exclusion of leukodystrophy (adrenoleukodystrophy, metachromatic leukodystrophy, etc.)
	Genetic criteria:
	NOTCH3 mutations localize in exons 2–24 and result in the gain or loss of cysteine residues in the epidermal growth factor-like repeat domain. Cysteine-sparing variants should be carefully evaluated by skin biopsy and segregation studies
	Pathological criteria:
	The pathological hallmark of CADASIL is GOM detected by electron microscopy. Immunostaining of NOTCH3 extracellular domain is also useful
	Definite:
	CADASIL is definite when the individual fulfils:
	• White matter lesions by MRI or CT
	• Clinical criteria 5
	• Genetic criteria and/or pathological criteria
	Probable:
	CADASIL is probable when the individual fulfils clinical criteria 1–5
	Possible:
	CADASIL is possible when the individual has abnormal white matter lesions (Fazekas grade ≥2) and fulfils either of:
	• ≤55 years old
	• At least one of the symptoms in clinical criteria 2, Fazekas grade was reported
		• This study involved Japanese subjects and aimed to develop new diagnostic criteria for CADASIL
		• Two groups of CADASIL patients were recruited: Group 1 diagnosed before 2011 and Group 2 diagnosed after 2011
		• Additionally, young stroke patients and NOTCH3-negative CADASIL-like patients were included as controls. The research committee discussed and established the new criteria, which were then validated for sensitivity and specificity
		• The results showed that the new criteria had a high sensitivity (97.3%) and specificity (80.6%) for distinguishing CADASIL
		• Group 1 patients from young stroke controls. However, when comparing CADASIL Group 2 patients to NOTCH3-negative controls, the specificity was much lower (7.5%)

Continued

Continued

Study	Criteria or scale			Salient features of the study

Bersano et al., 2018[52]	• Subcortical lacunar T2 sequence lesions at MRI
	• At least one of the following signs/symptoms:
	  ○ History of recurrent stroke/TIA
	  ○ Migraine with aura
	  ○ Dementia
	  ○ Major mood disorders
	  ○ Familial history of stroke/mood disorders, and/or migraine, and/or dementia
				• Patients with lacunar stroke or TIA were evaluated
				• Demographic and clinical data were collected, and MRI images were analyzed for various features including lacunar infarcts, microbleeds, temporal lobe involvement, global atrophy, and white matter hyperintensities
				• Out of the 128 patients included, 12.5% had a *NOTCH3* mutation associated with CADASIL
				• The presence of a family history of stroke, dementia, and external capsule lesions on MRI were significantly associated with the diagnosis of CADASIL
				• While other features like thalamic gliosis, temporal pole gliosis, and severe white matter hyperintensities were less specific, combining them with a familial history of stroke increased the positive predictive value and specificity for CADASIL diagnosis

	Lacunar lesions (cut-off: Diameter >2 mm)	Yes	No	
	Lacunar lesions site:			
	• Thalamic lacunae	Yes	No	
	• Basal ganglia lacunae	Yes	No	
	• Internal capsule lacunae	Yes	No	
	• External capsule lacunae	Yes	No	
	Leukoaraiosis (Fazekas scale):			
	0: Absent			
	1: Punctate foci			
	2: Beginning confluence			
	3: Large confluent areas			
	Temporal pole lesions	Yes	No	
	Capsule external lesions	Yes	No	
	Microbleeds	Yes	No	
	Temporo-mesial atrophy (Scheltens scale):			
	0: No CSF is visible around the hippocampus			
	1: Choroid fissure is slightly widened			
	2: Moderate widening of the choroid fissure, mild enlargement of the temporal horn, and mild loss of hippocampal height			
	3: Marked widening of the choroid fissure, moderate enlargement of the temporal horn, and moderate loss of hippocampal height			
	4: Marked widening of the choroid fissure, marked enlargement of the temporal horn, and the hippocampus is markedly atrophied, and internal structure is lost			
	Global cortical atrophy (Pasquier scale):			
	0: Normal volume/no ventricular enlargement			
	1: Opening of sulci/mild ventricular enlargement			
	2: Volume loss of gyri/moderate ventricular enlargement			
	3: A knife blade atrophy/severe ventricular enlargement			

(CADASIL: cerebral autosomal dominant arteriopathy with subcortical infarcts and leukoencephalopathy; CT: computed tomography; GOM: granular osmiophilic material; MRI: magnetic resonance imaging; NOTCH3: neurogenic locus notch homolog protein 3; TIA: transient ischemic attack)

CSF. These lesions are mostly located in the subcortical white matter, but they may also be present in other brain regions, such as the brainstem and subcortical gray matter. Although the brain lesions associated with CADASIL are typically bilateral, there have been reports of atypical cases of unilateral leukoencephalopathy. The onset and rate of progression of these MRI-visible lesions are variable, but by the age of 35 years, all carriers of pathogenic variants in NOTCH3 develop such lesions. In younger individuals, small irregular T2 hyperintensities in the periventricular and deep white matter are usually the first signs of CADASIL.[53,54]

The following MRI signs may help to identify patients with CADASIL **(Figs. 1A to F)**:

- *Temporal lobe and external capsule hyperintensities*: Anterior temporal lobe (temporal pole) white matter hyperintensities seen on T2-weighted sequences are found in approximately 90% of patients with CADASIL. External capsule and corpus callosum hyperintensities seen on T2-weighted sequences are also characteristic findings.[55,56]
- *Subcortical lacunar lesions*: These lesions are linearly arranged groups of rounded circumscribed lesions

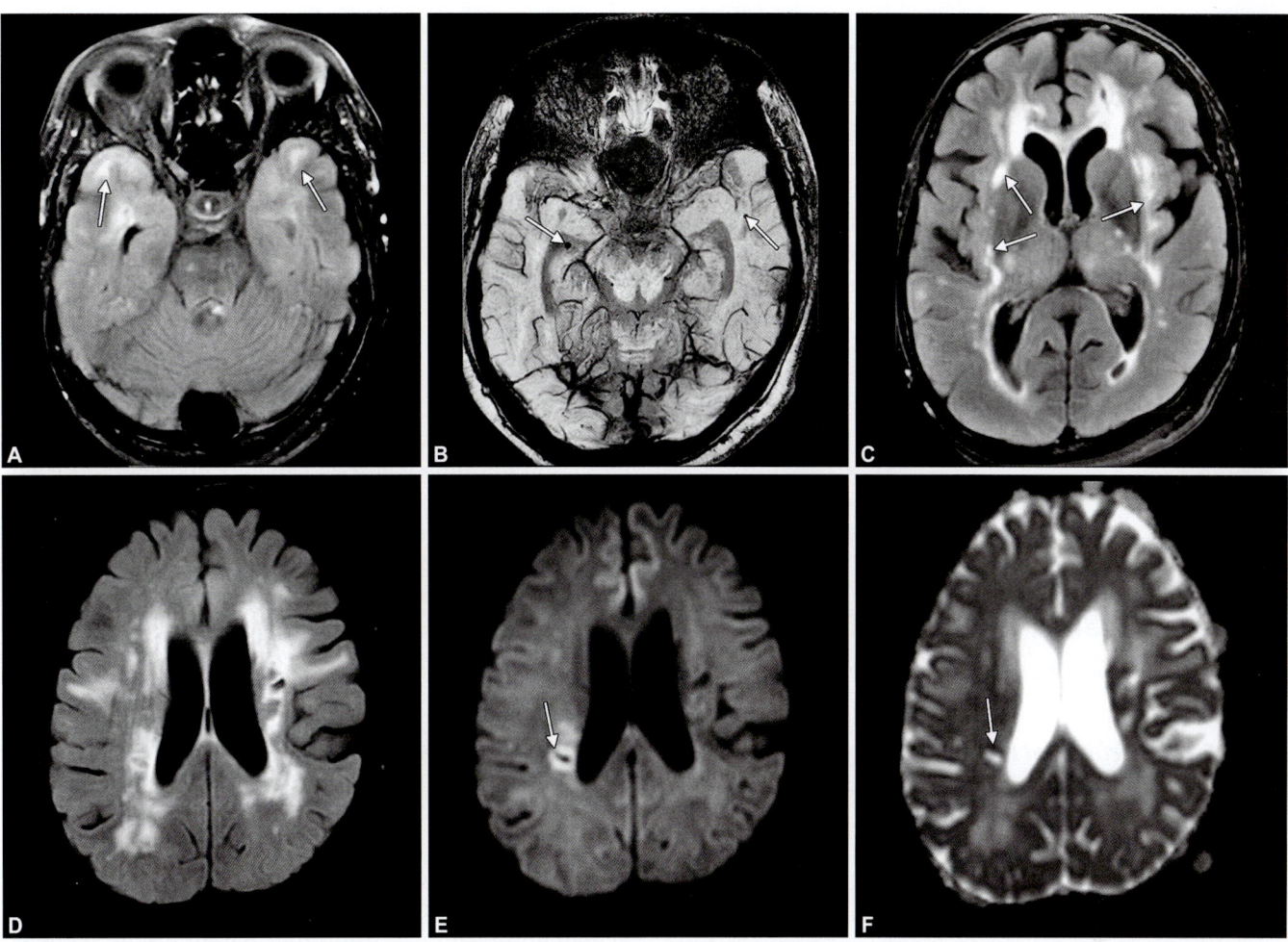

FIGS. 1A TO F: Typical imaging findings in CADASIL. Axial FLAIR images (A, C, and D) show a symmetric subcortical high signal in the anterior temporal lobes (arrows in A), internal and external capsules (arrows in B), and confluent involvement of the periventricular cerebral white matter and pons. Two distinct foci of hypointensities (arrows in C) are seen in SWI (B), suggestive of microhemorrhages. Axial diffusion-weighted (E) and ADC (F) images show a cavitating lesion in the right corona radiata (arrow in E and F), with central facilitated diffusion and peripheral diffusion restriction.
(ADC: apparent diffusion coefficient; CADASIL: cerebral autosomal dominant arteriopathy with subcortical infarcts and leukoencephalopathy; FLAIR: fluid-attenuated inversion recovery; SWI: susceptibility-weighted imaging)

that are just below the cortex at the gray–white matter junction with a signal intensity identical to CSF.[56]
- *Brain atrophy*: Brain atrophy as measured on MRI is another important feature of CADASIL. Brain atrophy may be due in part to secondary neurodegeneration of cortical regions caused by ischemic lesions in subcortical regions that disrupt connecting fibers.[57]
- *Cerebral microbleeds*: Cerebral microbleeds have been reported in 31–69% of patients. Conventional angiography is not helpful for patients with CADASIL.[58]

Confirming the Diagnosis

The diagnosis of CADASIL can be established in a proband through two approaches.
1. *Single-gene testing* involves sequencing *NOTCH3* and can identify small intragenic deletions/insertions, missense, nonsense, and splice site variants, but may not detect exon or whole-gene deletions/duplications. Biallelic *NOTCH3* pathogenic variants have been reported in individuals with CADASIL, so gene-targeted deletion/duplication analysis may be considered if a pathogenic variant is identified.
2. A *multigene panel* that includes *NOTCH3* and other genes of interest can be used to identify the genetic cause, while minimizing identification of variants of uncertain significance and pathogenic variants in genes that do not explain the phenotype. If the phenotype is like many other inherited disorders characterized by stroke and/or dementia, comprehensive genomic testing such as exome sequencing or genome sequencing is the preferred approach as it does not require the clinician to determine which gene(s) are likely involved.

Skin Biopsy

Confirmation of the CADASIL diagnosis can be achieved using ultrastructural analysis of small arterioles, which can be obtained from a skin biopsy.[59] Characteristic GOM is observed within the vascular media located near VSMCs, as shown by electron microscopy. While the detection of GOM is considered pathognomonic for CADASIL, the reported sensitivity can vary.[60] Additionally, NOTCH3 immunostaining of a skin biopsy reveals a positive granular NOTCH3 staining of the vessel wall.[16] The combined analysis of electron microscopy and immunohistochemistry usually leads to a conclusive CADASIL diagnosis.[61]

MANAGEMENT

Currently, there is no known disease-modifying treatment for CADASIL. Management of the disorder is mainly symptomatic and supportive.

Treatment and Prevention of Clinical Manifestations

Stroke

Acute Stroke/Transient Ischemic Attacks

In patients with CADASIL, acute TIAs and acute strokes are managed based on the general principles of stroke medicine. Although systemic intravenous thrombolysis has not been shown to improve outcomes after a stroke caused by small vessel occlusion in CADASIL patients, it may still be considered in cases where there is a thromboembolic large vessel occlusion unrelated to CADASIL, and the potential benefit of thrombolysis and/or mechanical thrombectomy outweighs the potential risk of intracerebral hemorrhage.[9,44]

Secondary Prevention

Individuals with CADASIL should be managed with all available risk-reduction measures, which include controlling hypertension, hyperlipidemia treatment with statins, glucose control, and antiplatelet therapy. However, there is insufficient evidence to suggest that these interventions are specifically effective for CADASIL. Of particular importance is smoking cessation, as active smoking has been found to increase the risk of stroke and dementia in CADASIL patients. Additionally, lifestyle changes may reduce risk.[34,62]

Antithrombotic Treatment

It is generally recommended to use low-dose aspirin alone or in combination with clopidogrel for secondary stroke prevention. However, the specific benefit of antiplatelet therapy in CADASIL is yet to be evaluated. It is important to carefully weigh the potential benefits and risks of therapy for each individual patient, considering their specific clinical characteristics and comorbidities.[63]

Managing the Risk Factors

Although there are no specific studies on blood pressure control in CADASIL, hypertension may increase the risk of ischemic stroke, brain atrophy progression, and the presence of cerebral microbleeds.[64] Therefore, controlling blood pressure may have additional benefits for patients with CADASIL. However, excessively low blood pressure has been linked to an increased risk of dementia. Therefore, caution should be exercised when implementing measures to control blood pressure in these patients.[65]

Migraine

For acute migraine attacks, triptans and ergot derivatives should be used with caution due to their vasoconstrictive effect and harmful action on capillary endothelium.[66] For prophylaxis, amitriptyline, beta-blockers, flunarizine, and topiramate may be used, but they may worsen mood and cognitive symptoms.[67] For CADASIL patients with migraine, it has been observed that they have higher blood homocysteine levels, and B12 vitamin supplementation that lowers homocysteine can decrease migraine severity and frequency.[68]

Cognitive Impairment and Dementia

No drugs have been found to provide clear benefits in terms of cognitive function. In a randomized controlled trial, donepezil did not demonstrate improved cognition in CADASIL patients compared to the control group, despite better executive functions in the donepezil group.[69] Another acetylcholinesterase inhibitor, galantamine, showed some benefit for behavior and caregiver burden in a small study of four CADASIL patients, suggesting the existence of a cholinergic deficit in CADASIL.[69] The treatment of psychiatric symptoms in CADASIL should be based on the best general clinical practice.

CLINICAL COURSE AND LONG-TERM PROGNOSIS

Cerebral autosomal dominant arteriopathy with subcortical infarcts and leukoencephalopathy is a progressive disorder, and the clinical course and prognosis may vary among individuals. The onset of symptoms usually occurs in mid-adulthood, typically between 30 and 50 years of age. The prognosis for CADASIL is generally poor, with a high risk of disability and mortality. The risk of stroke and other cardiovascular events is also increased in individuals with CADASIL, which can further worsen the prognosis.[1,33,37]

A large study of 411 individuals conducted by Opherk et al. in 2004 reported that the median age at which individuals were unable to walk without assistance was approximately 60 years, while the median age at which they became bedridden was 64 years. The median age at death was 68 years, and the disease progressed more rapidly in men than in women. The most common cause of death was pneumonia, followed by sudden unexpected death and asphyxia. In the later stages of the disease, 78% of individuals were completely dependent and 63% were confined to bed.[31]

In another prospective study of 290 adults with CADASIL, it was found that over a period of 3 years, a significant number of patients experienced clinical deterioration. The study conducted in Europe found that the most common clinical manifestations of the cohort at baseline included TIA or stroke, migraine with aura, and gait disturbance. At the 3-year follow-up, 47% of participants experienced incident stroke, incident dementia, moderate or severe disability, or death. Factors independently associated with the composite endpoint included gait disturbance, active smoking, a history of stroke, and the presence of more than three lacunar strokes or brain atrophy on MRI.[70]

GENETIC COUNSELING

The risk to the siblings of an affected individual depends on the genetic status of the parents. If one parent is affected, the risk to siblings is 50%. If the proband has biallelic *NOTCH3* pathogenic variants and both parents are heterozygous, the risk to the siblings is 75%. If the pathogenic variant cannot be detected in either parent, the risk to siblings is presumed to be slightly higher than in the general population due to the possibility of parental germline mosaicism.[71,72]

Predictive testing for at-risk relatives is possible once the pathogenic variant has been identified, but potential consequences and limitations of testing should be discussed in the context of formal genetic counseling prior to testing. Predictive testing in minors is generally considered inappropriate for adult-onset conditions with no early treatment options, as it may have negative effects on family dynamics and increase the risk of discrimination and anxiety.[73]

Prenatal testing and preimplantation genetic testing are two options for families at increased risk of having a child with a genetic condition such as CADASIL. It is important to note that there may be different perspectives among medical professionals and within families regarding the use of prenatal testing and preimplantation genetic testing.

CONCLUSION

Cerebral autosomal dominant arteriopathy with subcortical infarcts and leukoencephalopathy is the most important cause of inherited stroke and vascular cognitive impairment in middle-aged adults. However, the mechanisms behind the disease are not yet fully comprehended. Nonetheless, the identification of NOTCH3 mutations as the culprit of the disorder has led to various experimental investigations that may shed light on CADASIL. There are ongoing studies that are showing promise in terms of developing new treatment strategies in the years to come. MRI neuroimaging techniques are also improving, providing better markers to track disease progression. Since CADASIL can be viewed as a prototype for researching SVD, consistent efforts should be made to comprehend the pathogenesis of this genetic disease. As we move forward, translational research combining basic science and clinical findings will be essential to fully understand the disease's pathophysiology, identify biomarkers, and develop effective treatments. Large clinical studies involving patients at different disease stages will also be critical in this regard.

REFERENCES

1. Chabriat H, Joutel A, Dichgans M, et al. Cadasil. Lancet Neurol. 2009;8(7):643-53.
2. Viswanathan A, Gschwendtner A, Guichard JP, et al. Lacunar lesions are independently associated with disability and cognitive impairment in CADASIL. Neurology. 2007;69(2):172-9.
3. Moreton FC, Cullen B, Delles C, et al. Vasoreactivity in CADASIL: Comparison to structural MRI and neuropsychology. J Cereb Blood Flow Metab. 2018;38(6):1085-95.
4. Rutten JW, Hack RJ, Duering M, et al. Broad phenotype of cysteine-altering NOTCH3 variants in UK Biobank: CADASIL to nonpenetrance. Neurology. 2020;95(13):e1835-43.
5. Narayan SK, Gorman G, Kalaria RN, et al. The minimum prevalence of CADASIL in northeast England. Neurology. 2012;78(13):1025-7.
6. Razvi SSM, Davidson R, Bone I, et al. The prevalence of cerebral autosomal dominant arteriopathy with subcortical infarcts and leucoencephalopathy (CADASIL) in the west of Scotland. J Neurol Neurosurg Psychiatry. 2005;76(5):739-41.
7. Hack RJ, Rutten JW, Person TN, et al. Cysteine-altering NOTCH3 variants are a risk factor for stroke in the elderly population. Stroke. 2020;51(12):3562-9.
8. Moreton FC, Razvi SSM, Davidson R, et al. Changing clinical patterns and increasing prevalence in CADASIL. Acta Neurol Scand. 2014;130(3):197-203.
9. Di Donato I, Bianchi S, De Stefano N, et al. Cerebral Autosomal Dominant Arteriopathy with Subcortical Infarcts and Leukoencephalopathy (CADASIL) as a model of small vessel disease: Update on clinical, diagnostic, and management aspects. BMC Med. 2017;15(1):41.
10. Ferrante EA, Cudrici CD, Boehm M. CADASIL: New advances in basic science and clinical perspectives. Curr Opin Hematol. 2019;26(3):193-8.
11. Wang Z, Yuan Y, Zhang W, et al. NOTCH3 mutations and clinical features in 33 mainland Chinese families with CADASIL. J Neurol Neurosurg Psychiatry. 2011;82(5):534-9.
12. Ihalainen S, Soliymani R, Iivanainen E, et al. Proteome analysis of cultivated vascular smooth muscle cells from a CADASIL patient. Mol Med. 2007;13(5):305-14.
13. Takahashi K, Adachi K, Yoshizaki K, et al. Mutations in NOTCH3 cause the formation and retention of aggregates in the endoplasmic reticulum, leading to impaired cell proliferation. Hum Mol Genet. 2010;19(1):79-89.

14. Hase Y, Chen A, Bates LL, et al. Severe white matter astrocytopathy in CADASIL. Brain Pathol. 2018;28(6):832-43.
15. Pescini F, Donnini I, Cesari F, et al. Circulating biomarkers in Cerebral Autosomal Dominant Arteriopathy with Subcortical Infarcts and Leukoencephalopathy patients. J Stroke Cerebrovasc Dis. 2017;26(4):823-33.
16. Joutel A, Andreux F, Gaulis S, et al. The ectodomain of the Notch3 receptor accumulates within the cerebrovasculature of CADASIL patients. J Clin Invest. 2000;105(5):597-605.
17. Lesnik Oberstein SAJ, van Duinen SG, van den Boom R, et al. Evaluation of diagnostic NOTCH3 immunostaining in CADASIL. Acta Neuropathol. 2003;106(2):107-11.
18. Dichgans M, Mayer M, Uttner I, et al. The phenotypic spectrum of CADASIL: Clinical findings in 102 cases. Ann Neurol. 1998;44(5):731-9.
19. Peters N, Opherk C, Bergmann T, et al. Spectrum of mutations in biopsy-proven CADASIL: Implications for diagnostic strategies. Arch Neurol. 2005;62(7):1091-4.
20. Hu Y, Sun Q, Zhou Y, et al. (2021) NOTCH3 Variants and Genotype–Phenotype Features in Chinese CADASIL Patients. Frontiers in Genetics. [online] Available from https://www.frontiersin.org/articles/10.3389/fgene.2021.705284 [Last accessed June, 2023].
21. Cho BPH, Jolly AA, Nannoni S, et al. Association of NOTCH3 Variant Position With Stroke Onset and Other Clinical Features Among Patients With CADASIL. Neurology. 2022;99(5):e430-9.
22. Gravesteijn G, Hack RJ, Mulder AA, et al. NOTCH3 variant position is associated with NOTCH3 aggregation load in CADASIL vasculature. Neuropathol Appl Neurobiol. 2022;48(1):e12751.
23. Almeida MR, Elias I, Fernandes C, et al. NOTCH3 mutations in a cohort of Portuguese patients within CADASIL spectrum phenotype. Neurogenetics. 2022;23(1):1-9.
24. Tang Z, Wang A, Yuan F, et al. Differentiation of multipotent vascular stem cells contributes to vascular diseases. Nat Commun. 2012;3(1):875.
25. Gatti JR, Zhang X, Korcari E, et al. Redistribution of Mature Smooth Muscle Markers in Brain Arteries in Cerebral Autosomal Dominant Arteriopathy with Subcortical Infarcts and Leukoencephalopathy. Transl Stroke Res. 2019;10(2):160-9.
26. Carare RO, Hawkes CA, Jeffrey M, et al. Review: Cerebral amyloid angiopathy, prion angiopathy, CADASIL and the spectrum of protein elimination failure angiopathies (PEFA) in neurodegenerative disease with a focus on therapy: Protein elimination failure angiopathy (PEFA). Neuropathol Appl Neurobiol. 2013;39(6):593-611.
27. Granild-Jensen J, Jensen UB, Schwartz M, et al. Cerebral autosomal dominant arteriopathy with subcortical infarcts and leukoencephalopathy resulting in stroke in an 11-year-old male. Dev Med Child Neurol. 2009;51(9):754-7.
28. Hartley J, Westmacott R, Decker J, et al. Childhood-onset CADASIL: Clinical, imaging, and neurocognitive features. J Child Neurol. 2010;25(5):623-7.
29. Benabu Y, Beland M, Ferguson N, et al. Genetically proven cerebral autosomal-dominant arteriopathy with subcortical infarcts and leukoencephalopathy (CADASIL) in a 3-year-old. Pediatr Radiol. 2013;43(9):1227-30.
30. Tan RYY, Traylor M, Megy K, et al. How common are single gene mutations as a cause for lacunar stroke? A targeted gene panel study. Neurology. 2019;93(22):e2007-20.
31. Opherk C, Peters N, Herzog J, et al. Long-term prognosis and causes of death in CADASIL: A retrospective study in 411 patients. Brain. 2004;127(11):2533-9.
32. Liem MK, Lesnik Oberstein SAJ, van der Grond J, et al. CADASIL and migraine: A narrative review. Cephalalgia. 2010;30(11):1284-9.
33. Guey S, Mawet J, Hervé D, et al. Prevalence and characteristics of migraine in CADASIL. Cephalalgia. 2016;36(11):1038-47.
34. Adib-Samii P, Brice G, Martin RJ, et al. Clinical spectrum of CADASIL and the Effect of Cardiovascular Risk Factors on Phenotype. Stroke. 2010;41(4):630-4.
35. Reyes S, Viswanathan A, Godin O, et al. Apathy: A major symptom in CADASIL. Neurology. 2009;72(10):905-10.
36. Valenti R, Pescini F, Antonini S, et al. Major depression and bipolar disorders in CADASIL: A study using the DSM-IV semistructured interview. Acta Neurol Scand. 2011;124(6):390-5.
37. Tan RYY, Markus HS. CADASIL: Migraine, Encephalopathy, Stroke and Their Inter-Relationships. PLoS One. 2016;11(6):e0157613.
38. Haan J, Lesnik Oberstein SAJ, et al. Epilepsy in cerebral autosomal dominant arteriopathy with subcortical infarcts and leukoencephalopathy. Cerebrovasc Dis. 2007;24(2-3):316-7.
39. Desmond DW, Moroney JT, Lynch T, et al. The natural history of CADASIL: A pooled analysis of previously published cases. Stroke. 1999;30(6):1230-3.
40. Donnini I, Rinnoci V, Nannucci S, et al. Pregnancy in CADASIL. Acta Neurol Scand. 2017;136(6):668-71.
41. Lesnik Oberstein SAJ, Jukema JW, Van Duinen SG, et al. Myocardial infarction in cerebral autosomal dominant arteriopathy with subcortical infarcts and leukoencephalopathy (CADASIL). Medicine (Baltimore). 2003;82(4):251-6.
42. Cumurciuc R, Henry P, Gobron C, et al. Electrocardiogram in cerebral autosomal dominant arteriopathy with subcortical infarcts and leukoencephalopathy patients without any clinical evidence of coronary artery disease: A case-control study. Stroke. 2006;37(4):1100-2.
43. Lackovic V, Bajcetic M, Lackovic M, et al. Skin and sural nerve biopsies: Ultrastructural findings in the first genetically confirmed cases of CADASIL in Serbia. Ultrastruct Pathol. 2012;36(5):325-35.
44. Khan MT, Murray A, Smith M. Successful Use of Intravenous Tissue Plasminogen Activator as Treatment for a Patient with Cerebral Autosomal Dominant Arteriopathy with Subcortical Infarcts and Leukoencephalopathy: A Case Report and Review of Literature. J Stroke Cerebrovasc Dis. 2016;25(4):e53-7.
45. Cumurciuc R, Massin P, Pâques M, et al. Retinal abnormalities in CADASIL: A retrospective study of 18 patients. J Neurol Neurosurg Psychiatry. 2004;75(7):1058-60.
46. Alten F, Motte J, Ewering C, et al. Multimodal retinal vessel analysis in CADASIL patients. PLoS One. 2014;9(11):e112311.
47. Fang XJ, Yu M, Wu Y, et al. Study of Enhanced Depth Imaging Optical Coherence Tomography in Cerebral Autosomal Dominant Arteriopathy with Subcortical Infarcts and Leukoencephalopathy. Chin Med J (Engl). 2017;130(9):1042-8.
48. Lorenzi T, Ragno M, Paolinelli F, et al. CADASIL: Ultrastructural insights into the morphology of granular osmiophilic material. Brain Behav. 2017;7(3):e00624.
49. Bergmann M, Ebke M, Yuan Y, et al. Cerebral autosomal dominant arteriopathy with subcortical infarcts and leukoencephalopathy (CADASIL): A morphological study of a German family. Acta Neuropathol. 1996;92(4):341-50.
50. Pescini F, Nannucci S, Bertaccini B, et al. The Cerebral Autosomal-Dominant Arteriopathy With Subcortical Infarcts and Leukoencephalopathy (CADASIL) Scale: A screening tool to select patients for NOTCH3 gene analysis. Stroke. 2012;43(11):2871-6.
51. Mizuta I, Watanabe-Hosomi A, Koizumi T, et al. New diagnostic criteria for cerebral autosomal dominant arteriopathy with subcortical infarcts and leukoencephalopathy in Japan. J Neurol Sci. 2017;381:62-7.

52. Bersano A, Bedini G, Markus HS, et al. The role of clinical and neuroimaging features in the diagnosis of CADASIL. J Neurol. 2018;265(12):2934-43.
53. Roine S, Pöyhönen M, Timonen S, et al. Neurologic symptoms are common during gestation and puerperium in CADASIL. Neurology. 2005;64(8):14413.
54. Wang MM. CADASIL. In: Geschwind DH, Paulson HL, Klein C (Eds). Handbook of Clinical Neurology. Philadelphia: Elsevier; 2018. pp. 733-43.
55. Dichgans M, Filippi M, Brüning R, et al. Quantitative MRI in CADASIL: Correlation with disability and cognitive performance. Neurology. 1999;52(7):1361-7.
56. O'Sullivan M, Jarosz JM, Martin RJ, et al. MRI hyperintensities of the temporal lobe and external capsule in patients with CADASIL. Neurology. 2001;56(5):628-34.
57. Jolly AA, Nannoni S, Edwards H, et al. Prevalence and Predictors of Vascular Cognitive Impairment in Patients With CADASIL. Neurology. 2022;99(5):e453-61.
58. Lesnik Oberstein SAJ, van den Boom R, van Buchem MA, et al. Cerebral microbleeds in CADASIL. Neurology. 2001;57(6):1066-70.
59. Ruchoux MM, Maurage CA. CADASIL: Cerebral autosomal dominant arteriopathy with subcortical infarcts and leukoencephalopathy. J Neuropathol Exp Neurol. 1997;56(9):947-64.
60. Morroni M, Marzioni D, Ragno M, et al. Role of electron microscopy in the diagnosis of cadasil syndrome: A study of 32 patients. PLoS One. 2013;8(6):e65482.
61. Rutten JW, Haan J, Terwindt GM, et al. Interpretation of NOTCH3 mutations in the diagnosis of CADASIL. Expert Rev Mol Diagn. 2014;14(5):593-603.
62. Singhal S. The influence of genetic and cardiovascular risk factors on the CADASIL phenotype. Brain. 2004;127(9):2031-8.
63. Bersano A, Bedini G, Oskam J, et al. CADASIL: Treatment and Management Options. Curr Treat Options Neurol. 2017;19(9):31.
64. Viswanathan A, Guichard JP, Gschwendtner A, et al. Blood pressure and haemoglobin A1c are associated with microhaemorrhage in CADASIL: A two-centre cohort study. Brain. 2006;129(Pt 9):2375-83.
65. Verghese J, Lipton RB, Hall CB, et al. Low blood pressure and the risk of dementia in very old individuals. Neurology. 2003;61(12):1667-72.
66. Goldstein J, Hagen M, Gold M. Results of a multicenter, double-blind, randomized, parallel-group, placebo-controlled, single-dose study comparing the fixed combination of acetaminophen, acetylsalicylic acid, and caffeine with ibuprofen for acute treatment of patients with severe migraine. Cephalalgia. 2014;34(13):1070-8.
67. Ferrari MD, Roon KI, Lipton RB, et al. Oral triptans (serotonin 5-HT1B/1D agonists) in acute migraine treatment: A meta-analysis of 53 trials. Lancet. 2001;358(9294):1668-75.
68. Bousser MG, Lasserve ET. Cerebral autosomal dominant arteriopathy with subcortical infarcts and leukoencephalopathy: From stroke to vessel wall physiology. J Neurol Neurosurg Psychiatry. 2001;70(3):285-7.
69. Schneider LS. Does donepezil improve executive function in patients with CADASIL? Lancet Neurol. 2008;7(4):287-9.
70. Verdura E, Hervé D, Scharrer E, et al. Heterozygous HTRA1 mutations are associated with autosomal dominant cerebral small vessel disease. Brain. 2015;138(Pt 8):2347-58.
71. Mukai M, Mizuta I, Ueda A, et al. A Japanese CADASIL patient with homozygous NOTCH3 p.Arg544Cys mutation confirmed pathologically. J Neurol Sci. 2018;394:38-40.
72. Al-Shaar HA, Qadi N, Al-Hamed MH, et al. Phenotypic comparison of individuals with homozygous or heterozygous mutation of NOTCH3 in a large CADASIL family. J Neurol Sci. 2016;367:239-43.
73. Hack RJ, Rutten J, Lesnik Oberstein SAJ. CADASIL. In: Adam MP, Mirzaa GM, Pagon RA, et al. (Eds). GeneReviews®. Seattle: University of Washington; 1993.

CHAPTER 7

Cerebral Vasospasm and Delayed Cerebral Ischemia Following Aneurysmal Subarachnoid Hemorrhage: Current Concepts

Ajay Hegde, Girish Menon

ABSTRACT

Delayed cerebral ischemia (DCI) secondary to cerebral vasospasm (CV) is the most dreaded complication responsible for significant morbidity and mortality following aneurysmal subarachnoid hemorrhage (aSAH). Exclusively seen in aSAH, the exact pathogenesis remains a postulate. Affecting only one-third of patients with aSAH symptomatic vasospasm defies early prediction. Spread over a couple of weeks, risk of vasospasm remains a diagnostic challenge. Catheter angiography is the gold standard, yet close neurological monitoring combined with transcranial Doppler (TCD) studies remain the most practical approach for routine clinical diagnosis. Nimodipine continues to remain the only effective pharmacological strategy to improve functional outcomes in patients with SAH at risk for developing vasospasm. Conventional triple-H therapy has been replaced by euvolemia and judicious use of the pharmacologically induced hypertension. Interventional angioplasty techniques for rescue therapy following refractory vasospasm have shown promising results. Multiple novel molecules have been tried but are still experimental. This review provides a general overview on CV and DCI with a focus on current management strategies.

Keywords: Cerebral aneurysm, Subarachnoid hemorrhage, Vasospasm, Delayed cerebral ischemia, Nimodipine.

INTRODUCTION

The overall prevalence of cerebral aneurysms is estimated to be around 3% (1.9–5.2%) of the adult population, and the estimated annual incidence of aneurysmal subarachnoid hemorrhage (aSAH) is around 6–10/100,000 population.[1] The outcome following aSAH is unpredictable where nearly 35% succumb and of the survivors approximately one-third remain severely disabled and functionally dependent.[1,2] Adverse outcomes following aSAH are primarily related to two main complications—rebleeding and cerebral vasospasm (CV)-induced delayed cerebral ischemia (DCI). The risk of rebleeding is maximum soon after the bleed and can be prevented by timely intervention either through coiling or clipping. With modern SAH management routines, the combined risk for death and permanent disability from vasospasm alone has shrunk to <10%, but it remains one of the most difficult challenges following aSAH and has been aptly referred to as a "riddle wrapped in a mystery inside an enigma."

PATHOGENESIS

Subarachnoid hemorrhage-induced CV and DCI represent a sophisticated multistep process, but the exact pathogenesis of CV is still unclear. The initial trigger is the extravasation of blood and its breakdown products such as methemoglobin, oxyhemoglobin, heme, and hemin into the subarachnoid space. Blood breakdown products alter endothelial cell function by triggering entry of calcium and subsequent activation of calcium calmodulin-dependent myosin light chain kinase. Damage to the endothelium also results in loss of endothelial nitric oxide (NO), which is an important vasodilator and regulator of vascular tone. This coupled with overproduction of endothelin-1 (ET1) is a powerful vasoconstrictor, which sets the tone for vasoconstriction in the brain.[3,4] In addition, activation of inflammatory cascades after SAH produces several mediators, which act as catalyst for vasospasm. These include bilirubin oxidation products (BOXes), adhesion molecules such as intercellular adhesion molecule 1 (ICAM-1), vascular cell adhesion molecule 1 (VCAM-1), E-selectin, and cytokines including tumor necrosis factor alpha (TNF-α), interleukin-1 (IL-1), IL-6, and IL-8.[4] Moreover, there is increasing evidence that pathophysiologic processes such as upregulation of genes involved with inflammation and extracellular matrix remodeling, oxidative stress and free radical damage to smooth muscle, lipid peroxidation of cell membranes, cortical spreading depression, sympathetic activation resulting in the failure of cerebral autoregulation, and micro thrombosis result in cerebral ischemia and delayed neurological deterioration.[5]

CLINICAL PRESENTATION

Cerebral vasospasm is defined as reversible narrowing of blood vessels that typically develops a few days after SAH, peaks around 7–10 days, and resolves by 21 days.[6] CV may remain as angiographic vasospasm, which refers to arterial narrowing seen on vascular imaging—computed tomography angiogram (CTA) or digital subtraction angiogram (DSA). Angiographic spasm occurs in 50–90% of aneurysmal SAH patients, but manifests clinically in only one-third of patients.[7] CV manifests clinically as DCI, which may progress to delayed cerebral infarction. DCI refers to the clinical manifestations of vasospasm, and is defined as the presence of focal neurological deficit or a decrease of at least 2 points on the Glasgow Coma Scale (GCS), score lasting longer than 1 hour with no other identifiable cause.[8] DCI can result in delayed cerebral infarction, defined as radiologic evidence of an infarct present after the time of DCI within 6 weeks of SAH and 24–48 hours after aneurysm repair.[9]

The clinical manifestation of delayed ischemia/infarction depends on the vascular territory involved and may vary from focal neurological deficits to fluctuating levels of consciousness. Subtle signs such as impaired conscious levels, decrease in eye opening, decreased verbal output, and pronator drift can be early signs of vasospasm. CV, being a systemic inflammatory state, can also initially manifest clinically as a low-grade fever and a slight elevation in white blood cells.[10]

RISK AND PREDICTORS OF VASOSPASM

Characteristically seen following aneurysmal bleeds, CV is seldom seen following traumatic SAH, spontaneous parenchymal bleeds, or brain tumor surgery. CV is similarly uncommon following rupture of arteriovenous malformations brain tumor surgery or surgery for unruptured intracranial aneurysms. CV is surprisingly uncommon in perimesencephalic hemorrhage and nonaneurysmal SAH.[11] Prediction of vasospasm is thus difficult, and is based on certain clinical, radiological, and treatment-related factors.

Poor GCS on arrival, history of cigarette smoking, hypertension, hyperglycemia, hyponatremia, and meningitis during treatment are important clinical predictors for CV. For reasons yet unclear, pediatric and adolescent patients with aSAH have a low risk of vasospasm. Radiologically, the volume of SAH as quantified by the Fisher scale and the modified Fisher rating scale remains the strongest predictor for CV **(Table 1)**.[12] Hijdra et al. later proposed a revised scale incorporating volume of intraventricular blood and observed that the Hijdra score along with a history of smoking to be a strong risk factor for CV.[13] A novel color-coded risk stratification VASOGRADE score has also been designed to classify patients to low, medium, and high risk of developing DCI based on the World Federation of Neurosurgical Societies (WFNS) clinical grade and Fisher CT grade **(Table 2)**.[14]

Despite common belief, higher risk of intraoperative aneurysm rupture on development of vasospasm has not been conclusively established.[15] Among treatment-related factors, patients undergoing endovascular treatment have been reported to have lesser risk of CV compared to the surgical group.[16-18]

TABLE 1: Modified Fisher score and risk of DCI.		
Modified Fisher score	CT scan findings	Risk for DCI (%)
0	No SAH or IVH	0
1	Minimal/thin SAH, no IVH	6
2	Minimal/thin SAH, with IVH in both lateral ventricles	15
3	Dense SAH, no IVH	35
4	Dense SAH, with IVH in both ventricles	34
(CT: computed tomography; DCI: delayed cerebral ischemia; IVH: intraventricular hemorrhage; SAH: subarachnoid hemorrhage)		

TABLE 2: VASOGRADE score.					
VASOGRADE	WFNS	Modified Fisher scale	Sensitivity	Specificity	Correctly classified
Green	1–2	1–2	100%	0%	21.6%
Yellow	1–3	3–4	63.5%	57.6%	58.9%
Red	4–5	Any	49.1%	74.7%	69.2%
(WFNS: World Federation of Neurosurgical Societies)					

DIAGNOSIS

Regular neurological monitoring of patients in the intensive care remains the simplest and most effective means of detecting vasospasm. However, all patients with neurological worsening may not be related to symptomatic vasospasm. The first step, therefore, in diagnosing symptomatic vasospasm is to rule out other causes of delayed neuro worsening such as fever, infection, hydrocephalus, seizures, and electrolyte disturbances.

Transcranial Doppler Ultrasonography

In an unconscious patient, continuous monitoring with transcranial Doppler (TCD) can diagnose vasospasm. TCD examinations are noninvasive, carried out at the bedside, and can easily be performed on a regular basis. A mean flow velocity in the middle cerebral artery (MCA) or anterior cerebral artery (ACA) of >120 cm/s is suspicious, but aggressive management is initiated when the value exceeds 200 cm/s, or there is a serial increase of flow velocity by 50 cm/s/24 hours.[19] The ratio of velocity in the MCA and internal carotid artery (ICA) can be used to differentiate hyperemic circulation. A Lindegaard ratio (LR) of VMCA/VICA >3 is consistent with vasospasm, and severe vasospasm can lead to an LR >6.[20] TCD does not consistently detect vasospasm in more peripheral branches, which could explain why perfusion deficits found in cerebral blood flow (CBF) investigations are not always correlated with TCD results.[21] Although TCD is an important and useful tool in detection and surveillance of vasospasm, it is highly operator-dependent, results can be affected by high intracranial pressure or hydrocephalus, and results do not always correlate with risk for developing DCI.[22]

Catheter Angiography

Digital subtraction angiogram remains the gold standard for the detection of angiographic CV. DSA is, however, invasive and best limited to selected patients with significant vasospasm diagnosed by TCD/transcranial color-coded sonography (TCCS). CV can be focal, segmental, or diffuse, and can be graded as mild (25%), moderate (25–50%), and severe (>70%) based on DSA findings. Although routine vascular imaging is not routinely recommended to predict vasospasm, a screening on day 4 for high-risk patients and day 8 for low-risk patients is recommended.[23] An alternate is to perform CTA and in the TACTICS study comparing Doppler and CT angiogram to detect DCI, CTA had a greater sensitivity and specificity.[24] However, cerebral angioplasty and intra-arterial calcium channel antagonist administration are just two of the specific therapies that can be performed during catheter angiography to treat CV.

Newer Technologies

Newer techniques such as near-infrared spectroscopy (NIRS) and continuous electroencephalography (EEG) monitoring have been to predict DCI.[25] NIRS is a noninvasive and relatively low-cost optical technique for measuring tissue oxygen saturation, changes in hemoglobin volume, and, indirectly, CBF. Continuous EEG monitoring coupled with spectral analysis, including decreasing alpha-to-delta power ratio, relative alpha power variability, epileptiform discharges, rhythmic and periodic ictal–interictal continuum patterns, and isolated alpha suppression is able to detect DCI with good sensitivity of 96%.[19] Cortical spreading depolarizations (SDs) are self-propagating waves in the grey matter monitored by invasive subdural strip electrodes, and in brain injured patients, SDs are associated with DCI. A decrease in Neurological Pupil Index (NPi) as assessed by pupillometry is another useful tool which aids in early diagnosis of DCI. CBF can be measured by using thermal-diffusion flowmetry or by imaging modalities such as computed tomography perfusion (CTP), magnetic resonance (MR) perfusion, positron emission tomography (PET), and Xenon CT. Diminished brain perfusion as detected by CTP precedes DCI and vasospasm and can help in timely intervention.[19] However, increased radiation exposure, allergic reaction to contrast agent, and restricted temporal resolution limit the general and repeated use of CTP. Invasive monitoring of brain oxygenation levels and cerebral micro dialysis have been shown to have good prediction value for DCI and a brain tissue oxygen ($P_{bt}O_2$) <20 mm Hg warrants intervention, whereas levels below 10 mm Hg are judged critical. Cerebral microdialysis (CMD) and detection of increased levels of CMD-glutamate and CMD-lactate, elevated CMD-lactate-to-pyruvate-ratio (LPR), and CMD-glycerol levels can also help in detecting impending DCI.[19] These ancillary tests are not cost effective, user friendly, and practical in a day-to-day clinical setting.

TREATMENT

The first step following aSAH is to secure the aneurysm either through surgery or through interventional neuroradiology techniques. Post securing, management of CV can be either prophylactic or rescue management. Prophylactic treatment refers to certain blanket regimen initiated in all patients, whereas rescue management is administered after radiographic or clinical evidence of vasospasm.

Prophylaxis

Prophylaxis is administered in the acute period after aSAH, before the occurrence of vasospasm and includes certain general measures and one pharmacological agent.

Basic Interventions (Applied in All Patients)

These include avoidance of fever, maintenance of euvolemia, correction of dysnatremia, tight glycemic control (130–180 g/dL), cerebral perfusion pressure (CPP) maintenance at least 60 mm Hg and titration to higher levels, partial pressure of arterial carbon dioxide ($PaCO_2$) levels between 35 and 45 mm Hg, and avoidance of hypoxemia [partial pressure of arterial oxygen (PaO_2) <60 mm Hg] or hyperoxemia (>150 mm Hg).[26]

Volume Optimization (Euvolemia)

Earlier used widely, the triple-H therapy (hypertension, hypervolemia, and hemodilution) regimen has been discontinued due to lack of favorable evidence and higher risk of associated complications. Morbidity due to hypervolemia (anemia, hyponatremia, pulmonary edema, and circulatory overload), and cardiac complications from induced hypertension led to the discontinuation of this regimen. With euvolemia maintenance using crystalloids, DCI was observed in 13% of the patients in the goal-directed therapy group and in 32% of the patients in the control group {odds ratio (OR) 0.324 [95% confidence interval (CI) 0.11–0.86]; $p = 0.021$} in one study.[27] A similar study was observed that initiation of the euvolemic protocol reduced DCI from 44.2 to 7.7% [OR 0.10 (95% CI 0.04–0.23); $p < 0.001$].[28] Current guidelines recommend euvolemia and hemodynamic augmentation using pressors and inotropes to augment blood pressure and cardiac output for prophylaxis and treatment.[19,26,29,30]

Augmenting Cerebrospinal Fluid Flow by Clot Clearance (Surgery and Intrathecal Therapies)

Different techniques have been investigated to reduce the risk of CV by prompt evacuation of blood and blood products from the subarachnoid space. Surgical clearance post clipping and post clipping cisternal administration of fibrinolytics such as recombinant tissue plasminogen activator (rTPA) and urokinase have shown favorable results but need larger studies for validation.[29,31] Fenestration of the lamina terminalis during aneurysm clipping has been found to lower the risk of subsequent hydrocephalus and vasospasm by facilitating clot clearance and CSF flow in the basal cisterns.[32] Global clot clearance as achieved by lumbar CSF replacement or drainage therapies has also shown a significant decrease in vasospasm.[33,34] Lumbar infusion therapies with a variety of drugs including calcium channel blockers, fibrinolytics, and other vasodilators have shown promising results in experimental and small group studies warranting larger randomized controlled trials (RCTs).[35] Intrathecal drug distribution of higher drug concentrations to the spasmodic arteries while reducing systemic toxicity is the primary advantage of this method of drug delivery. A recent meta-analysis which included 29 studies reported beneficial effects with intrathecal therapy using rTPA, nimodipine, and magnesium.[35] In order to deliver nimodipine, particles are injected through an external ventricular drain (EVD) and circulate through the basal cisternal subarachnoid space. The results of the clinical trial known as NEWTON (Nimodipine Microparticles to Enhance Recovery While Reducing Toxicity After Subarachnoid Hemorrhage) were promising, but the subsequent NEWTON-2 trial had to be terminated early.[29]

Nimodipine

Nimodipine is the only drug used today world over consistently as a prophylactic agent with the intention to reduce vasospasm.[36,37] Several large RCTs with over 1,700 patients analyzed have consistently shown nimodipine to reduce poor outcome and mortality.[38] Nimodipine is a dihydropyridine calcium channel blocker, which acts by blocking the flux of extracellular calcium via L-type voltage-gated calcium channels. Neuroprotective mechanisms are postulated through inhibition of SDs, decrease of microthrombic emboli, and enhancing fibrinolytic activity. It is preferable to other calcium channel antagonists because of its relative selectivity for the cerebral vasculature as a result of its lipophilic nature and capacity to cross the blood brain. A dose of 60 mg 4 hourly for 21 days is the standard dose with dose adjustments possible to maintain normotension.

■ First-line Treatment for New Onset-delayed Cerebral Ischemia-tiered Approach (in the Setting of Delayed Cerebral Ischemia)

- Nimodipine acts both as prophylaxis and first line of treatment for patients with suspected vasospasm and early DCI.
- Volume optimization—euvolemia acts both as prophylaxis and first line of treatment for patients with suspected vasospasm and early DCI.
- Vasopressors—permissive hypertension and hemodynamic augmentation
It is widely believed that hypertensive therapy induced through different methods, including intravenous colloids or various vasopressor medications (dobutamine, norepinephrine, milrinone, and phenylephrine) improves cerebral perfusion, thereby preventing vasospasm or DCI. The HIMALAIA (Hypertension Induction in the Management of Aneurysmal Subarachnoid Hemorrhage with Secondary Ischemia), trial which studied the role of induced hypertension in aSAH, was prematurely stopped due to poor enrolment and a lack of benefit for cerebral perfusion, with no improvement in functional outcome.[39] However, observational research, including extensive, multicenter retrospective data, shows that 80% of symptomatic patients improved after being subjected to induced hypertension.[39,40] Death, myocardial infarction, and cardiac arrhythmia were serious adverse events that were more common but not statistically significant in the treatment group.[39] A reactive approach to hemodynamic augmentation is now preferred to a prophylactic approach, and induced hypertension may be reasonable

in patients with evolving or established DCI. In a recent German randomized, controlled, single-center study, goal-directed hemodynamic therapy (GDHT) patients had significantly lower rates of DCI (13%) as compared to patients treated according to standard clinical care (32%). Stepwise increases in blood pressure levels can be achieved by vasopressors or fluid administration.[41]

- *Arteriolar vasodilators*: Milrinone has been observed to reduce radiographic vasospasm in a small number of investigations and demonstrates both inotropic and vasodilatory effects by specifically inhibiting low-Km cyclic adenosine monophosphate (cAMP)-specific phosphodiesterase.[26,29] Recent research suggests that intrathecal milrinone injection through a lumbar catheter is a safer alternative to systemic delivery; however, additional randomized controlled studies are required to establish the effectiveness.[29] Cyclic guanosine monophosphate (cGMP)-specific phosphodiesterase-5 inhibitor sildenafil has apparently also demonstrated beneficial outcomes in lowering DCI.[29]

Rescue Therapy for Medically Refractory Vasospasm

Chemical Angioplasty Intra-arterial Calcium Channel Antagonists

Intra-arterial administration of calcium channel antagonists (papaverine, nimodipine, milrinone, verapamil, or nicardipine) may alleviate CV if neurological impairments caused by it are resistant to induced hypertension. The time and intensity, on the other hand, have not been thoroughly established, and the impact could be transient, requiring repeated administration. A new study contrasted conservative endovascular therapy (EVT), which is triggered by persistent neurologic impairments despite induced hypertension, with aggressive EVT, which is activated by higher TCD velocities or suspicion of neurologic deficit, reported better outcomes with an aggressive strategy.

Transluminal Balloon Angioplasty

A number of studies have described transluminal balloon angioplasty (TBA) as effective for the treatment of CV both for prophylaxis and treatment.[42,43] TBA was found to be effective in improving the spasm in nearly 80% of patients, especially in large capacitance proximal arteries with thick muscular walls like the ICA or vertebral arteries. Success rate is >90%, especially if done early. Complications include thrombosis, vessel rupture, and dissection, and a risk of recurrence especially in patients with a moderate or poor angiographic response initially. Novel techniques, such as stent retriever angioplasty with the ability to simultaneously apply intra-arterial calcium channel antagonists, are also under evaluation.

Cardiac Output Augmentation

By boosting CBF and maximizing mean arterial pressure, cardiac output augmentation aims to maintain a suitable CPP. Due to tachyarrhythmias, slowed ventricular filling time, and peripheral vasoconstriction, the administration of inotropic or vasopressor drugs might aggravate cardiogenic shock. As a therapeutic option, the use of intra-aortic balloon counterpulsation pumps (IABPs) is growing in acceptance. It reduces afterload and lowers coronary perfusion during diastole, which lessens left ventricular strain and myocyte oxygen demand.

Hemoglobin Optimization

The ideal hemoglobin (Hb) level needed to prevent vasospasm and the association between anemia and the condition are less certain. Current critical care recommendations take a step-by-step approach to transfusion trigger limitations. The criterion is 8 g/dL for people without DCI, but 9–10 g/dL has been suggested as a more aggressive threshold for DCI patients who are not responding to first-line therapy. A suitable trigger limit for Hb resuscitation will be determined by the Aneurysmal Subarachnoid Hemorrhage: Red Blood Cell Transfusion and Outcome (SAHaRA Pilot) randomized controlled study, which is now taking place.[44]

Sympatholytic Therapy

The cerebral vasculature enlarges when the sympathetic nerve fibers that leave the superior cervical ganglion and proceed via the ICA are disrupted, which can assist relieve vasospasm. In order to prevent CV and DCI, it has been tried to block the stellate ganglion, which is made up of the inferior cervical and first thoracic ganglia.[45]

Newer Drugs and Techniques

Fasudil, a strong Rho-kinase inhibitor, has been approved for use in various nations in patients with aSAH due to evidence that it improves clinical outcomes. Other medications, such as cilostazol, clazosentan, magnesium, heparin, and dantrolene, have been predicted to improve DCI, but there is not enough data to back up their routine usage in patients with aSAH.[46] Statins alter cholesterol synthesis pathways, and in addition to their cholesterol-lowering effects are known to improve endothelial function, modulate inflammatory response, and maintain plaque stability. They are known to improve CBF by upregulation of endothelial nitric oxide synthase (NOS), increasing NO synthesis and availability.[47] The international, randomized, double-blind trial STASH (Simvastatin in Aneurysmal Subarachnoid Haemorrhage) failed to detect any benefit from simvastatin 40 mg/day, started within 96 hours of ictus and then continued for up to 3 weeks, for either short- or long-term outcome.[48] According to a recent meta-analysis by Shen and colleagues[49], vasospasm was decreased in the six randomized aSAH studies for statin medication, but neither DCI nor mortality showed any discernible benefits. Statins are not advised as standard therapy in this population due to the lack of benefit in outcomes based on earlier dose techniques suggested by the available evidence.[50]

A stepwise flowchart assisted evidence-based management recommendation protocol for CV-induced DCI has been recently proposed by the AHA[50] and is shown in **Flowchart 1**.

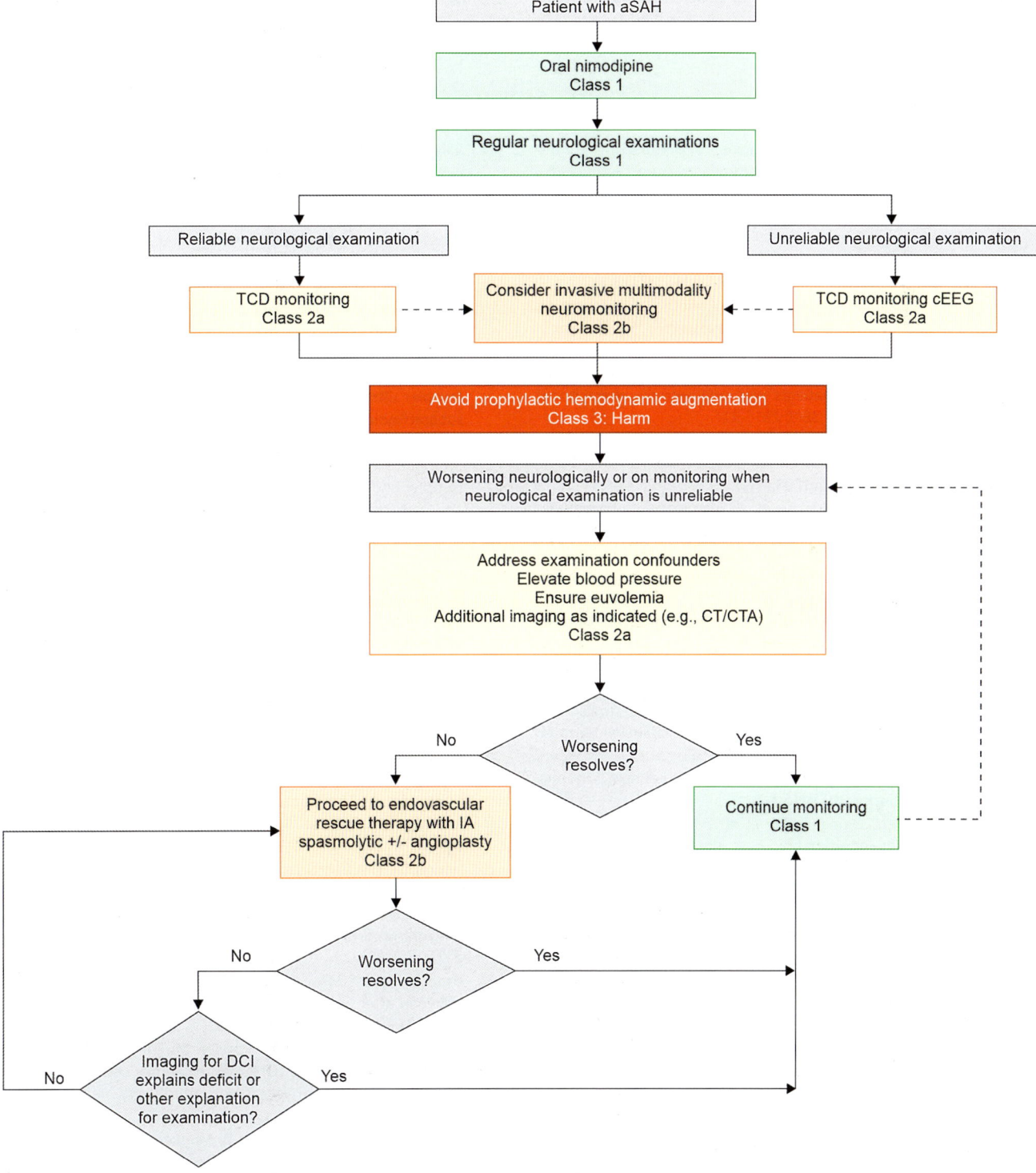

FLOWCHART 1: An evidence-based approach to the management of patients with cerebral vasospasm and DCI after aSAH.[50]
(aSAH: aneurysmal subarachnoid hemorrhage; cEEG: continuous electroencephalography; CT/CTA: computed tomography/computed tomography angiography; DCI: delayed cerebral ischemia; TCD: transcranial Doppler)

CONCLUSION

Vasospasm and ensuing DCI are significant causes of poor morbidity and mortality after aSAH. Quantum of subarachnoid blood on CT scan remains the best predictor for vasospasm but an astute clinical acumen to detect early neurological deterioration is the key diagnostic tool. Catheter angiography is the gold standard for diagnostic confirmation, but TCD remains the best bedside diagnostic modality for routine clinical practice. Management includes nimodipine, euvolemia, and induced hypertension for all patients followed by a tiered stepwise approach for rescue management once DCI steps in. A blanket approach considering all aSAH patients to be potential candidates for DCI needs to be adopted to avoid delayed detection and late intervention.

REFERENCES

1. Thompson BG, Brown RD, Amin-Hanjani S, et al. Guidelines for the Management of Patients with Unruptured Intracranial Aneurysms: A Guideline for Healthcare Professionals from the American Heart Association/American Stroke Association. Stroke. 2015;46(8):2368-400.
2. Lantigua H, Ortega-Gutierrez S, Schmidt JM, et al. Subarachnoid hemorrhage: Who dies and why? Crit Care. 2015;19(1):309.
3. Iuliano BA, Pluta RM, Jung C, et al. Endothelial dysfunction in a primate model of cerebral vasospasm. J Neurosurg. 2004;100(2):287-94.
4. Rosengart AJ, Schultheiss KE, Tolentino J, et al. Prognostic factors for outcome in patients with aneurysmal subarachnoid hemorrhage. Stroke. 2007;38(8):2315-21.
5. Viderman D, Tapinova K, Abdildin YG. Mechanisms of cerebral vasospasm and cerebral ischaemia in subarachnoid haemorrhage. Clin Physiol Funct Imaging. 2023;43(1):1-9.
6. Burns SK, Brewer KJ, Jenkins C, et al. Aneurysmal Subarachnoid Hemorrhage and Vasospasm. AACN Adv Crit Care. 2018;29(2):163-74.
7. Dorsch NW, King MT. A review of cerebral vasospasm in aneurysmal subarachnoid haemorrhage Part I: Incidence and effects. J Clin Neurosci. 1994;1(1):19-26.
8. Dority JS, Oldham JS. Subarachnoid Hemorrhage: An Update. Anesthesiol Clin. 2016;34(3):577-600.
9. Vergouwen MDI, Vermeulen M, van Gijn J, et al. Definition of delayed cerebral ischemia after aneurysmal subarachnoid hemorrhage as an outcome event in clinical trials and observational studies: Proposal of a multidisciplinary research group. Stroke. 2010;41(10):2391-5.
10. Macdonald RL. History and definition of delayed cerebral ischemia. Acta Neurochir Suppl. 2013;115:3-7.
11. Raya A, Zipfel GJ, Diringer MN, et al. Pattern Not Volume of Bleeding Predicts Angiographic Vasospasm in Nonaneurysmal Subarachnoid Hemorrhage. Stroke. 2014;45(1):265-7.
12. Jung SW, Lee CY, Yim MB. The Relationship Between Subarachnoid Hemorrhage Volume and Development of Cerebral Vasospasm. J Cerebrovasc Endovasc Neurosurg. 2012;14(3):186-91.
13. Hijdra A, Brouwers PJ, Vermeulen M, et al. Grading the amount of blood on computed tomograms after subarachnoid hemorrhage. Stroke. 1990;21(8):1156-61.
14. de Oliveira Manoel AL, Jaja BN, Germans MR, et al. The VASOGRADE. Stroke. 2015;46(7):1826-31.
15. Sheth SA, Hausrath D, Numis AL, et al. Intraoperative rerupture during surgical treatment of aneurysmal subarachnoid hemorrhage is not associated with an increased risk of vasospasm. J Neurosurg. 2014;120(2):409-14.
16. Imamura H, Tani S, Adachi H, et al. Comparison of Symptomatic Vasospasm after Surgical Clipping and Endovascular Coiling. Neurol Med Chir (Tokyo). 2022;62(5):223-30.
17. Rabinstein AA, Pichelmann MA, Friedman JA, et al. Symptomatic vasospasm and outcomes following aneurysmal subarachnoid hemorrhage: A comparison between surgical repair and endovascular coil occlusion. J Neurosurg. 2003;98(2):319-25.
18. Gross BA, Rosalind Lai PM, Frerichs KU, et al. Treatment modality and vasospasm after aneurysmal subarachnoid hemorrhage. World Neurosurg. 2014;82(6):e725-30.
19. Rass V, Gaasch M, Kofler M, et al. Fluid Intake but Not Fluid Balance Is Associated With Poor Outcome in Nontraumatic Subarachnoid Hemorrhage Patients. Crit Care Med. 2019;47(7):e555-62.
20. Lindegaard KF, Bakke SJ, Sorteberg W, et al. A noninvasive Doppler ultrasound method for the evaluation of patients with subarachnoid hemorrhage. Acta Radiol Suppl. 1986;369:96-8.
21. Minhas PS, Menon DK, Smielewski P, et al. Positron emission tomographic cerebral perfusion disturbances and transcranial Doppler findings among patients with neurological deterioration after subarachnoid hemorrhage. Neurosurgery. 2003;52(5):1017-22; discussion 1022-4.
22. Washington CW, Zipfel GJ. Participants in the International Multidisciplinary Consensus Conference on the Critical Care Management of Subarachnoid Hemorrhage. Detection and monitoring of vasospasm and delayed cerebral ischemia: A review and assessment of the literature. Neurocrit Care. 2011;15(2):312-7.
23. Francoeur CL, Mayer SA. Management of delayed cerebral ischemia after subarachnoid hemorrhage. Crit Care. 2016;20(1):277.
24. van der Harst JJ, Luijckx GR, Elting JWJ, et al. Transcranial Doppler Versus CT-Angiography for Detection of Cerebral Vasospasm in Relation to Delayed Cerebral Ischemia After Aneurysmal Subarachnoid Hemorrhage: A Prospective Single-Center Cohort Study: The Transcranial doppler and CT-angiography for Investigating Cerebral vasospasm in Subarachnoid hemorrhage (TACTICS) study. Crit Care Explor. 2019;1(1):e0001.
25. Hänggi D. The Participants in the International Multi-disciplinary Consensus Conference on the Critical Care Management of Subarachnoid Hemorrhage. Monitoring and Detection of Vasospasm II: EEG and Invasive Monitoring. Neurocrit Care. 2011;15(2):318-23.
26. Ikram A, Javaid MA, Ortega-Gutierrez S, et al. Delayed Cerebral Ischemia after Subarachnoid Hemorrhage. J Stroke Cerebrovasc Dis. 2021;30(11):106064.
27. Anetsberger A, Gempt J, Blobner M, et al. Impact of Goal-Directed Therapy on Delayed Ischemia After Aneurysmal Subarachnoid Hemorrhage: Randomized Controlled Trial. Stroke. 2020;51(8):2287-96.
28. Duangthongphon P, Souwong B, Munkong W, et al. Results of a Preventive Rebleeding Protocol in Patients with Ruptured Cerebral Aneurysm: A Retrospective Cohort Study. Asian J Neurosurg. 2019;14(3):748-53.

29. Al-Mufti F, Amuluru K, Damodara N, et al. Novel management strategies for medically refractory vasospasm following aneurysmal subarachnoid hemorrhage. J Neurol Sci. 2018;390:44-51.
30. Gelder CL, Bautista M, Awan SA, et al. Unaccounted for enteral volume loss linked to delayed cerebral ischemia after subarachnoid hemorrhage. Neurosurgical Focus. 2022;52(3):E5.
31. Amin-Hanjani S, Ogilvy CS, Barker FG. Does intracisternal thrombolysis prevent vasospasm after aneurysmal subarachnoid hemorrhage? A meta-analysis. Neurosurgery. 2004;54(2):326-34; discussion 334-5.
32. Andaluz N, Zuccarello M. Fenestration of the lamina terminalis as a valuable adjunct in aneurysm surgery. Neurosurgery. 2004;55(5):1050-9.
33. Geng L, Ma F, Liu Y, et al. Massive Cerebrospinal Fluid Replacement Reduces Delayed Cerebral Vasospasm After Embolization of Aneurysmal Subarachnoid Hemorrhage. Med Sci Monit. 2016;22:2404-8.
34. Borkar SA, Singh M, Kale SS, et al. Spinal Cerebrospinal Fluid Drainage for prevention of Vasospasm in Aneurysmal Subarachnoid Hemorrhage: A Prospective, Randomized controlled study. Asian J Neurosurg. 2018;13(2):238-46.
35. Grossen AA, Ernst GL, Bauer AM. Update on intrathecal management of cerebral vasospasm: A systematic review and meta-analysis. Neurosurg Focus. 2022;52(3):E10.
36. Allen GS, Ahn HS, Preziosi TJ, et al. Cerebral Arterial Spasm—A Controlled Trial of Nimodipine in Patients with Subarachnoid Hemorrhage. N Engl J Med. 1983;308(11):619-24.
37. Pickard JD, Murray GD, Illingworth R, et al. Effect of oral nimodipine on cerebral infarction and outcome after subarachnoid haemorrhage: British aneurysm nimodipine trial. BMJ. 1989;298(6674):636-42.
38. Hao G, Chu G, Pan P, et al. Clinical effectiveness of nimodipine for the prevention of poor outcome after aneurysmal subarachnoid hemorrhage: A systematic review and meta-analysis. Front Neurol. 2022;13:982498.
39. Gathier CS, van den Bergh WM, van der Jagt M, et al. Induced Hypertension for Delayed Cerebral Ischemia After Aneurysmal Subarachnoid Hemorrhage: A Randomized Clinical Trial. Stroke. 2018;49(1):76-83.
40. Haegens NM, Gathier CS, Horn J, et al. Induced Hypertension in Preventing Cerebral Infarction in Delayed Cerebral Ischemia After Subarachnoid Hemorrhage. Stroke. 2018;49(11):2630-6.
41. Dushianthan A, Knight M, Russell P, et al. Goal-directed haemodynamic therapy (GDHT) in surgical patients: Systematic review and meta-analysis of the impact of GDHT on postoperative pulmonary complications. Perioper Med (Lond). 2020;9:30.
42. Schacht H, Küchler J, Boppel T, et al. Transluminal balloon angioplasty for cerebral vasospasm after spontaneous subarachnoid hemorrhage: A single-center experience. Clin Neurol Neurosurg. 2020;188:105590.
43. Zwienenberg-Lee M, Hartman J, Rudisill N, et al. Effect of Prophylactic Transluminal Balloon Angioplasty on Cerebral Vasospasm and Outcome in Patients with Fisher Grade III Subarachnoid Hemorrhage. Stroke. 2008;39(6):1759-65.
44. English SW, Fergusson D, Chassé M, et al. Aneurysmal Subarachnoid Hemorrhage-Red Blood Cell Transfusion and Outcome (SAHaRA): A pilot randomised controlled trial protocol. BMJ Open. 2016;6(12):e012623.
45. Salvagno M, Gouvea Bogossian E, Halenarova K, et al. Cervical Ganglion Sympathectomy to Treat Cerebral Vasospasm in Subarachnoid Hemorrhage. Neurocrit Care. 2023.
46. Maruhashi T, Higashi Y. An overview of pharmacotherapy for cerebral vasospasm and delayed cerebral ischemia after subarachnoid hemorrhage. Expert Opin Pharmacother. 2021;22(12):1601-14.
47. O'Driscoll G, Green D, Taylor RR. Simvastatin, an HMG-coenzyme A reductase inhibitor, improves endothelial function within 1 month. Circulation. 1997;95(5):1126-31.
48. Kirkpatrick PJ, Turner CL, Smith C, et al.; STASH Collaborators. Simvastatin in aneurysmal subarachnoid haemorrhage (STASH): A multicentre randomised phase 3 trial. Lancet Neurol. 2014;13(7):666-75.
49. Shen J, Huang KY, Zhu Y, et al. Effect of statin treatment on vasospasm-related morbidity and functional outcome in patients with aneurysmal subarachnoid hemorrhage: A systematic review and meta-analysis. J Neurosurg. 2017;127(2):291-301.
50. Hoh BL, Ko NU, Amin-Hanjani S, et al. 2023 Guideline for the Management of Patients with Aneurysmal Subarachnoid Hemorrhage: A Guideline from the American Heart Association/American Stroke Association. Stroke. 2023;54(7):e314-70.

CHAPTER 8

Diagnosis and Management of Intracranial Dural Arteriovenous Fistulae

Akshaya Saravanan, Aravinda HR, Padmasri Gorantla, Vipul Gupta

ABSTRACT

Dural arteriovenous malformations (AVMs) are abnormal communications between dural arterial feeders and dural, meningeal or cortical veins with occasional pial arterial supply. They account for 10–15% of intracranial AVMs and frequently presently in fifth or sixth decade. Symptoms depend on site of fistula, pattern of venous drainage, and presence or absence of cortical venous reflux. Most widely used classification systems are Borden and Cognard and types IIb to V can have aggressive symptoms and warrant prompt treatment. Spontaneous closure of type 1 fistulae can occur rarely. Digital subtraction angiography (DSA) is the gold standard for diagnosis, classifying, and understanding the angioarchitecture of dural arteriovenous fistulas (DAVFs). Endovascular embolization is the mainstay of treatment with other less commonly used options being microsurgical disconnection and gamma knife radiosurgery. Transarterial embolization with liquid embolic agents is the widely used approach; however, transvenous or combined approaches can be used in complex cases. Detailed understanding of angioanatomy, dangerous external carotid artery–internal carotid artery (ECA–ICA) anastomosis and cranial nerve blood supply help in avoiding nontarget embolization and complications. High index of suspicion and timely intervention can help in mitigating the symptoms.

Keywords: Intracranial DVAF, Cortical venous reflux, Embolization, Transarterial, Transvenous, Liquid embolic.

INTRODUCTION

Intracranial dural arteriovenous fistulas (DAVFs) are the abnormal vascular communications involving the dura mater between dural arteries and dural venous sinuses, meningeal veins, or cortical veins accounting for 10–15% of intracranial arteriovenous malformations (AVMs). Most DAVFs present in adulthood and are located in relation to the transverse, sigmoid, and cavernous sinuses. Occasionally, they are seen in pediatric population that tend to be complex, often having bilateral arterial feeders and large venous lakes, and frequently involving the torcular herophili and superior sagittal sinus.[1,2]

ETIOPATHOGENESIS

Intracranial dural arteriovenous fistulae are predominantly idiopathic, though a small percentage of patients have a history of previous craniotomy, trauma, or dural sinus thrombosis. Heritable risk factors for venous thrombosis, such as deficiencies of antithrombin, protein C, and protein S, have been associated with DAVF occurrence and this implicates the role of an underlying hypercoagulability as a causative factor.

Two etiologic hypotheses based around sinus thrombosis have been put forward. The first is that physiologic arteriovenous shunts between meningeal arteries and dural venous sinuses enlarge in response to elevated local venous pressure, resulting in a pathologic shunt. The second is that venous hypertension due to outflow obstruction causes decreased cerebral perfusion and promotes neoangiogenesis.

It has been noted that dura mater is composed of two layers, an internal layer dura propria, and an outer layer osteal dura (periosteal dura). They are derived from the mesoderm or neural crest cells.

Neural crest group: The dura mater of the olfactory groove, falx cerebri, inferior sagittal sinus, tentorium cerebelli, and falx cerebelli, and the dura mater at the level of the spinal cord are composed only of dura propria, and these areas are derived from neural crest cells.

This group of DAVFs are at a distance from the main dural sinuses; therefore, almost 100% of the shunt flow with DAVFs located on this group usually drains into the adjacent pial vein directly. Thus, the natural course of this group is usually aggressive and malignant.

Mesenchymal group: The dura mater of the cavernous sinus, transverse sinus, sigmoid sinus, and anterior condylar confluence surrounding the hypoglossal canal are composed of both dura propria and osteal dura; this group is derived from mesoderm. The DAVFs located in this group are close and mostly on the surface of dural sinuses. This proximity allows the shunt flow to drain into the adjacent main dural sinuses. Therefore, the cortical venous reflux is not so significant unless there is thrombosis or a pathological steno-occlusive lesion in the affected dural sinuses.[3,4]

Dural fistulae are usually fed by multitude of dural feeding arteries, draining veins, and sinuses with shunt in between them. Arterial supply may be composed of a single feeder or multiple feeders. The supplying arteries most often originate external to the dura mater (e.g., the middle meningeal, occipital, ascending pharyngeal, and superficial temporal arteries) but can less commonly arise from intradural pial artery branches. Secondary induced pial supply from vessels that do not normally supply the dura is well described in the literature (**Table 1**); however, this is not the sole supply in DAVFs. Venous drainage can be directly into cortical veins, or into the meningeal veins and in turn into dural venous sinuses, or into dural venous sinuses with reflux into the cortical veins.

Understanding angioarchitecture of DAVFs is important for guiding accurate endovascular therapy and preventing percolation of liquid embolic agents into nontarget vascular structures. A multitude of concepts with nomenclature of "parallel venous channel," "venous septation/pouch," and "common arterial collector" at the fistulous point of DAVF exist. A "shunted pouch" (SP) that is independent and outside the lumen of the sinus proper is the bottom line to pathoanatomy. Discrete shunting domains exist between this vessel and the lumen proper of the sinus. Superselective embolization and exclusion of such a common collector is desirable to minimize hazards of collateral/nontarget embolization and preserve sinus patency and function.

CLASSIFICATION

Different classification systems exist for DAVF; however, the most widely used are proposed by Borden et al. [based on cortical venous drainage (CVD)] and Cognard et al. (based on shunt location and venous outflow angioarchitecture) (**Table 2**).

NATURAL HISTORY

■ Low-grade Dural Arteriovenous Fistulae (Fistulae without Cortical Venous Drainage)

Annual rate of new neurological events for DAVFs without CVD is 0.0–0.6%, and the annual mortality rate for these lesions is 0.0%. DAVFs without CVD can convert to DAVFs with CVD over time and the annual rate of this upconversion is around 0.8%. Angiographic re-evaluation is warranted when any change in the patient symptoms are observed.

TABLE 1: Various pial–dural connections.	
Intracranial pial artery	**Dural arterial feeder**
Internal cerebral artery	Artery of Bernasconi–Cassinari
Anterior cerebral artery	Olfactory branches and pericallosal branches, anterior falcine artery
Posterior cerebral artery	Artery of Davidoff and Schechter
Superior cerebellar artery	Medial dural tentorial branch
Anterior inferior cerebellar artery	Subarcuate artery
Posterior inferior cerebellar artery	Posterior meningeal artery
Vertebral artery	Posterior meningeal artery

TABLE 2: Borden and Cognard classification of DAVF.							
	Borden classification			**Cognard classification**			
Natural course	Type	Venous drainage site	CVR	Type	Venous drainage site	Flow pattern in sinus	CVR
Benign	I	Dural sinus	No	I	Dural sinus	Antegrade	No
Benign				IIa	Dural sinus	Retrograde	No
Aggressive	II	Dural sinus	Yes	IIb	Dural sinus	Antegrade	Yes
Aggressive				IIa+b	Dural sinus	Retrograde	Yes
Aggressive	III	Cortical vein	Yes	III	Cortical vein		Yes without venous ectasia
Aggressive				IV	Cortical vein		Yes with venous ectasia
Aggressive				V	Cortical vein with spinal medullary drainage		Yes
(CVR: cortical venous reflux; DAVF: dural arteriovenous fistula)							

High-grade Dural Arteriovenous Fistulae (Fistulae with Cortical Venous Drainage)

Annual neurological event rate is 15.0% and an annual mortality rate is 10.4%. They are at substantial risk of intracranial hemorrhage (ICH), nonhemorrhagic neurological deficits (NHNDs), death, and treatment is warranted. Symptomatic CVD has a higher likelihood of suffering hemorrhagic or nonhemorrhagic neurological injury compared with those presenting incidentally or with symptoms of increased sinus drainage (i.e., asymptomatic CVD).

The natural history of patients with aggressive symptoms such as ICH and NHND is poor and correspondingly annual rate of such aggressive symptoms is 7.4–19.0% and the annual rate of mortality is 3.8%. Statistically significant increase in hemorrhagic risk is noted in patients with DAVFs having venous ectasia. Approximately 20–33% of DAVFs present with ICH.

CLINICAL PRESENTATION

A majority of patients with DAVFs present in the fifth and sixth decades with symptoms related to lesion location and pattern of venous drainage.

Most common site of DAVFs is along transverse and sigmoid sinus (45%), followed by cavernous sinus (24%), superior sagittal sinus (12%), tentorium cerebelli (10%), anterior cranial fossa (ACF) (8%), and foramen magnum (1%).[5] DAVF patients primarily present in three ways:

1. Aggressive symptoms such as ICH and NHND related to cortical venous hypertension, which only develop in DAVFs with CVD
2. Benign symptoms such as tinnitus and ophthalmologic phenomenon related to increased sinus drainage can occur in any DAVF having venous sinus drainage.
3. Incidental

Intracranial hemorrhage is more frequent in high-grade (Borden types II and III; Cognard types IIb to IV) DAVFs and occurs due to rupture of delicate, arterialized leptomeningeal veins or hemorrhagic transformation of cortical venous congestion. Fistulae located in the ACF base, along the foramen magnum and along the falx and tentorium cerebelli, usually present with hemorrhagic symptoms.

Nonhemorrhagic neurological deficit occurs in type IIb and type IIa+b fistulae and develops more gradually over days to weeks resulting from focal or global cortical venous hypertension that produces varying degrees of cerebral ischemia. These include seizures, parkinsonism, cerebellar symptoms, apathy, failure to thrive, dementia, and cranial nerve abnormalities including rare cases of trigeminal neuralgia and symptoms related to increased pressure including headache, nausea, and vomiting. Pressure symptoms, including dementia and cognitive decline, are likely to improve after treatment.

Cavernous sinus DAVFs can present with ophthalmoplegia, proptosis, chemosis, retro-orbital pain, or decreased visual acuity.

IMAGING

Skull Radiograph

Skull radiograph is infrequently advised in recent times. However, it may show secondary features of raised ICT or chronic venous congestion such as impressions of arterial or venous channels, silver-beaten appearance (**Figs. 1A to D**).

Computed Tomography

Plain computed tomography (CT) can show prominent and hyperdense vessels and may help in identifying the complications such as hemorrhage and edema secondary to venous hypertension (**Fig. 1**). Dilated and tortuous transosseous channels may also be appreciated, especially

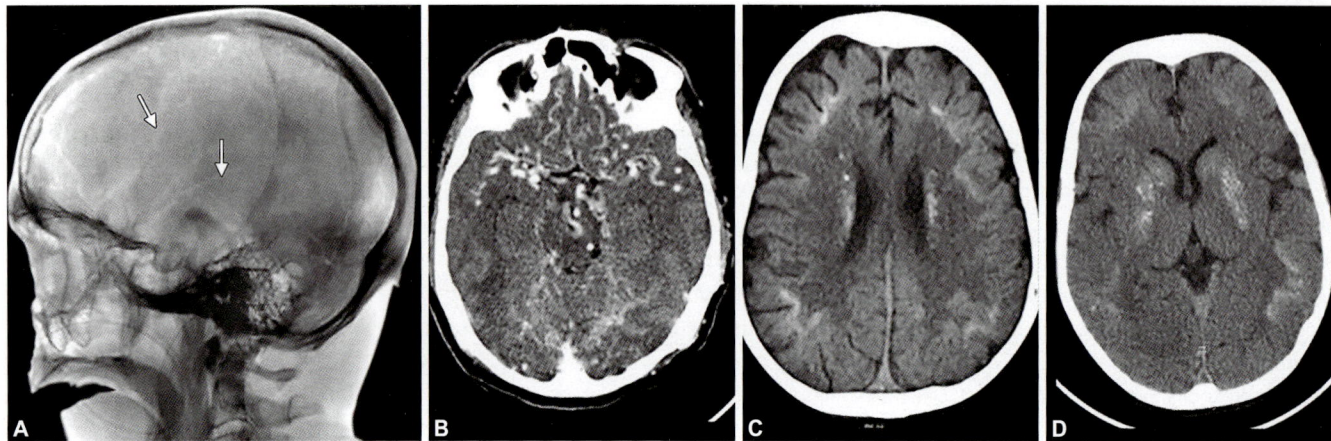

FIGS. 1A TO D: (A) X-ray lateral view showing prominent linear markings in the calvarium suggesting enlarged vascular channels (arrows); (B) Contrast computed tomography (CT) showing abnormal multiple dilated tortuous vessels; (C and D) Plain CT images show calcifications along subcortical white matter and bilateral basal ganglia secondary to chronic venous congestion in a case of dural arteriovenous fistula.

on bone window images. Subcortical and basal ganglia calcifications can be seen in cases with chronic venous hypertension **(Figs. 1A to D)**.

Computed tomography angiogram helps in identifying abnormal vessels in relation to bony anatomy. However, CTA has reduced sensitivity as compared to magnetic resonance angiography (MRA) in detecting DAVFs (15.4% vs. 50%).

Four-dimensional (4D) CTA provides hemodynamic information and helps in classification and treatment planning of AVMs and dural fistulae. It features all cranial vascular territories simultaneously and is helpful in follow-up imaging.[6]

■ Magnetic Resonance Imaging

Conventional magnetic resonance imaging (MRI) sequences show multiple abnormal prominent flow voids and help in identifying the associated features of venous hypertension, venous sinus thrombosis, and hemorrhage **(Figs. 2A to H)**.

Chronic venous hypertension may lead to white matter signal changes and parenchymal calcifications, typically at the cortical–subcortical junction **(Figs. 2A to H)** and in deep gray nuclei, especially in patients presenting with dementia.[7] Pattern of hemorrhage can be single or multicompartmental including intraparenchymal, subarachnoid, intraventricular, and even subdural hemorrhage.

Lesions in cavernous sinus region may show proptosis, enlarged superior ophthalmic vein (SOV) (flow void), and bulging of the cavernous sinus in the involved side.

Susceptibility-weighted imaging shows the prominence of the linear hypointense signals in the transmedullary veins and in the cortical veins due to chronic venous hypertension **(Figs. 2A to H)**. This phenomenon results from the increased transit time of the venous blood (deoxyhemoglobin) in the presence of venous hypertension.

Time-of-flight (TOF)-MRA is more sensitive in identifying the possible site of fistula, arterial feeders. Venous reflux in the superior sagittal sinus is identified as an arterial signal due

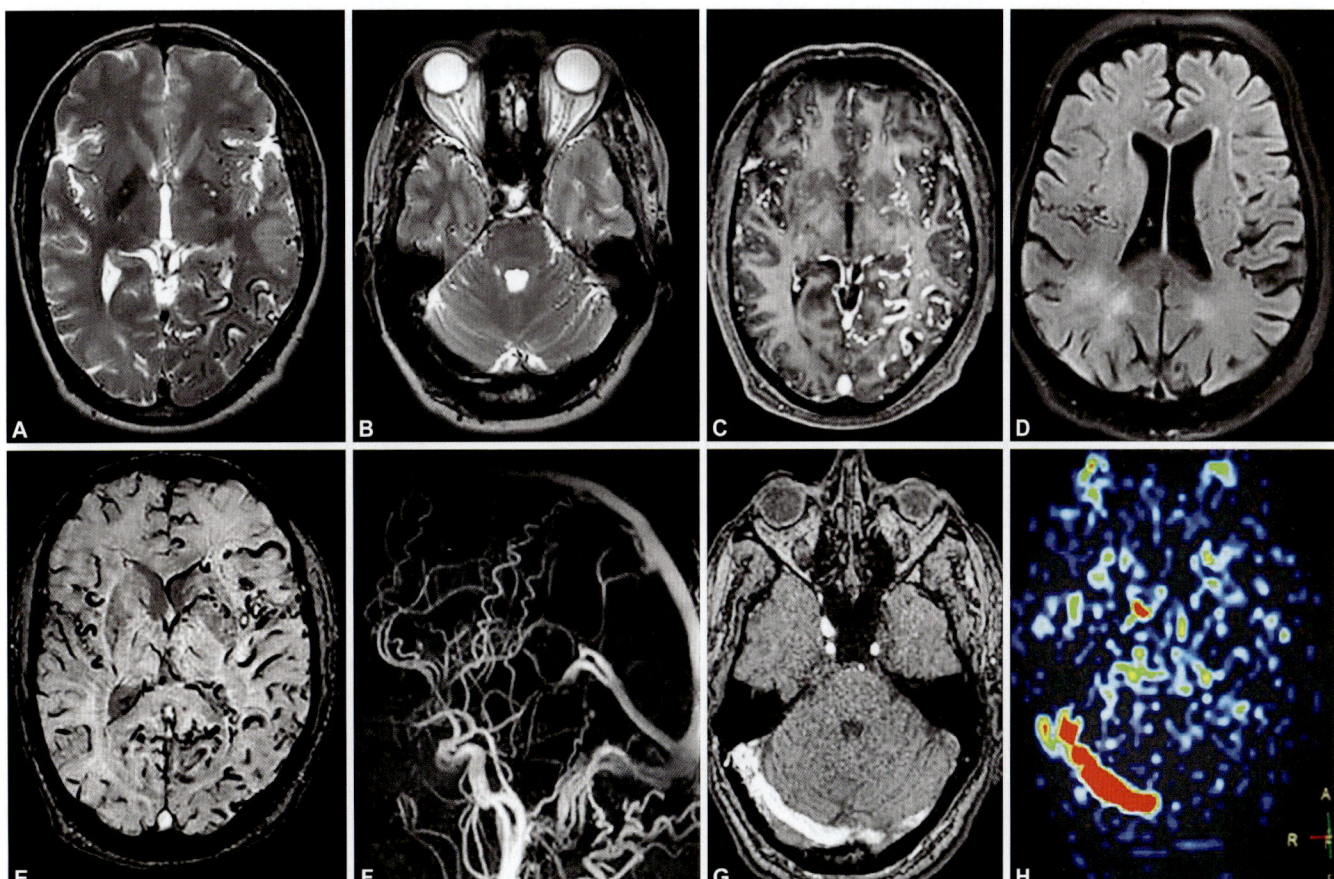

FIGS. 2A TO H: Dural arteriovenous fistula (DAVF) MRI features (images from different patients). (A and B) T2 axial images showing multiple flow voids with raised ICP features (prominent perioptic CSF sheaths and papilledema); (C) Postcontrast T1 axial image showing enhancement of the corresponding dilated vessels; (D) FLAIR showing white matter edema and (E) SWI showing prominent hypointensity involving the trans medullary and cortical veins due to increased venous transit time secondary to chronic venous hypertension; (F and G) TOF-MRA in a case of right transverse-sigmoid DAVF with signals in the superior sagittal, transverse, and straight sinuses identified as arterialized signal due to retrograde flow; (H) Corresponding ASL shows labeled arterial signals within the right transverse sinus.

(ASL: arterial spin labeling; CSF: cerebrospinal fluid; ICP: intracranial pressure; FLAIR: fluid-attenuated inversion recovery; MRI: magnetic resonance imaging; MRA: magnetic resonance angiography; SWI: susceptibility-weighted imaging; TOF: time-of-flight)

to retrograde flow (in sync with the direction of arterial flow) **(Figs. 2A to H)**. However, normal MRA does not completely rule out the presence of underlying DAVF. Contrast MRI shows engorged and dilated arterial feeders and venous channels. Engorged pial veins may suggest cortical venous reflux.

Arterial spin labeling (ASL) is useful in detecting the presence and site of shunting. Multidelay ASL helps in noninvasively identifying the presence of fistula and in assessing the cortical venous or sinus reflux **(Figs. 2A to H)**. This is based on the principle of direct transit of the labeled arterial blood signals into the venous channels without passing through the capillaries due to the presence of fistulae. Normally these signals are dampened when the blood passes through the capillaries. Added, this technique is used in follow-up of benign variety of DAVF and also cases of completely or partially treated DAVF as it mitigates the usage of contrast and radiation-related risks associated with DSA.

Digital Subtraction Angiography

Digital subtraction angiography remains the gold standard in diagnosing and classifying the DAVFs into low-risk versus high-risk fistulae. It gives the hemodynamic information and further assists in precisely identifying the fistula point, arterial feeders, and status of draining veins, helping in taking appropriate management decisions.

Imaging protocol includes six-vessel angiograms with high frame rate (six or more frames per second), acquiring till late venous phase to determine the pattern of venous drainage. Selective injections, especially of external carotid artery (ECA) feeders, help in improved detection of the fistulous points and assessing the risk of inadvertent nontarget embolization via dangerous internal carotid artery (ICA) ECA anastomosis. 3D rotational angiography with volume reconstitution may help in precise identification of fistulous point in complex cases with multiple arterial feeders.

Competitive angiogram allows superimposition of venous drainage of fistula and normal venous drainage of brain parenchyma. It requires selective injection of ICA followed by selective injection of ECA dural feeder and eventually resubtracting and changing the mask runs. This technique helps in identifying the functional status of the sinus or the enlarged veins (if it is draining the normal parenchyma) and deciding, if it (vein or sinus) can be sacrificed or not during embolization **(Fig. 3A)**.

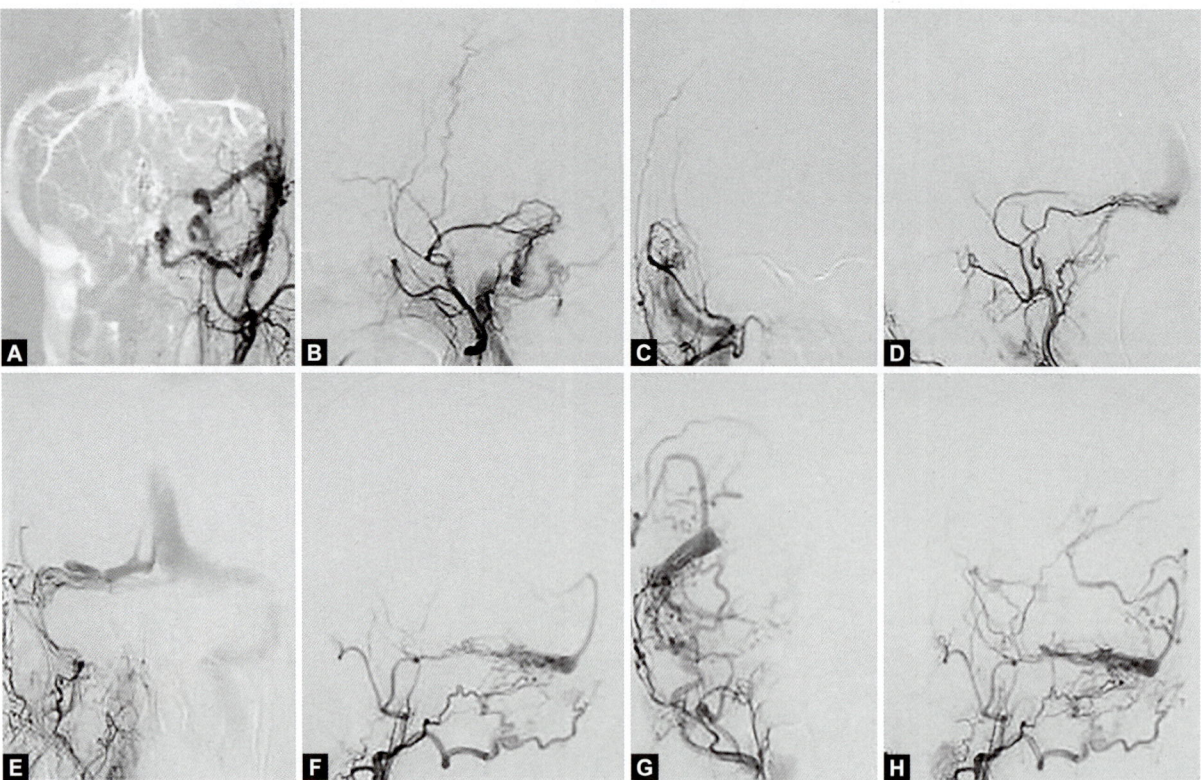

FIGS. 3A TO H: (A) Competitive angiography shows superimposed image of drainage of fistula and normal parenchyma, obtained by sequential selective injection of ICA followed by ECA and resubtraction and changing of the mask runs; (B and C) Right ECA lateral and AP views showing Cognard type 1 DAVF along right transverse-sigmoid sinus with antegrade venous outflow flow supplied by hypertrophied petrosquamous branch of MMA and occipital branches; (D and E) Cognard type IIa DAVF along right transverse-sigmoid sinus with retrograde venous outflow into torcula, SSS, and left transverse sinus and nonfunctioning right transverse-sigmoid; (F to H) Cognard type IIa+b DAVF along right transverse-sigmoid sinus with retrograde venous outflow into transverse sinus and cortical venous reflux.
(AP: anteroposterior; ECA: external carotid artery; ICA: internal carotid artery; DAVF: dural arteriovenous fistula; MMA: middle meningeal artery; SSS: superior sagittal sinus)
Courtesy: Sree Chitra Tirunal Institute for Medical Sciences and Technology, Kerala.

Features identified on DSA include:
- Arterial feeders, their course, relation to ECA-ICA anastomosis and tortuosity to determine the access for embolization
- Exact point of fistula
- Venous drainage pattern of fistula and of normal brain parenchyma to determine route and methods of embolization (transarterial vs. transvenous)
- Presence or absence of CVD
- Circulation time
- Status of draining vein—stenosis or ectasia of venous channel, compartmentalization, isolated sinus, functional status of sinus
- Drainage and site
- Direction of dural sinuses drainage—antegrade versus retrograde

*Representative DSA images of various subtypes of DAVFs are depicted in **Figures 3 and 4**.*

DIAGNOSIS AND DIFFERENTIAL DIAGNOSES

Any high-flow AVM like pial arteriovenous fistula (AVF) or parenchymal AVMs can mimic DAVFs on cross-sectional imaging. On MRI, prominence of the alternate venous channels secondary to cerebral venous/sinus thrombosis can also mimic the dural AV fistula. However, main differentiating features of DAVFs are predominant presence of dural arterial supply and absent nidus. Prominent transosseous feeders may also help in differentiating DAVFs from other vascular malformations.[8]

TREATMENT

Decision to treat and determine the modality of treatment is mainly based on pattern of venous drainage, presenting symptoms, and natural history of the DAVFs.

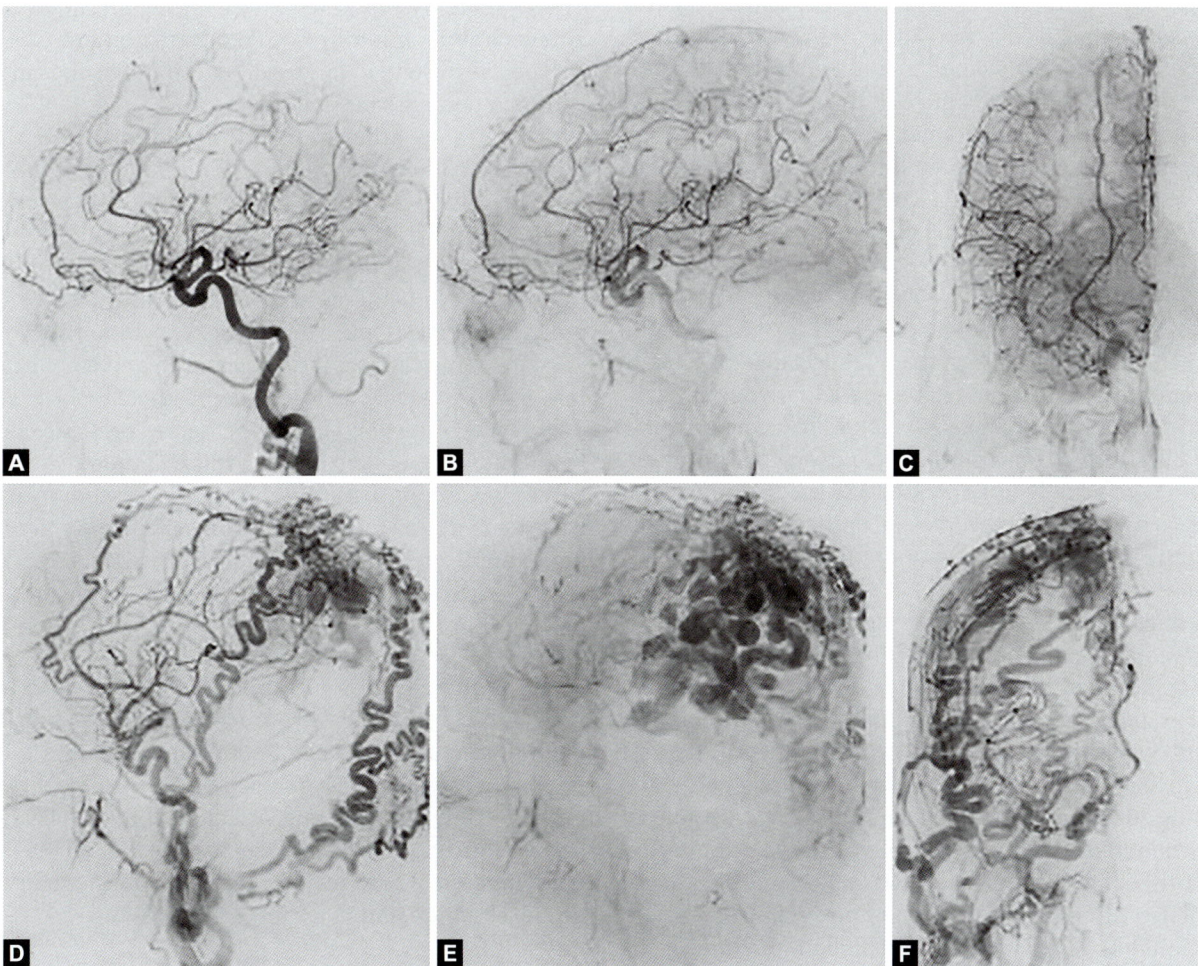

FIGS. 4A TO F: (A to C) Cognard type III DAVF along right ACF base with direct drainage into right frontal cortical vein, which in turn drains into mid third of SSS. Arterial feeders are from ethmoid branches of ophthalmic artery; (D to F) Cognard type IV DAVF along right parietal region with direct drainage into ectatic cortical veins.
(ACF: anterior cranial fossa; DAVF: dural arteriovenous fistula; SSS: superior sagittal sinus)

Treatment modalities include:
- Conservative management
- Endovascular embolization
- Microsurgical disconnection
- Stereotactic radiosurgery

Conservative Management

It is a mainstay of the management of low-grade DAVFs without any disabling symptoms keeping the patient on close follow-up. This can be followed in type I and type IIa fistulae. There are reports of spontaneous resolution of DAVFs.[9] Any new-onset symptoms or change of pattern/severity of symptoms in such fistulae indicate change in the underlying venous drainage pattern requiring immediate intervention. This conversion may be seen in approximately 2–4% of patients.[2]

Endovascular Management

Endovascular management is the first line and mainstay of management of intracranial DAVFs. Various embolic agents are injected or deployed at the site of fistulae either through the transarterial, transvenous, and combined routes. Liquid embolic agents used include EVOH (ethylene-vinyl alcohol) copolymers (Onyx, Squid, Menox) or Glue (n-butyl cyanoacrylate), and they remain the mainstay of treatment of the fistulae. Occasionally, coils are also used when fistulae is accessed through the venous route (especially in cavernous dural fistulae).

Transarterial Approach

It is the most widely used approach, especially for dorsally and laterally located fistulas (superior sagittal sinus, torcula, and transverse-sigmoid sinuses). Ventrally located fistulas (along cavernous sinus, petrous, condylar, and foramen magnum) are usually not accessed via transarterial route as they may pose higher risk of cranial nerve palsies and inadvertent embolization of dangerous ECA–ICA anastomosis.[10]

The main goal of treatment is to obliterate the fistula point and proximal portion of draining vein to ensure complete cure rate. In majority of the time, middle meningeal artery is used as an access to approach the site of the fistula. This artery is favorable as it has short trans-osseous course and the tortuosity of the artery usually gets straightened while accessing the shunt point. The microcatheter tip has to be positioned as distal as possible in the feeding artery toward the site of fistula to avoid reflux, and to ensure good penetration and percolation of the embolizing agent. Care should be taken to avoid percolation into dangerous ECA–ICA anastomosis and premature occlusion of feeding artery, which in turn may result in loss of access in further attempts.

Techniques of transarterial approach:
- Plug formation
- Pressure cooker (dual microcatheter)
- Dual-lumen balloon
- Balloon sinus protection

Plug Formation

It is the most commonly used technique, which allows controlled injections to form a stable plug **(Figs. 5A to E)**. Liquid embolic agent is slowly injected via microcatheter tip intermittently within the anatomic constraints to form a plug, preventing the reflux. Further injections will allow forward course toward fistula, with long injection time.[11] In case of microcatheter sticking within the plug, attempt may be done to remove it via snare or may be left within the vessel cutting it at the skin entry site. This technique is preferred in convexity DAVFs and in small diameter vessels. In case of large diameter vessels, longer segment of reflux is required to form a stable plug.

Pressure Cooker (Dual Microcatheter)

This technique minimizes reflux during embolization and is especially useful in large caliber arterial feeders and with shorter anatomic safety margins.

Two microcatheters, one with detachable tip and other for coiling, are required. Initially detachable tip microcatheter is placed close to fistula point. Coiling microcatheter is placed close to the detachable segment of first microcatheter and the feeder is blocked via coiling microcatheter using coils and glue. Alternatively, liquid embolic agent alone can be used to block the feeding vessel. Coiling catheter is then removed and embolization is performed via detachable tip microcatheter, which helps in forced antegrade flow (hence the name "pressure cooker"). Eventually the detachable tip microcatheter is removed carefully without dislodging the plug adjacent to it.[12] The advantage of this technique is longer injection time, good penetration, and percolation of the liquid embolic agent with minimal risk of microcatheter to get stuck within the vessel.

Dual-lumen Balloon Technique

It is a modified version of pressure cooker technique to limit the extent of reflux. It uses only one dual-lumen balloon microcatheter and balloon inflation as alternative to coiling microcatheter to occlude the proximal segment of the feeding artery during simultaneous embolization via second lumen. Disadvantage includes balloon may provide inadequate seal at times that can result in the reflux of the liquid embolic agent.[13]

Balloon Sinus Protection

When the fistula is directly draining into a patent dural sinus, which is also draining the normal brain parenchyma,

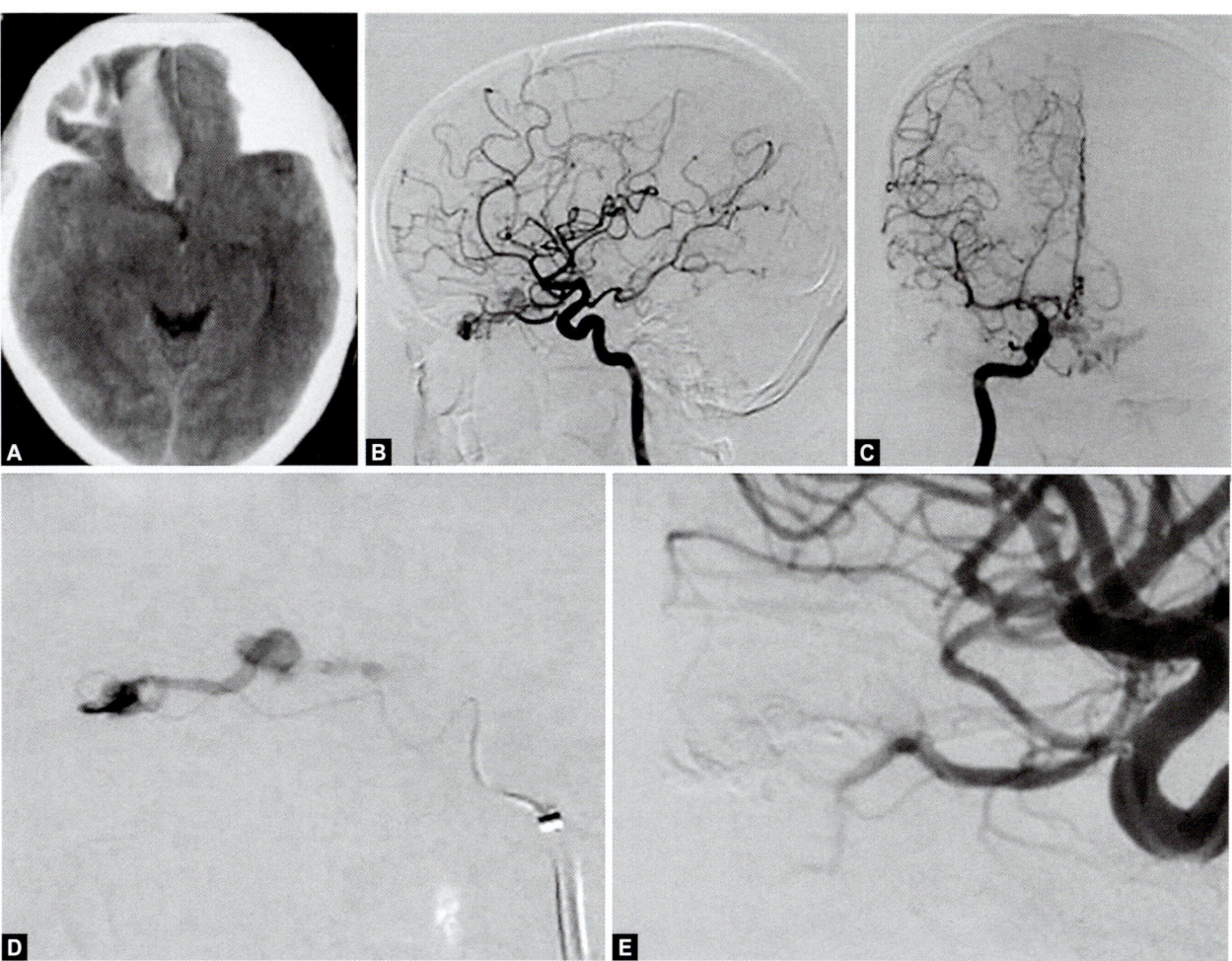

FIGS. 5A TO E: Noncontrast computed tomography (NCCT) (A) reveals gyrus rectus and right orbitofrontal hematoma; (B and C) frontal and lateral projections of right ICA injection reveal Cognard type 4 DAVF at the anterior cranial fossa base with feeders from the anterior ethmoidal branches of the right ophthalmic artery and extensive cortical venous reflux; (D) Microcatheter run of trans arterial access via ophthalmic artery showing catheter close to fistula point; (E) Postembolization reveals complete exclusion of fistula.
(DAVF: dural arteriovenous fistula; ICA: internal carotid artery)

the sinus needs to be preserved to prevent sinus thrombosis, venous hypertension (due to occlusion), and hemorrhage **(Figs. 6A to D)**.

Use of balloons (~8–10 mm diameter) is recommended to temporarily occlude the sinus (8–10 minutes) via transvenous route to maintain the patency of the dural sinus, preserving the antegrade venous outflow in the sinuses. Apart from preserving the sinus, in case of complex fistulae, balloon inflation helps in forming a tunnel along the sinus wall allowing controlled reflux into multiple adjacent arterial feeders, thereby resulting into complete obliteration of fistula.[14] Additionally, use of balloon helps in decreasing the quantity of liquid embolic agent used to obliterate the fistula.

Complications of transarterial route include occlusion of the artery, vessel perforation and hemorrhage, venous thrombosis, cranial nerve palsies, and microcatheter related (perforation or stuck within the artery).

In depth review of angiographic anatomy prior to procedure, sound knowledge of cranial nerve blood supply and dangerous ECA–ICA anastomosis (predominantly along orbit, petrocavernous, and upper cervical) may help in mitigating the above said complications.

Transvenous Approach

This approach is predominantly used for ventral DAVFs (along ACF base, cavernous sinus, petrous, condylar, and foramen magnum), which helps in reducing the risk of inadvertent embolization occurring via transarterial route or difficult transarterial access. Majority of the times, ACF-DAVFs are also treated through the transarterial route.

Main goal is to retrogradely occlude the proximal aspect of the draining vein and allowing the liquid agent to retrogradely percolate and penetrate into the feeding arteries. 80–90% angiographic cure rate can be seen in transvenous access. Access routes can be via inferior petrosal sinus, facial

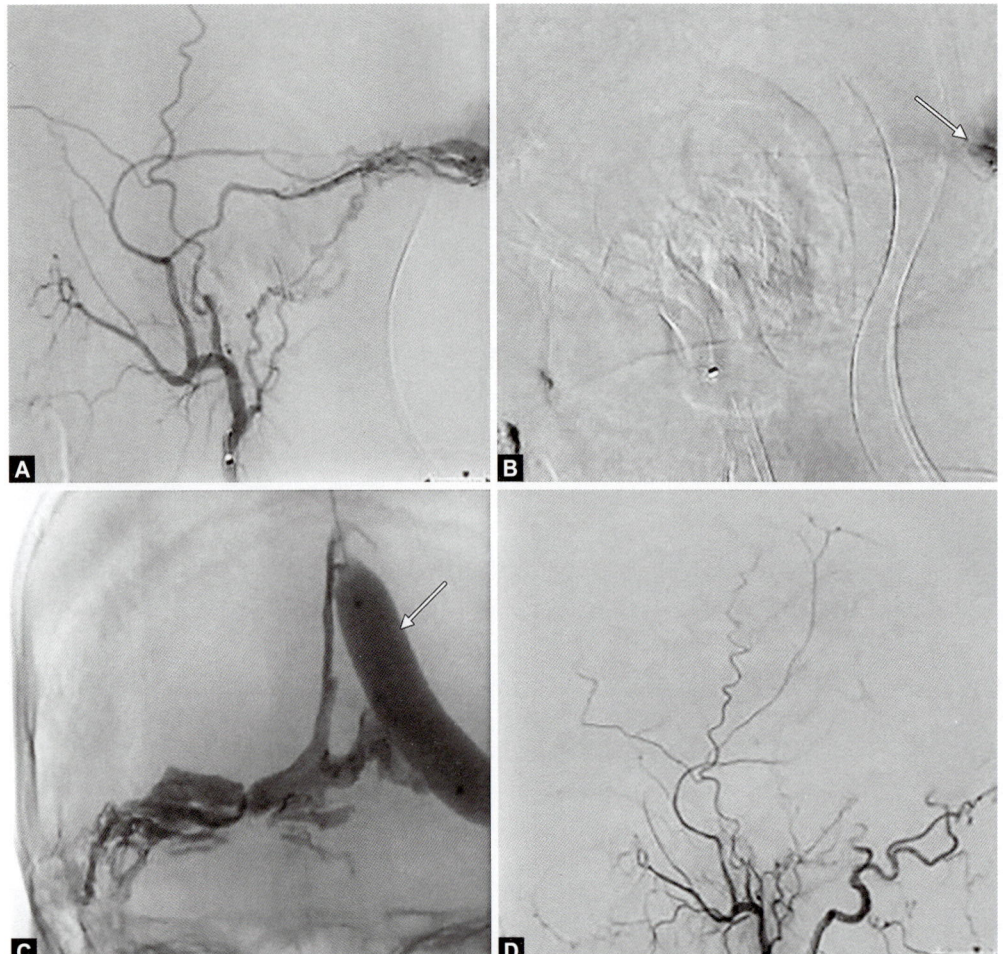

FIGS. 6A TO D: Transarterial embolization with balloon sinus protection of right transverse-sigmoid DAVF. (A) Right ECA injection lateral view showing arterial feeders from petrosquamosal branch of MMA; (B) Selective microcatheter injection close to the fistula point; (C) AP view of skull X-ray showing glue cast along the draining venous channel and balloon inflated along left side venous sinuses; (D) Postembolization right ECA lateral view showing complete obliteration of the fistula.
(AP: anteroposterior; ECA: external carotid artery; DAVF: dural arteriovenous fistula; MMA: middle meningeal artery)

vein, or even SOV or other venous channels depending on the site of the fistulae.

Materials and techniques of transvenous approach:
- Coil occlusion
- EVOH (with or without coil) occlusion
- Reverse pressure cooker (RPC) technique
- Reverse dual-lumen balloon microcatheter

Coil Occlusion

It is used for indirect carotico-cavernous fistulas (CCFs) and transverse-sigmoid sinus DAVFs. Coil mass is placed within the sinus, which eventually forms sinus thrombosis and occlusion. With the promising results of transarterial embolization, coil embolization of the transverse-sigmoid dural AVF has become obsolete except in residual/recurrent cases.

EVOH Occlusion

It is used for indirect CCFs, condylar DAVFs, or transverse sigmoid DAVFs with isolated sinus and help to occlude the fistula in a retrograde and controlled manner.

Reverse Pressure Cooker Technique

It is similar to transarterial pressure cooker technique where the two microcatheters are placed in the draining vein, which is occluded and forces the embolic agent to occlude the fistula point retrogradely.

Reverse Dual-lumen Balloon Microcatheter

It is similar to arterial dual lumen balloon microcatheter technique with balloon inflated within the draining vein via transvenous access. However, inadequate seal is often noted to achieve controlled retrograde embolization.[15]

Complications of transvenous approach are usually due to cortical vein rupture or occlusion, venous rerouting, venous congestion, and secondary hemorrhage. Detailed preprocedure assessment of venous drainage pathways is important. Cavernous sinus DAVFs especially may pose a risk of SOV thrombosis and proptosis postembolization, due to intraluminal stasis secondary to shunt obliteration. Postprocedure anticoagulation and corticosteroids may help reduce the symptoms.

Combined Transarterial and Transvenous Approach

Complex cases, especially fistulae along the falx/tentorium cerebelli, may require combination of transarterial and transvenous approaches to achieve desired angiographic cure rate.

Surgery

It is particularly opted for ACF-based DAVFs with feeders from ophthalmic artery and petrous AVFs involving the facial nerve arterial arcade. Main goal is to disconnect the draining vein via ligation or aneurysmal clip placement. In some cases, it may at least convert high-risk AVF into low-risk AVF by downgrading the fistula and reducing the cortical venous reflux.[16]

Gamma Knife Radiosurgery

Gamma knife radiosurgery (GKRS) is an alternative option to endovascular and surgical disconnection, especially in low-risk fistulas. Approximate dose is 20–30 Gy. The mechanism includes thrombosis of vessel and closure of fistula. It is not indicated in high-risk DAVFs because of long latency period and persisting risk of hemorrhage during the latent period, which may range from months to years.[17]

When used alone, it has incomplete cure rates with only up to 50% angiographic cure in long-term follow ups, further requiring additional modality for complete cure. However, it may be used in complex or recurrent fistulas to reduce the symptom severity (pulsatile tinnitus in transverse sinus fistulas).[18]

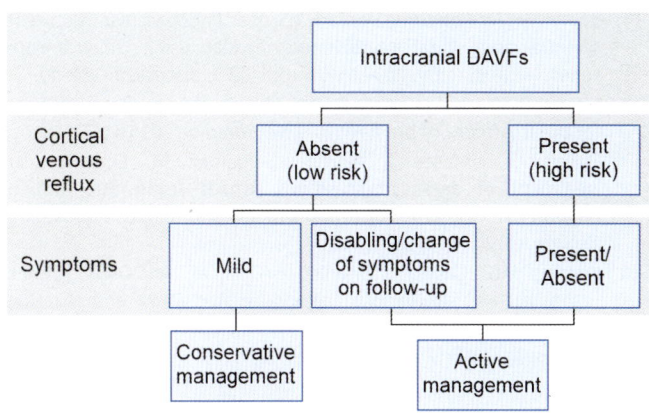

FLOWCHART 1: Treatment evaluation.
(DAVF: dural arteriovenous fistula)

TREATMENT EVALUATION

Flowchart 1 depicts the treatment evaluation.

CONCLUSION

Intracranial dural arteriovenous fistulas are the complex vascular malformations, resulting in features of venous hypertension and hemorrhage. They are associated with venous thrombosis and acquired in majority of cases and potentially treatable. Assessing the pattern of venous drainage is crucial for the type of clinical presentation and plan of management. Mainstay of the management is endovascular embolization completely obliterating the site of fistula. High index of suspicion with timely imaging and intervention can help in mitigating the symptoms.

REFERENCES

1. Bhatia KD, Lee H, Kortman H, et al. Endovascular Management of Intracranial Dural AVFs: Principles. AJNR. 2022;43(2):160-6.
2. Gandhi D, Chen J, Pearl M, et al. Intracranial dural arteriovenous fistulas: classification, imaging findings, and treatment. AJNR Am J Neuroradiol. 2012;33(6):1007-13.
3. Tanaka M. Embryological Consideration of Dural AVFs in Relation to the Neural Crest and the Mesoderm. Neurointervention. 2019;14(1):9-16.
4. Geibprasert S, Pereira V, Krings T, et al. Dural arteriovenous shunts: a new classification of craniospinal epidural venous anatomical bases and clinical correlations. Stroke. 2008;39(10):2783-94.
5. Elhammady MS, Ambekar S, Heros RC. Epidemiology, clinical presentation, diagnostic evaluation, prognosis of cerebral dural arteriovenous fistulas. Handb Clin Neurol. 2017;143:99-105.
6. Brouwer PA, Bosman T, van Walderveen MA, et al. Dynamic 320-section CT angiography in cranial arteriovenous shunting lesions. AJNR Am J Neuroradiol. 2010;31:767-70.
7. Brito A, Tsang AC, Hilditch C, et al. Intracranial dural arteriovenous fistula as a reversible cause of dementia: case series and literature review. World Neurosurg. 2019;121:e543-53.
8. Alatakis S, Koulouris G, Stuckey S. CT-demonstrated transcalvarial channels diagnostic of dural arteriovenous fistula. AJNR Am J Neuroradiol. 2005;26:2393-6.
9. Barrow DL, Spector RH, Braun IF, et al. Classification and treatment of spontaneous carotid cavernous sinus fistulas. J Neurosurg. 1985;62:248-56.
10. Bhatia KD, Lee H, Kortman H, et al. Endovascular Management of Intracranial Dural Arteriovenous Fistulas: Transarterial Approach. AJNR Am J Neuroradiol. 2022;43(3):324-331.

11. Stiefel MF, Albuquerque FC, Park MS, et al. Endovascular treatment of intracranial dural arteriovenous fistulae using Onyx: a case series. Neurosurgery. 2009;65(6 Suppl);32-9; discussion 139-40.
12. Chapot R, Stracke P, Velasco A, et al. The pressure cooker technique for the treatment of brain AVMs. J Neuroradiol. 2014;41:87-91.
13. Dabus G, Linfante I, Martínez-Galdámez M. Endovascular treatment of dural arteriovenous fistulas using dual lumen balloon microcatheter: technical aspects and results. Clin Neurol Neurosurg. 2014;117:22-7.
14. Kerolus MG, Chung J, Munich SA, et al. An Onyx tunnel: reconstructive transvenous balloon-assisted Onyx embolization for dural arteriovenous fistula of the transverse-sigmoid sinus. J Neurosurg. 2018;129:922-7.
15. Bhatia KD, Lee H, Kortman H, et al. Endovascular Management of Intracranial Dural AVFs: Transvenous Approach. AJNR Am J Neuroradiol. 2022;43(4): 510-6.
16. Jandial R, McCormick P, Black P (Eds). Core Techniques in Operative Neurosurgery. Elsevier Health Sciences; 2019.
17. Guo WY, Pan DH, Wu HM, et al. Radiosurgery as a treatment alternative for dural arteriovenous fistulas of the cavernous sinus. AJNR Am J Neuroradiol. 1998;19:1081-7.
18. Dmytriw AA, Schwartz ML, Cusimano MD, et al. Gamma knife radiosurgery for the treatment of intracranial dural arteriovenous fistulas. Interv Neuroradiol. 2017;23:211-20.

CHAPTER 9

Headache in Stroke and Transient Ischemic Attacks

Surendra Kumar, Amit Kumar, Kameshwar Prasad

ABSTRACT

Headache is a common symptom of stroke and transient ischemic attacks (TIAs). Its incidence and prevalence vary depending on the type of stroke. In subarachnoid hemorrhage (SAH), its prevalence is nearly 100%, except in patients who lose consciousness at the onset. Typical features of headache in SAH are sudden onset, and unusually severe. Sudden, severe headache of intensity never experienced before in life should warrant a computed tomography (CT) head to rule out SAH, even though there are other causes mimicking SAH. Prevalence of headache in intracerebral hemorrhage (ICH) is approximately 50%, depending on the size and location of ICH. Prevalence of headache in TIA (~25%) is higher than in ischemic stroke (~20%). In venous stroke, the prevalence of headache is variable and the characteristics of headache associated with venous stroke may mimic SAH, and may sometimes be the only symptom even in the absence of raised intracranial pressure. The characteristics of headache may help in raising clinical suspicion of the type of stroke.

Keywords: Headache, Stroke, Headache attributed to stroke, Headache in ICH, Headache in subarachnoid hemorrhage.

INTRODUCTION

Headache is something we all like to avoid, but there is one situation in which headache can be lifesaving, and doctors as well as patients feel grateful to this headache. We start this chapter from this situation. Such a headache due to the so-called "warning leak" may precede headache due to a major catastrophic subarachnoid hemorrhage (SAH), and proper identification of "warning leak" as a harbinger of major SAH may help avoid loss of life or limb due to the hemorrhage from a ruptured aneurysm.

The prevalence of headache in acute cerebrovascular events is highest in SAH, followed by cortical venous sinus thromboses (50–68%), intracranial hemorrhage (21–100%), transient ischemic attack (TIA) (16–44%), and ischemic stroke (16–38%).[1] The prevalence of headaches in different types of acute stroke is shown in **Table 1**.

HEADACHE IN SUBARACHNOID HEMORRHAGE

Sentinel headaches due to "warning leaks" of saccular intracranial aneurysm is unusually severe and lasts several hours. The International Classification of Headache Disorders, 3rd edition (ICHD-3) diagnostic criteria[2] for headache attributed to SAH are given in **Box 1**. Any headache that is sudden, severe, and unusual should be referred to a hospital and evaluated with computed tomography (CT) scan of head. This may avoid the patient developing "rebleed" or another secondary complication due to SAH. Headache is the primary clinical manifestation of SAH. It is the only symptom in approximately one-third of patients, but occurs in 85–100% of patients at some point **(Table 1)**.[3] Only patients who become suddenly unconscious or develop SAH during sleep may not have headache as the

TABLE 1: Prevalence of headaches in different types of strokes in acute phase.

Study	Year	TIA (%)	Ischemic stroke (%)	ICH (%)	SAH (%)
Andre C[31]	1996	24			
Arboix A[33]	1993	26	32		100
Ferro et al.[14]	1995a	29	34		
Grindal AB[34]	1974	25			
Koudstall PJ[20]	1991	18			
Tentchert S[18]	2005	27			
Gorelick PB[35]	1986		17	55	100
Kumral E[36]	1995		16	36	
Mitsias PD[37]	2006		31		
Vestergaard K[21]	1993		26		
Oliveira FAA[27]	2023		25		
Shigematsu K[38]	2013		12		94
Pollak L[39]	2017		8	21	
Leira R[40]	2005			34	
Vestergaard K[21]	1993			50	
Shigematsu K[38]	2013			30	

(ICH: intracerebral hemorrhage; SAH: subarachnoid hemorrhage; TIA: transient ischemic attack)

BOX 1: Diagnostic criteria for headache attributed to subarachnoid hemorrhage as per ICHD-3.

A. Any new headache fulfilling criteria C and D
B. Subarachnoid hemorrhage (SAH) in the absence of head trauma has been diagnosed
C. Evidence of causation demonstrated by at least two of the following:
   1. Headache has developed in close temporal relation to other symptoms and/or clinical signs of SAH, or has led to the diagnosis of SAH
   2. Headache has significantly improved in parallel with stabilization or improvement of other symptoms or clinical or radiological signs of SAH
   3. Headache has sudden or thunderclap onset
D. Either of the following:
   1. Headache resolves within 3 months
   2. Headache has not yet resolved but 3 months have not yet passed
E. Not better accounted for by another ICHD-3 diagnosis

(ICHD-3: International Classification of Headache Disorders, 3rd edition)

---

first symptom. In a consecutive series of 92 patients with SAH caused by a ruptured aneurysm in whom the onset of headache was recorded, 62 patients (67%) had headache as the initial symptom, whereas the remaining patients had lost consciousness immediately.[4] The headache appears abruptly and reaches its peak within seconds. A total of 54 (87%) of the 62 patients listed earlier with headache as the primary symptom experienced an abrupt onset of headache. In the remaining eight patients, the discomfort developed over minutes rather than within seconds. Patients with nonaneurysmal perimesencephalic SAH are more likely to experience headaches of progressive onset than patients with aneurysmal SAH.[5] Patients with vertebral artery dissection may experience a biphasic headache; first, a severe occipital headache radiating from the neck, followed by a less severe holocranial headache exacerbation a few hours or a day later.

In SAH, the headache is typically diffuse and inadequately localized, spreading over time to the head, neck, and back. Occasionally, the headache is most severe beneath the eyes. Patients frequently characterize the headache as the most severe headache of their lifetime, but a few cases may have mild headache. It is the suddenness of onset which is most important for diagnosis.

Typically, the headache lasts 1–2 weeks, but can last longer. If there has been a minor blood leak, the headache may last only a few hours or even lesser, and there may be no other symptoms, such as neck stiffness. Nonetheless, it is possible for this to occur; therefore, it is prudent to think SAH in somebody with sudden, severe headache with or without change in sensorium, even if it resolves within minutes. A study showed that a persistent headache is a long-term complication of an SAH, which may persist for years with gradual improvement with time.[6]

In clinical practice, some patients had a history of severe headache with a sudden onset few weeks (or more) ago, which looks familiar to SAH, but resolved within a short period of few hours or days.

INTRACEREBRAL HEMORRHAGE

Headache is reported by 21–100% of intracerebral hemorrhage (ICH) patients at presentation.[1] The frequency of headaches differs greatly based on the location and the size of the hemorrhage. The headache associated with ICH is typically unilateral, focal, and mild to severe in intensity. The ICHD-3 diagnostic criteria for headache[2] attributed to ICH are given in **Box 2**. In case of a small-sized bleed, the probability of headache is lower than in moderate or large-sized bleed. In putaminal and thalamic hemorrhages, the presumably intraventricular and subarachnoid extension of the hematoma causes the typically severe headache. Frequently, the headache is bilateral and excruciating, similar to a ruptured saccular aneurysm.

In cerebellar hemorrhage, the headache is frequently acute, severe, and maximal at onset, mimicking an SAH. Headache is reported in 13% of patients with putaminal hemorrhage, 46–68% with lobar hemorrhage, 30% with thalamic hemorrhage, 35% with pontine hemorrhage, and 48–80% with cerebellar hemorrhage.[1] A study observed that presence of headache at acute phase was significantly associated with mortality at 30 days in ICH patients.[7]

ISCHEMIC STROKE

Ischemic stroke results from occlusion of an artery supplying blood to the brain. The area of brain fed by the artery suffers from lack of blood supply. To compensate for the lack, collateral arteries open up in an attempt to bring blood to the area. These collaterals may dilate to an extent that pain-sensitive structures in the wall of the arteries may get stimulated to cause headaches. Some collaterals open up immediately after the occlusion, possibly even before stroke symptoms appear, while others may take some time. Accordingly, the headache may start at the onset or even before the commencement of symptoms of ischemic stroke or after few hours and days. The collaterals may resume their previous state if the cause of occlusion resolves, while they may persist in dilated state if the occlusion persists. Accordingly, the headache may last only few hours to days, or become persistent. The ICHD-3 diagnostic criteria for headache attributed to ischemic stroke[2] are given in **Box 3**.

PREVALENCE, TIME OF ONSET, AND DURATION OF HEADACHE IN RELATION TO STROKE SYMPTOM ONSET

As explained in the earlier paragraph, headache may be acute or persistent in case of ischemic stroke. A meta-analysis involving 20 studies showed that the pooled prevalence of headache after ischemic stroke was 22% [95% confidence interval (CI) 17–27%].[8]

BOX 2: Diagnostic criteria for headaches attributed to intracerebral hemorrhage.

A. Any new acute headache fulfilling criterion C and D
B. Intracerebral hemorrhage (ICH) in the absence of head trauma has been diagnosed
C. Evidence of causation demonstrated by at least two of the following:
  1. Headache develops simultaneously with or in very close temporal relation to intracerebral hemorrhage
  2. Headache has developed in close temporal relation to other symptoms and/or clinical signs of ICH, or has led to the diagnosis of ICH
  3. Headache has significantly improved in parallel with stabilization or improvement of other symptoms or clinical or radiological signs of ICH
  4. Headache has at least one of the following three characteristics:
    i. Sudden or thunderclap onset
    ii. Maximal on the day of its onset
    iii. Localized in accordance to the site of the hemorrhage
D. Either of the following:
  1. Headache has resolved within 3 months
  2. Headache has not yet resolved but 3 months have not yet passed
E. Not better accounted for by another ICHD-3 diagnosis

(ICHD-3: International Classification of Headache Disorders, 3rd edition)

BOX 3: Diagnostic criteria for headache attributed to ischemic stroke.

A. Any new headache fulfilling criteria C and D
B. Acute ischemic stroke has been diagnosed
C. Evidence of causation demonstrated by either or both of the following:
  1. Headache has developed in very close temporal relation to other symptoms and/or clinical signs of ischemic stroke, or has led to the diagnosis of ischemic stroke
  2. Headache has significantly improved in parallel with stabilization or improvement of other symptoms or clinical or radiological signs of ischemic stroke
D. Either of the following:
  1. Headache has resolved within 3 months
  2. Headache has not yet resolved but 3 months have not yet passed
E. Not better accounted for by another ICHD-3 diagnosis

(ICHD-3: International Classification of Headache Disorders, 3rd edition)

A study observed that in patients who had headache in association with ischemic stroke, the headache occurred in 86% of subjects on the day of stroke symptoms, while the rest experienced headaches between 2 and 5 days later.[9] Another study conducted in patients with lacunar infarct observed that 93% of the participants reported headache at the time of onset, while 7% reported headache prior to stroke.[10] Another study reported 31% of the subjects had headache before, 11% during and 45% after the commencement of stroke symptoms (1% within seconds, 10% within minutes, and 34% within hours). In the rest 13% of patients, the timing of onset was not clear.[11] These findings suggest that a majority of patients experience headache at the time of onset of symptoms. Poststroke headache timing varied from 1 to 4 days.[9-11] Approximately 1–23% of stroke survivors experience headaches lasting longer than 3 months.[12,13] A cohort study with 3 years follow-up in 222 subjects observed that a total of 12% subjects reported persistent headache; of these, 81.2% had on an average of 2–14 days headache per month and 18.8% reported daily headache.[13] A study conducted in 182 ischemic stroke patients demonstrated vertebrobasilar stroke [odds ratio (OR) 6.9], and past history of migraine (OR 6.7) were significant predictors for headache.[14]

HEADACHE CHARACTERISTICS

In approximately 50–80% of patients, tension-type headaches were reported.[15] A cohort study reported bilateral and pressure-like headache in 80% of subjects, while 16% had throbbing and 10% had stabbing pain.[16] This study reported 30% photophobia, 24% phonophobia, and 28% nausea or vomiting. Another cohort study reported tension-type headache in 50% subjects and migraine-like headache in 31.3% subjects.[13] Sentinel headache occurs in approximately 10–43% in patients with ischemic stroke, and is more common in cardioembolic stroke (22%) as compared to TIAs and other types of ischemic stroke.[17] Sentinel headache is unilateral, of sudden onset, and usually leads to neurological deficit within 24–72 hours. In case of ischemic stroke, it is unilateral, focal, and mild to moderate.

INFLUENCE OF AGE AND GENDER

Gender and young age have been shown to be associated with occurrence of headache in stroke. A study showed that females are more likely to have headache at the onset of stroke than males in ischemic stroke.[18] A meta-analysis of 11 studies involving 23,614 patients showed that females have greater odds (OR 1.25) of occurrence of headache than males with ischemic stroke.[8] Another study indicated that the frequency of headache was 1.3 times higher in females than in males.[18]

INFLUENCE OF STROKE LOCATION AND ETIOLOGY OF HEADACHE ASSOCIATED WITH ISCHEMIC STROKE

The headaches, if localized, are often related to the location of the brain/eye lesion. They are more prevalent in vertebrobasilar distribution than carotid distribution and less prevalent in lacunar stroke.[19-21] A meta-analysis of seven studies estimated that there is 1.92 higher odds of headache associated with posterior circulation stroke than anterior circular stroke.[8] Severe unilateral pain in the head, face, neck, or eye that occurs at the time or before the onset of a stroke should raise a strong suspicion of carotid dissection. Patients with cerebral autosomal dominant arteriopathy with subcortical infarcts and leukoencephalopathy (CADASIL) commonly suffer from migraine. Although intracranial venous thrombosis typically presents as an isolated intracranial hypertension syndrome or a subacute loss of consciousness, a focal onset can be seen, and headaches may be the presenting feature.[22] Vasculitis is considered when stroke or TIA occurs in a patient who had refractory headaches of acute to subacute onset.

Headache is more frequently observed in larger ischemic lesions (OR 2.62) in ischemic stroke of vertebrobasilar system.[23] Patients with ischemic stroke exhibited a higher incidence of headaches with cortical involvement than with subcortical involvement.[23] Headache are more prevalent in the deep gray matter or brainstem than supratentorial white matter in patients with lacunar infarction.[10] The trigeminovascular system innervates the vertebrobasilar system more densely than it innervates the carotid system, which may contribute to this difference in frequency.[10]

There are several hypotheses regarding the cause of headaches in stroke patients, but the precise etiology remains unknown. Most studies corroborate that headaches are more frequently associated with posterior cerebral circulation strokes. One possible explanation is the presence of densely innervated pain-sensitive vessels at the base of the brain,[21] which turn on the nociceptive trigeminovascular pathway. Headache in vertebrobasilar stroke is commonly migraine-like, implying that migraine and stroke have a common pathogenic neural mechanism as their underlying etiology.

Alternately, the pain may be caused by vasodilation of arteries as a result of emboli/thrombus formation at the base of the brain or occlusion of several arterial branches, resulting in alterations in vascular perfusion. This mechanism could explain migraines associated with embolic or thrombotic strokes, but does not apply in case of TIA. Ischemic stroke in acute phase might cause headache due to the production of prothrombotic, inflammatory, and excitotoxic chemicals. A study showed that as cerebral ischemic event activates platelets, which cause release of vasoactive substances such as serotonin and prostaglandin leading to headache.[24]

In elderly individuals, new-onset headache along with other neuropsychiatric symptoms such as seizures, psychoses, hyponatremia, and faciobrachial dystonia may mimic stroke, but with proper clinical suspicion, they are clearly diagnosed as autoimmune encephalitis.[25] In young individuals, headache and recurrent stroke may be the presenting features of mitochondrial encephalomyopathy, lactic acidosis, and stroke-like episodes (MELAS) if there are other associated features like hemianopia, cortical blindness, hemiparesis, and sensorineural hearing loss in presence of mitochondrial genetic abnormality. Headache is commonly present in MELAS as repeated episodes mimicking migraine or may be the presenting symptom of stroke-like episodes.

ASSOCIATION WITH OUTCOME IN PATIENTS WITH ISCHEMIC STROKE

In a retrospective cohort study involving 11,523 Taiwanese people who have previously experienced an ischemic stroke, headache was associated with a more favorable outcome.[26] The study observed that patients with headache were less likely to deteriorate in the hospital [risk ratio (RR) 0.62; 95% CI 0.52–0.79] and associated with better National Institutes of Health Stroke Scale (NIHSS) (0.08 vs. 0.2, $p = 0.02$).[26] The prognosis measured by favorable outcome modified Rankin Scale (mRS) 0–2 was observed to be higher in patients having headache following ischemic stroke at 1 month (RR 0.85; 95% CI 0.72–0.95). There was also a trend of better functional outcome in 3–6 months follow-up.[26] Another study also found that patients with headaches during ischemic stroke or TIA had a better prognosis.[27] A prospective cohort of 2,473 patients with cerebral ischemic of noncardioembolic origin with median follow-up 14.1 years found a reduced risk of vascular death in patients who had concomitant headache than no headache [adjusted hazard ratio (HR) 0.73, 95% CI 0.68–0.91].[28] A second cohort of 1,185 stroke patients found no correlation between ischemic stroke symptoms including headache and a 30-day mortality (RR 1.01; 95% CI 0.53–1.92).[29] The occurrence of headache was found to be strongly linked with an early deterioration in neurologic function in a cohort of 241 stroke patients in Spain who were prospectively evaluated with the Canadian Stroke Scale during the first 48 hours after hospital admission (OR 16.01; 95% CI 5.40–47.48).[30] More well-designed studies are needed to confirm the association of headache in prognosis of ischemic stroke.

TRANSIENT ISCHEMIC ATTACK

Approximately 24% of patients experience headaches at the onset of TIA. Headache is more frequently associated with TIAs than ischemic stroke with incidence rates of 25–44%.[22] The prevalence of headaches is higher in TIAs that occur in the basilar territory compared to those in the carotid territory. The ICHD-3 diagnostic criteria for headache attributed to TIA[2] are given in **Box 4**. It is difficult to distinguish between TIA with headache and an attack of migraine with aura. The mode of onset is important; the focal deficit is commonly sudden in TIA, while it is more frequently progressive in migraine with aura. A study conducted in 49 patients with single or multiple TIAs observed that the patients with multiple TIAs had stereotyped headaches.[31]

VENOUS STROKE

No specific headache characteristics associated with cerebral venous thrombosis (CVT) have been identified. However, it is typically diffuse, progressive, and severe and accompanied by other signs of intracranial hypertension. **Box 5** provides ICHD-3 diagnostic criteria[2] for headaches attributable to venous thrombosis. The prevalence of headache in CVT is approximately 80%. It may have a sudden onset and be unilateral, but it can be extremely misleading, mimicking any of the following: (1) Migraine without aura, (2) migraine with aura, (3) cluster headache,

---

BOX 4: Diagnostic criteria for headache attributed to TIA.

A. Any new headache fulfilling criterion C
B. A transient ischemic attack (TIA) has been diagnosed
C. Evidence of causation demonstrated by both of the following:
 1. Headache has developed simultaneously with other symptoms and/or clinical signs of TIA
 2. Headache resolves within 24 hours
D. Not better accounted for by another ICHD-3 diagnosis

(ICHD-3: International Classification of Headache Disorders, 3rd edition)

BOX 5: Diagnostic criteria for headache attributed to venous stroke.

A. Any new headache fulfilling criterion C
B. Cerebral venous thrombosis (CVT) has been diagnosed
C. Evidence of causation demonstrated by both of the following:
 1. Headache has developed in close temporal relation to other symptoms and/or clinical signs of CVT, or has led to the discovery of CVT
 2. Either or both of the following:
   a. Headache has significantly worsened in parallel with clinical or radiological signs of extension of the CVT
   b. Headache has significantly improved or resolved after improvement of the CVT
D. Not better accounted for by another ICHD-3 diagnosis

(ICHD-3: International Classification of Headache Disorders, 3rd edition)

(4) thunderclap headache, and (5) headache associated with low cerebrospinal fluid pressure. Occasionally, headache is the only symptom of CVT, but in approximately 90% of patients, the headache is accompanied by focal signs (neurological deficits or seizures) and/or may indicate intracranial hypertension, subacute encephalopathy, or cavernous sinus syndrome. Neuroimaging [magnetic resonance imaging (MRI) with T2-weighted images plus magnetic resonance venography (MRV) or CT scan plus CT venography and digital subtraction angiography should be used for diagnosis. Treatment should be started as soon as it is possible and should consist of treating symptoms, taking heparin, then using oral anticoagulation for atleast 6 months and in selected cases even for lifetime, and treating the underlying cause when it is required. A retrospective single center study that recruited 49 patients with CVT observed that the most common symptoms were acute unilateral headaches of high intensity, whereas patients without headaches had more severe symptoms.[32] To standardize the criteria for diagnosis and treatment of this disease, large, well-designed cohort studies are required.

CONCLUSION

Headache may be the presenting feature of stroke or TIA. Its prevalence is variable depending on the type of stroke, but also according to study design (prospective versus retrospective), inclusion criteria, methodology, and intensity of questioning in various studies. As a rough approximation, prevalence of headache in stroke or TIA is 100% in SAH, 75% in CVT, 50% in ICH, 25% in TIA, and 20% in ischemic stroke. Headache may be the sole symptom in SAH and CVT. The characteristic of headache in many cases may point to the diagnosis of stroke type. Sudden severe headache of intensity never experienced before in life warrants exclusion of SAH. New-onset headache in association with neck pain and stroke should raise suspicion of arterial dissection as the cause of stroke. In ischemic stroke, patients with headache at onset have better prognosis than those without headache. More well-planned prospective studies are required to characterize headache in various stroke types and TIA, also to establish the etiologic, diagnostic, and prognostic value of the headache and its treatment.

REFERENCES

1. Carolei A, Sacco S. Headache attributed to stroke, TIA, intracerebral haemorrhage, or vascular malformation. Handb Clin Neurol. 2010;97:51728.
2. Headache Classification Committee of the International Headache Society (IHS). The International Classification of Headache Disorders, 3rd edition. Cephalalgia. 2018;38:1-211.
3. Davenport R. Acute Headache in the Emergency Department. J Neurol Neurosurg Psychiatry. 2002;72:ii33-7.
4. van Gijn J, van Dongen KJ, Vermeulen M, et al. Perimesencephalic hemorrhage: A nonaneurysmal and benign form of subarachnoid hemorrhage. Neurology. 1985;35:493-7.
5. Rinkel GJ, Wijdicks EF, Vermeulen M, et al. The clinical course of perimesencephalic nonaneurysmal subarachnoid hemorrhage. Ann Neurol. 1991;29:463-8.
6. Gaastra B, Carmichael H, Galea I, et al. Duration and characteristics of persistent headache following aneurysmal subarachnoid hemorrhage. Headache. 2022;62:1376-82.
7. Puthik M, Tuan LV. Headache in acute phase of intracerebral hemorrhage. Joint Event on International Conference on Neuroimmunology, Neurological disorders, and Neurogenetics & 28th World Summit on Neurology, Neuroscience and Neuropharmacology. J Neurol Neurophysiol. 2018.
8. Harriott AM, Karakaya F, Ayata C. Headache after ischemic stroke. Neurology. 2020;94:e75-86.
9. Verdelho A, Ferro JM, Melo T, et al. Headache in acute stroke. A prospective study in the first 8 days. Cephalalgia. 2008;28:346-54.
10. Arboix A, García-Trallero O, García-Eroles L, et al. Stroke-related headache: A clinical study in lacunar infarction. Headache. 2005;45:1345-52.
11. van Os HJA, Mulder IA, van der Schaaf IC, et al. Role of atherosclerosis, clot extent, and penumbra volume in headache during ischemic stroke. Neurology. 2016;87:112430.
12. Paolucci S, Iosa M, Toni D, et al. Prevalence and Time Course of Post-Stroke Pain: A Multicenter Prospective Hospital-Based Study. Pain Med. 2016;17:924-30.
13. Hansen AP, Marcussen NS, Klit H, et al. Development of persistent headache following stroke: A 3-year follow-up. Cephalalgia. 2015;35:399-409.
14. Ferro JM, Melo TP, Oliveira V, et al. A multivariate study of headache associated with ischemic stroke. Headache. 1995;35:315-9.
15. Widar M, Ek AC, Ahlström G. Coping with long-term pain after a stroke. J Pain Symptom Manage. 2004;27:215-25.
16. Seifert CL, Schönbach EM, Magon S, et al. Headache in acute ischaemic stroke: A lesion mapping study. Brain. 2016;139:217-26.
17. Diener HC, Katsarava Z, Weimar C. Headache associated with ischemic cerebrovascular disease. Rev Neurol (Paris). 2008;164: 819-24.
18. Tentschert S, Wimmer R, Greisenegger S, et al. Headache at stroke onset in 2,196 patients with ischemic stroke or transient ischemic attack. Stroke. 2005;36:e1-3.
19. Nichols FT, Mawad M, Mohr JP, et al. Focal headache during balloon inflation in the internal carotid and middle cerebral arteries. Stroke. 1990;21:555-9.
20. Koudstaal PJ, van Gijn J, Kappelle LJ. Headache in transient or permanent cerebral ischemia. Dutch TIA Study Group. Stroke. 1991;22:754-9.
21. Vestergaard K, Andersen G, Nielsen MI, et al. Headache in stroke. Stroke. 1993;24:1621-4.
22. Edmeads J. Headache in cerebrovascular disease. A common symptom of stroke. Postgrad Med. 1987;81:191-3, 196-8.
23. Kropp P, Holzhausen M, Kolodny E, et al. Headache as a symptom at stroke onset in 4,431 young ischaemic stroke patients. Results from the "Stroke in Young Fabry Patients (SIFAP1) study." J Neural Transm (Vienna). 2013;120:1433-40.

24. Castillo J, Martínez F, Corredera E, et al. Amino acid transmitters in patients with headache during the acute phase of cerebrovascular ischemic disease. Stroke. 1995;26:2035-9.
25. Schankin CJ, Kästele F, Gerdes LA, et al. New-Onset Headache in Patients With Autoimmune Encephalitis Is Associated With anti-NMDA-Receptor Antibodies. Headache. 2016;56:995-1003.
26. Chen P-K, Chiu PY, Tsai IJ, et al. Onset headache predicts good outcome in patients with first-ever ischemic stroke. Stroke. 2013;44:1852-8.
27. Oliveira FAA, Rocha-Filho PAS. Headaches Attributed to Ischemic Stroke and Transient Ischemic Attack. Headache. 2019;59:469-76.
28. Maino A, Algra A, Koudstaal PJ, et al. Concomitant Headache Influences Long-term Prognosis After Acute Cerebral Ischemia of Noncardioembolic Origin. Stroke. 2013;44:2446-50.
29. Abadie V, Jacquin A, Daubail B, et al. Prevalence and prognostic value of headache on early mortality in acute stroke: The Dijon Stroke Registry. Cephalalgia. 2014;34:887-94.
30. Leira R, Dávalos A, Aneiros A, et al. Headache as a surrogate marker of the molecular mechanisms implicated in progressing stroke. Cephalalgia. 2002;22:303-8.
31. André C, Neves FF, Vincent MB. Headache in transient ischaemic attacks. Funct Neurol. 1996;11:195-200.
32. Petrović J, Švabić T, Zidverc-Trajković J, et al. Cerebral venous thrombosis: A retrospective unicentric analysis of clinical and neuroimaging characteristics. Neurol Sci. 2022;43:1839-47.
33. Arboix A, Massons J, Arribas MP, et al. Headache in acute cerebrovascular ischemic disease: A prospective clinical study of 195 patients. Med Clin (Barc). 1993;100:611-3.
34. Grindal AB, Toole JF. Headache and transient ischemic attacks. Stroke. 1974;5:603-6.
35. Gorelick PB, Hier DB, Caplan LR, et al. Headache in acute cerebrovascular disease. Neurology. 1986;36:1445-50.
36. Kumral E, Bogousslavsky J, Melle GV, et al. Headache at stroke onset: The Lausanne Stroke Registry. J Neurol Neurosurg Psychiatry. 1995;58:490-2.
37. Mitsias PD, Ramadan NM, Levine SR, et al. Factors determining headache at onset of acute ischemic stroke. Cephalalgia. 2006;26:150-7.
38. Shigematsu K, Nakano H, Watanabe Y, et al. Headache at the onset of stroke: Frequencies, background characteristics, and correlation with mortality. Health. 2013;5:89-95.
39. Pollak L, Shlomo N, Korn Lubetzki I; National Acute Stroke Israeli Survey Group. Headache in stroke according to National Acute Stroke Israeli Survey. Acta Neurol Scand. 2017;135:469-75.
40. Leira R, Castellanos M, Alvarez-Sabín J, et al. Stroke Project, Cerebrovascular Diseases Group of the Spanish Neurological Society. Headache in cerebral hemorrhage is associated with inflammatory markers and higher residual cavity. Headache. 2005;45:1236-43.

CHAPTER 10

Ditans and Gepants for Acute Migraine Treatment

George O Dickson, Sarah Miller, Alok Tyagi

ABSTRACT

A literature review was performed of seminal studies around the treatments known as Ditans and Gepants, outlining their efficacy against acute migraine and their adverse effects.

Migraine continues to be a disorder across the globe with significant health impact. Triptans have been considered the gold standard for the treatment of acute migraine attacks. However, up to 70% patients do not achieve pain freedom at 2 hours. Therefore, there is a clear unmet need for additional treatments for the acute migraine attacks. Significant advances in the understanding of migraine pathophysiology and numerous clinical trials have led to the development of two new classes of acute migraine treatments, namely the Ditans, which are 5HT1F receptor agonists and the Gepants, which are calcitonin gene-related peptide (CGRP) receptor antagonists.

Ubrogepant, rimegepant, and zavegepant are indicated for use in acute migraine with or without aura. Rimegepant and atogepant are indicated for use as prophylaxis for episodic migraine. These nonserotoninergic drugs are unique in the management of migraine with no vasoconstrictive action. This affords them greater opportunity to be used by a wider demographic of patients including those with vessel diseases, such as ischemic heart disease or cerebrovascular disease.

An alternative group of drugs undergoing clinical trials are Ditans. These are serotoninergic agonists targeted at 5HT1F receptors. Specifically, Lasmiditan has shown favorable effectiveness and safety profile in two randomized controlled trials (RCTs) and was approved by the Food and Drug Administration (FDA) in 2019.

Keywords: Ditans, Gepants, Primary headache, Acute migraine, CGRP.

INTRODUCTION

Migraine remains one of the top ten disorders across the globe, affecting one billion people every year. In one study looking at service use and lost work days, the average cost per migraine patient over a 4-month period was £857, and the average total cost including lost employment was £6,588. More severe symptoms were associated with higher costs. The annual cost to the country for people referred to migraine specialists was estimated at £835 million, including healthcare costs and lost productivity costs (2018 prices).[1] The global age-standardized years living with disability from migraine in 2019 was 525.5,[2] which represents a significant public health issue and calls for effective treatment strategies in the management of acute migraine.

Triptans have been considered the gold standard for the treatment of acute migraine attacks. Triptans are 5HT1B and 1D receptor agonists, activation of which results in a cascade of processes resulting in the release of inflammatory peptides, including calcitonin gene-related peptide (CGRP), by the trigeminal nerves resulting in inhibition of pain neurotransmission.[3]

The 5HT1B and 1D receptors are located in blood vessels throughout the body and the use of triptans can result in vasoconstriction of the cerebral and coronary arteries. Triptans are therefore relatively contraindicated in patients with active cerebrovascular and coronary artery disease. Triptans are very effective treatments for the acute migraine attack and have been used extensively in clinical practice for decades. However, up to 70% patients do not achieve pain freedom at 2 hours.[4] Triptans are associated with side effects in a significant proportion of patients and the discontinuation rates can be as high as 81.5%.[5] Frequent use of triptans can also result in the development of medication overuse headache, which is a common risk factor of chronic headache. Therefore, there is a clear unmet need for additional treatments for the acute migraine attacks.

Development of additional treatments to address this unmet needs dates back to at least two decades. Significant advances in the understanding of migraine pathophysiology and numerous clinical trials have led to the development of two new classes of acute migraine treatments, namely the Ditans, which are 5HT1F receptor agonists and the Gepants, which are CGRP receptor antagonists. This comes at the time when the preventive treatment of migraine has been revolutionized by the CGRP monoclonal antibodies and this is a generational advance in the treatment of migraine.

CALCITONIN GENE-RELATED PEPTIDE

Calcitonin gene-related peptide has a pivotal role in the initiation of migraine pain. It facilitates an increase in neurogenic inflammation through release of proinflammatory mediators, as well as allowing vasoconstriction through its vasoactive action.[6] CGRP and CGRP receptors are widely expressed in the central nervous system (CNS), especially within the trigeminovascular system. Binding studies show coexpression of CLR and RAMP-1 in the smooth muscle of cranial blood-vessels and CGRP and CGRP receptor expression in the dura mater and trigeminal ganglion. CGRP also acts on the second order neurons in the trigeminocervical complex. CGRP receptor localization supports a role for CGRP in trigeminal sensitization and migraine pathology.

The pathophysiology of migraine involves activation and sensitization of trigeminovascular pathways, as well as brainstem and diencephalic nuclei.[7] The crucial importance of the serotoninergic system in the genesis of migraine has led to the development of the 5HT1 receptor agonists. These include agonist actions on 5HT1B/D and 5HT1F receptors.

Triptans are likely to have such mechanisms with regards to the trigeminal pain pathway. 5HT1D receptors have been linked to trigeminal nociceptive neurons involved in CGRP release.[8] 5HT1F receptors are also present both inside and outside the CNS. Notably, they are activated in regions indicated during a migraine event (hypothalamus, trigeminal ganglia, and locus coeruleus).[9] These receptors are located in both peripheral and central trigeminal neurons, and through their activation, are able to block impulses from these neurons. In turn, this prevents subsequent release of CGRP.[8]

Figure 1 shows the initiation of signal in the brain. This, in turn, activates the trigeminal nerve via its ganglion, which acts as a migraine amplifier and triggers the headache phase. Gepants and anti-CGRP antibodies work at this level preventing activation of trigeminovascular pain pathway.

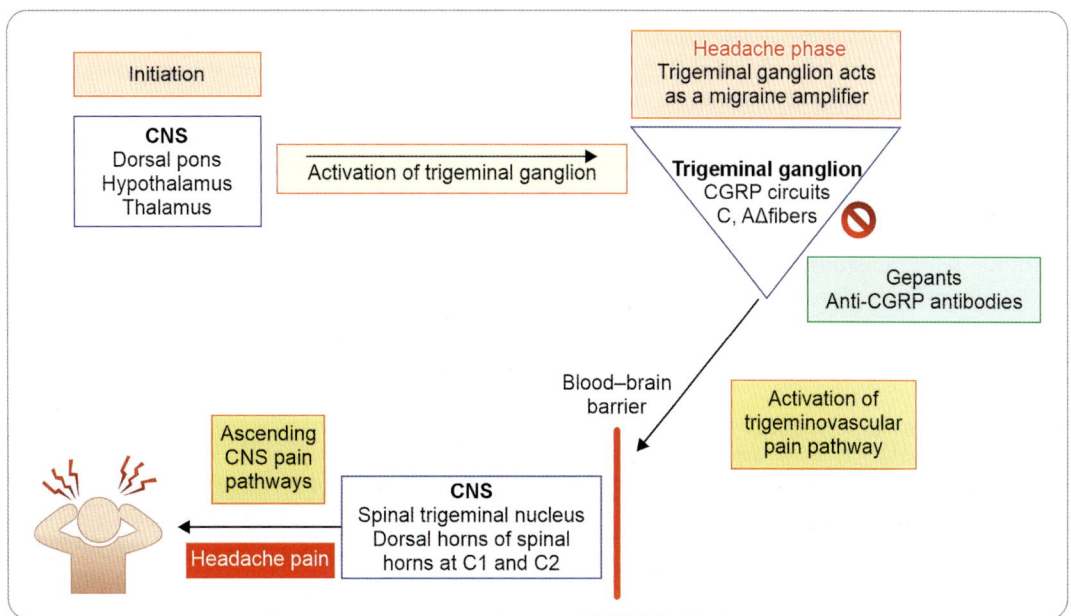

FIG. 1: The trigeminovascular pain pathway showing where CGRP targeted drugs act.
(CNS: central nervous system; CGRP: calcitonin gene-related peptide)

DITANS

Ditans are selective 5HT1F receptor agonists with low affinity for the 5HT1B/D receptors, resulting in significantly less cardiac and cerebrovascular vasoconstrictive side effects. The 5HT1F receptor is also found in arteries both inside and outside of the brain. However, they do not cause vasoconstriction at these sites.[9] Selected Triptans and Ditans are able to cross the blood–brain barrier due to their high lipophilicity. This enables Ditans to act peripherally on trigeminal afferents and ganglia, thus decreasing the activation of subsequent trigeminal neurons. They also work centrally on the trigeminovascular system. As of 2019, the Food and Drug Administration (FDA) has approved Lasmiditan as an acute treatment for migraine.[10] Two phase 3 trials showed Lasmiditan significantly increased the number of patients achieving freedom from headache pain.[11,12] It was also associated with relief from other migraine-associated sequelae, including photophobia, phonophobia, or nausea, without reported cardiovascular adverse events.[13]

Ditan Efficacy

Table 1 summarizes the efficacy of Lasmiditan in multiple studies with regards to pain freedom at 2 hours, and freedom from most bothersome symptom (MBS).

Lasmiditan has a good effect on migraine-related disability. The GLADIATOR study data showed that patients with severe migraine-related disability [a Migraine Disability Assessment (MIDAS) score of 29] showed significant improvement on each of the three assessments after the use of Lasmiditan 100 and 200 mg. A reduction of almost 50% in MIDAS scores was reported by 49% of participants in one group, and 53% in the other group. This reduction in score might be partly attributed to a reduction in disability reported by patients using Lasmiditan. The GLADIATOR study showed 64.5% of participants with no disability at 4 hours after the drug, and 85.7% had no disability at 24 hours. No significant differences were found between the two Lasmiditan groups (all $p > 0.43$).[14] Mean number of headache days (all $p > 0.31$) and mean headache pain in the last 3 months (all $p > 0.46$) achieved similar results.

Lasmiditan also had a significant impact on health-related quality of life indices. These include factors such as absenteeism, reduced productivity, and presenteeism (days of reduced productivity by at least 50% whilst attending work). For those taking Lasmiditan 100 mg, absenteeism days were reduced to 1.9 days in 3 months from 3.1 days. Those taking 200 mg, a reduction to 1.6 days from 3.2. ($p < 0.001$) was reported. Presenteeism days were reduced to 3.5 from 6.3 in the Lasmiditan 100 mg group and to 3.0 from 6.2 in the Lasmiditan 200 mg group.[15]

Ditan Adverse Effects

In randomized controlled trials (RCTs), Ditans cause nonsevere and short-term adverse events. Fatigue, nausea, dizziness, and paresthesia were the most frequently reported.[4,9] After ingestion, side effects had a variable onset time ranging from 40 minutes to 1 hour. Such effects ranged from 1.8 to 5.5 hours.[19]

Of these reported CNS side effects, some can be attributed to their action on the 5HT1F receptors located in the cortex and cerebellum.[10] Lasmiditan dosing studies using 50, 100, 200, and 400 mg doses showed that side effects were dose dependent.[4,18] However, even at a lower dosage, Lasmiditan showed a greater rate of CNS-related adverse events when compared with Triptans and Gepants {OR 3.12 [95% confidence interval (CI) 1.86–5.24] and OR 4.30 [95% CI 2.80–6.58]}, though most of these were mild to moderate in severity.[19] An indirect comparison of Gepants and each Lasmiditan dose revealed the highest significant incidence of mild adverse events were from 200 mg of Lasmiditan. This could potentially limit the use of Ditans in the migraine population due to their greater rate of CNS-related adverse events compared with other drugs.

Patients taking Lasmiditan over a 1-year period showed a significantly reduced incidence of adverse events. In the CENTURION study, there were limited examples of adverse incidents that were defined as treatment related. These included asthma in 0.2% of those taking 100 mg Lasmiditan, hemiplegic migraine, and serotonin syndrome

TABLE 1: Ditan efficacy across multiple studies.							
Study	Number of participants	Reporting pain freedom at 2 hours (%)			Reporting freedom of most bothersome symptom (%)		
		100 mg	200 mg	Placebo	100 mg	200 mg	Placebo
Samurai (2018)[16]	2,231	28.2	32.2	15.3	40.9	40.7	29.5
Spartan (2019)[17]	3,005	31.4	38.8	21.3	44.2	48.7	33.5
Gladiator (2019)[14]	2,171	26.7	32.2	–	37.2	40.8	–
Centurion (2021)[18]	1,633	25.8	29.3	8.4	40.4	39.0	28.0

in 0.4% of those taking 200 mg, and liver disorders and suicidal ideation in 0.4% of those taking placebo.[18] Among participants who experienced an adverse event at first intake, <45% experienced the same event with further doses. Of those participants who experienced no adverse event at first intake, very few had side effects with repeat usage.[20] This could prove beneficial in the detoxification process of medication overuse headache.

Some adverse events, however mild, did result in 12.8% of participants to drop out according to an interim analysis of the GLADIATOR study. Dizziness was the biggest culprit, causing 2.7% of patients taking 100 mg Lasmiditan, and 4.3% taking 200 mg Lasmiditan to leave the study.[14,15] There were no deaths related with the use of Ditans in any RCT.[21]

Despite these encouraging elements, the main limitation to the increased use of Ditans remains that of their adverse effects, and their potential implications on driving. Those taking Lasmiditan were instructed not to drive or operate machinery for at least 8 hours.[18] This could represent significant limitations for patients given the impact on quality of life.

In all studies involving Ditans, physiological testing, observation and vital assessments, and further monitoring including blood and urine parameters disclosed no variation or change after taking Lasmiditan.[18] It has also been revealed that Lasmiditan does not provoke QT prolongation, arrhythmia, or proarrhythmias. A cardiovascular risk assessment of Lasmiditan did not distinguish the drug from placebo [relative risk (RR) = 2:75; 95% CI (0.81, 9.37), $p = 0.11$].

GEPANTS

Table 2 represents different Gepant drugs, their indication, dosage, and any cautions.

Table 3 shows the efficacy of different Gepants across multiple studies for acute migraine treatment including their respective proportion of adverse events.

The first drug to competitively block the effect of CGRP was Olcegepant.[22] This represented a nonpeptide CGRP receptor antagonist showing high efficacy but low oral bioavailability. A proof-of-concept study was performed in 2004, which showed that intravenous Olcegepant was effectual in the treatment of acute migraine.[23] This guided the production and testing of many further CGRP receptor antagonists called Gepants for the acute treatment of migraine. All Gepants were significantly greater than placebo at accomplishing pain freedom or pain relief at 2 hours. Though these efficacy results were encouraging, development of some Gepants was ceased because of liver toxicity upon recurrent dosing.[24]

Since 2019 three Gepants, namely ubrogepant, rimegepant, and zavegepant have been approved by the FDA for the acute treatment of migraine. Rimegepant and atogepant are approved for preventive treatment of migraine.[25]

■ Ubrogepant

Ubrogepant is an oral CGRP receptor antagonist developed for the acute treatment of migraine. Its absorption is rapid

TABLE 2: Gepant drugs, their indications, posology, and cautions.

Drug	Indication	Dose	Regimen	Comment	Cautions
Ubrogepant	Treatment of acute migraine with/without aura	• 50 mg • 100 mg	• Oral • PRN	• A second dose may be administered at least 2 hours after the initial dose • Maximum daily dose 200 mg	• Contraindicated with strong inhibitors/inducers • Severe hepatic or renal impairment • Pregnancy or breastfeeding
Rimegepant	Treatment of acute migraine with/without aura	• 75 mg oral • 75 mg oral dissolving tablet	• Oral • Oral dissolving • PRN	Maximum dose 75 mg in a 24-hour period	• Severe renal or hepatic impairment • Pregnancy or breastfeeding
Zavegepant	Treatment of acute migraine with/without aura	10 mg	• Nasal spray • PRN	Maximum dose 10 mg in a 24-hour period	• Severe renal or hepatic impairment (dose reduction may be required) • Pregnancy or breastfeeding
Atogepant	Prophylaxis for episodic migraine with/without aura on >4 days per month	10 mg, 30 mg, 60 mg	• Oral • Once a day	(Not specified)	• Severe renal or hepatic impairment (dose reduction may be required) • Pregnancy or breastfeeding
Rimegepant	Prophylaxis for episodic migraine with/without aura on 4–14 days per month	• 75 mg oral • 75 mg oral dissolving tablet	• Oral • Oral dissolving • Alternate days	Maximum dose 75 mg in a 24-hour period	• Severe renal or hepatic impairment • Pregnancy or breastfeeding

TABLE 3: Gepants efficacy across multiple studies for acute migraine.					
Acute medications	Study	Dosage	Pain freedom at 2 hours	Absence of most bothersome symptom at 2 hours	Total % of adverse events
Ubrogepant	ACHIEVE I[26]	50 mg	19.2	38.6	9.4
		100 mg	21.2	37.7	16.3
		Placebo	11.8	27.8	12.8
	ACHIEVE II[27]	25 mg	20.7	34.1	9.2
		50 mg	21.8	38.9	12.9
		Placebo	14.3	27.4	10.2
Rimegepant	STUDY 301[31]	75 mg	19.2	36.6	12.6
		Placebo	14	27.7	10.7
	STUDY 302[32]	75 mg	19.6	37.6	17.1
		Placebo	12	25.4	14.2
	STUDY 303[33]	75 mg	21	35	13.2
		Placebo	11	27	10.5
Zavegepant	CROOP R, et al.[38]	10 mg	22.5	41.9	13.5
		20 mg	23.1	42.5	16.1
		Placebo	15.5	33.7	3.5

with a half-life of approximately 3 hours. It is metabolized through the liver, primarily via CYP3A4, and it is also a p-glycoprotein substrate.[26]

Two RCTs were performed to assess efficacy of ubrogepant for the treatment of acute migraine.[26,27] In the ACHIEVE I study, ubrogepant 50 mg, 100 mg, or placebo were administered to 1,327 patients. Pain freedom at 2 hours was 19.2% in the 50 mg group ($p = 0.0023$) versus 11.8% in the placebo group, and 21.2% in the 100 mg group ($p = 0.0003$). Freedom from MBS at 2 hours was reported by 38.6% in the 50 mg group ($p = 0.0023$) versus 27.8% in the placebo group and 37.7% in the 100 mg group ($p = 0.0023$).[24]

The ACHIEVE II trial involved 1,686 participants receiving 25 mg, 50 mg ubrogepant, or placebo. In the 25 mg group, 20.7% achieved pain freedom at 2 hours (vs. placebo, $p = 0.0285$). Those taking 50 mg, 21.8% achieved pain freedom (vs. placebo, $p = 0.0129$) and 14.3% in the placebo group. 34.1% achieved freedom from MBS at 2 hours of the 25 mg group (vs. placebo, $p = 0.0711$), 38.9% taking 50 mg (vs. placebo, $p = 0.0129$), compared to 27.4% of the placebo group. However, the 25 mg dose was not statistically significant compared to placebo.[27] Participants with moderate-to-severe cardiovascular risk factors were eligible. However, participants with clinically significant cardiovascular or cerebrovascular disease were excluded.

Another multicenter, randomized, open-label extension study included 1,254 patients who completed one of the ACHIEVE trials. Subjects were recruited to assess the efficacy of 50 mg ($n = 417$) and 100 mg ($n = 420$) doses of ubrogepant compared to a typical remedy ($n = 417$).[28] After 12 months, 24% of those treated with either 50 or 100 mg of ubrogepant reported pain freedom at 2 hours after an initial dose, and 67% reported pain relief at 2 hours postdose after a migraine attack.[29]

Significant improvements when compared to placebo were also seen for 50 mg ubrogepant concerning other outcomes. These included absence of photophobia and phonophobia at 2 hours, sustained pain freedom and sustained pain relief 2-24 hours and 2-48 hours, and total migraine freedom at 2 hours and at 2-24 hours. Further significant data were found for 25 mg ubrogepant concerning sustained pain freedom at 2-24 hours and at 2-48 hours. Similar data were also found for sustained pain relief at 2-48 hours and for total migraine freedom at 2 hours.[27]

■ Atogepant

Atogepant was approved by the FDA in September 2021 for the preventive treatment of episodic migraine based on the phase 3 ADVANCE study and the long-term safety study.[30] It has since also been approved for the preventive treatment of episodic and chronic migraine. In the ADVANCE study, 910 patients were recruited with 4-14 migraine days per month (baseline 7.5-7.9 days). The atogepant group saw a mean reduction in days with migraine when compared with placebo over 12 weeks. This was dose related, as those at an increased dosage experienced fewer days with migraine. Those receiving 10 mg atogepant saw a 55.6% reduction in migraine days per month; 58.7% for those taking 30 mg, and 60.8% reduction in migraine days for those with 60 mg atogepant, as compared to a 29.0% reduction for those taking placebo. There was also in an improvement to quality of life as per scores on Migraine-Specific Quality of Life Questionnaire (MSQ). All these results were statistically significant with $p < 0.001$.[30]

Rimegepant

Rimegepant is another oral CGRP antagonist, which was found to be effective in the treatment of acute migraine. Efficacy, safety, and tolerability have been demonstrated by several clinical studies—Study 301, 302, and 303.[31-33] A phase 3 study recruiting 3,019 subjects (NCT03461757)[34] administered 75 mg of rimegepant to patients and compared to placebo group. The primary outcomes analyzed were freedom from pain at 2 hours postdose, freedom from MBS at 2 hours postdose while the secondary outcomes included several parameters such as photophobia-free, pain relief, nausea-free, rescue medications sustained pain free, and pain relapse at 2 hours or 24-48 hours. The results showed a significant and durable clinical effect with a single dose of rimegepant in pain freedom, freedom from MBS, pain relief, and recovery of normal function and other outcome measures.

A phase 3 trial, (NCT03237845), evaluates the efficacy of rimegepant compared with placebo in migraine acute treatment. 1,499 participants were enrolled to receive rimegepant 75 mg oral tablet, or placebo 75 mg oral tablet. All primary endpoints were met. 19.6% of participants receiving rimegepant experienced pain freedom at 2 hours compared to 12% receiving placebo ($p = 0.0006$). 37.6% of participants receiving rimegepant experienced freedom from MBS at 2 hours compared to 25.2% receiving placebo ($p = <0.0001$). Benefit was sustained between 24 and 48 hours and more treated patients achieved normal function and used a lower number of rescue meds.[35]

The efficacy of rimegepant was assessed in a double-blind multicenter phase 3 RCT (NCT03461757) in those with acute migraine when compared to a placebo group. 1,811 participants were recruited to receive 75 mg rimegepant versus placebo. Results revealed that rimegepant orally disintegrating tablet was more effective than placebo at 2 hours after intake with regards to freedom from pain (21% vs. 11%, $p < 0.0001$) and freedom from the MBS (35% vs. 27%, $p = 0.0009$).[36]

In an open label trial (NCT03732638), treatment with rimegepant 75 mg was associated with greater improvement in health status during the 12-week double-blind treatment phase when compared to placebo. Patients originally randomized to placebo experienced a similar improvement in health status after switching to rimegepant during the open-label extension, demonstrating that benefits are realized within 12 weeks of active treatment. This preventive effect was durable out to 64 weeks and was associated with an additional increase in health-related quality of life over time.[37]

Zavegepant

Zavegepant (BHV3500-201), formerly known as vazegepant,[38] is a third-generation Gepant. Because of its structure, different routes of administration are under study, and these include subcutaneous, oral, and intranasal. A phase 3 RCT (NCT03872453) looked at the intranasal formulation and showed positive initial results. The intranasal formulation aims for a rapid onset of action. Zavegepant 10 mg and 20 mg reached the primary endpoints for efficacy; the 10 mg dose led to pain freedom at 2 hours in 22.5% of the patients as compared to 15.5% with the placebo ($p = 0.0113$) and the 20 mg was, similarly, superior to the placebo (23.1% vs. 15.5%; $p = 0.0055$).[38]

Of those participants taking 10 mg zavegepant 41.9% achieved freedom of MBS at 2 hours, and 42.5% of those taking 20 mg when compared to placebo ($p < 0.05$). Pain relief was reported as early as 15 minutes postdose with sustained efficacy at 2 hours. There is currently no published data on whether the efficacy is sustained after 48 hours, as with other Gepants. Dysgeusia was the most frequently reported adverse event in 13.5%, 16.1%, and 3.5% of patients in the 10 mg, 20 mg, and placebo groups, respectively. Similarly to other new generation Gepants, no hepatic issues were reported and no safety concerns have yet been discovered.[38]

Table 4 reflects the Gepants used in the prevention of acute migraine, their reduction in migraine days per month, and their respective proportion of adverse events.

Adverse Effects

Table 5 shows the most common adverse events experienced by each Gepant and their relatively proportions.

In the ACHIEVE I and II studies, adverse events were reported in <5% of patient uses **(Table 5)**.[26,27] One patient in the ubrogepant 50 mg group, with a previous history of supraventricular tachycardia with ablation, experienced a serious adverse event (sinus tachycardia) considered treatment related. The study also reported 20 cases of AST/ALT levels ≥3 × upper limit of normal in the two groups, two of which were considered treatment related.[29]

In the atogepant trials, there was a similar incidence of adverse events in treatment arm (18-54%) to those in the placebo group (16-57%) with the majority being mild to moderate. 3.1% discontinued the trial in the atogepant arm due to adverse events. Serious adverse events were observed in 3.4% of participants (none were treatment related), and there were no deaths. Adverse events leading to discontinuation occurring at >0.1% were nausea (0.4%) and abdominal pain, vomiting, weight decrease, dizziness, and migraine (0.3% each).[40]

TABLE 4: Gepants for prevention of migraine.				
Preventive medications	Study	Dosage	Migraines per month (days)	Total % of adverse events
Rimegepant	Croop R, et al.[39]	75 mg alternate days	−4.3	36
		Placebo	−3.5	36
Atogepant	Goadsby PJ, et al.[40]	10 mg QID	−4	18
		30 mg QID	−3.76	21
		60 mg QID	−3.55	23
		30 mg BD	−4.23	21
		60 mg BD	−4.14	26
		Placebo	−2.85	16

TABLE 5: Adverse effects of Gepants.		
Drug	Adverse events	Percentage of participants
Ubrogepant	Nausea	4
	Somnolence	3
	Dry mouth	2
Atogepant	Constipation	3.4
	Nausea	3.4
	URTI	5.5
	UTI	5.3
	Nasopharyngitis	4.8
	Sinusitis	3.6
Rimegepant	URTI	8.5
	Nasopharyngitis	6.4
	Sinusitis	4.8
	UTI	1.5
	Nausea	1.8
Zavegepant	Dysgeusia	13.5
		16.1
		3.5

(URTI: upper respiratory tract infection; UTI: urinary tract infection)

Phase 3 RCTs with regards to safety and tolerability of rimegepant were similar to placebo and better if compared to the past triptan experience.[35,36] No serious adverse events were reported. Two participants, one for each group, reported abnormal transaminase concentration of >3 times the upper limit, but it was deemed to be not related to study medication. Moreover, no elevations in bilirubin >2 times the upper limit of normal were reported.[36]

Table 6 summarizes the mechanisms of action, contraindications, and warnings of different classes of acute migraine treatments.

DISCUSSION

The currently available medical treatments for acute migraine are only able to provide complete sustained pain relief in a proportion of patients. Very often, the regular or excessive use of these medicines is associated with the worsening and chronification of headaches. In addition, the effectiveness of treatments is impeded by poor tolerability and contraindications. In recent years, clinical and preclinical research has largely focused on the pathophysiological basis of migraine and the role CGRP in triggering migraine attacks. CGRP has been confirmed as a powerful therapeutic target and the development of "Gepants" represents a huge opportunity for migraine therapy.

Gepants are selective CGRP receptor antagonists. These represent molecules that compete with endogenous CGRP at specific receptors. First-generation Gepants, Olcegepant and Telcagepant, showed good efficacy in the treatment of acute migraine; however, their production was halted by dissatisfactory adverse outcomes or cumbersome administration routes. Further clinical studies have been performed on more recent drugs at differing therapeutic dosages with encouraging results with all Gepants appearing to have comparable efficacy, few adverse events, and favorable safety profiles.

Ubrogepant, rimegepant, and zavegepant are indicated for use in acute migraine with or without aura. Rimegepant and atogepant are indicated for use as prophylaxis for episodic migraine. These nonserotoninergic drugs are unique in the management of migraine with no vasoconstrictive action. This affords them greater opportunity to be used by a wider demographic of patients including those with vessel diseases, such as ischemic heart disease or cerebrovascular disease.

An alternative group of drugs undergoing clinical trials are Ditans. These are serotoninergic agonists targeted at 5HT1F receptors. Specifically, Lasmiditan has shown favorable effectiveness and safety profile in two RCTS and was approved by the FDA in 2019.

TABLE 6: An outline of medications for acute migraine and their relevant and cautions.				
Drug	Lasmiditan	Sumatriptan	Rimegepant	Ubrogepant
Mechanism of action	Selective serotonin 5HT1F receptor agonist	Serotonin 5HT1B, 1D receptor agonist	CGRP receptor antagonist	CGRP receptor antagonist
Contraindications	Hypersensitivity	Hypersensitivity, coronary artery disease, cerebrovascular disease, peripheral vascular disease, Wolff–Parkinson–White syndrome, hemiplegic/basilar migraine, severe hepatic impairment, uncontrolled hypertension, peripheral vascular disease	Hypersensitivity	Hypersensitivity, concomitant use of strong CYP3A4 inhibitors or inducers, end-stage renal disease
Warnings	Driving impairment, CNS depression, serotonin syndrome, medication overuse headache	Ischemic heart disease, arrhythmias, cerebral hemorrhages, stroke, vascular disease, thromboembolic events, medication overuse headache, serotonin syndrome, seizures	Concomitant use of strong CYP3A4 inhibitors or inducers, concomitant administration of inhibitors of P-glycoprotein or breast cancer resistance protein	Dose reduction required in severe hepatic impairment

(CGRP: calcitonin gene-related peptide; CNS: central nervous system)

CONCLUSION

The latest drug therapies available for the acute, or preventive, treatment of migraine represent significant progression in the fight against this disease. The development of monoclonal antibodies in migraine management has led to the introduction of novel therapies with specific action for CGRP receptors. This has led to a much greater tool for migraine control for patients, giving the means for improved outcomes and quality of life. Future study only seeks to increase this arsenal against migraine attacks. The development of migraine-specific therapies based on basic science is an encouraging step forward for a group of patients previously neglected in the drug industry. These new therapies will allow us to get a step closer to precision targeted medicine for migraine, aiming for an individualized therapy for any individual patient and improving migraine care worldwide.

REFERENCES

1. Osumili B, McCrone P, Cousins S, et al. The economic costs of patients with migraine headache referred to specialist clinics. Headache. 2018;58(2):287-94.
2. Safiri S, Pourfathi H, Eagan A, et al. Global, regional, and national burden of migraine in 204 countries and territories, 1990 to 2019. PAIN. 2022;163(2):293-309.
3. Tepper SJ, Rapoport AM, Sheftell FD. Mechanisms of action of the 5-HT1B/1D receptor agonists. Arch Neurol. 2002;59:1084-8.
4. Ferrari MD, Goadsby PJ, Roon KI, et al. Triptans (serotonin, 5-HT1B/1D agonists) in migraine: detailed results and methods of a meta-analysis of 53 trials. Cephalalgia. 2002;22(8):633-8.
5. Dodick DW. Migraine. Lancet. 2018;391(10127):1315-30.
6. Karsan N, Goadsby PJ. CGRP Mechanism Antagonists and Migraine Management Curr Neurol Neurosci Rep 2015;15:25.
7. Vila-Pueyo M, Strother LC, Kefel M, et al. Divergent influences of the locus coeruleus on migraine pathophysiology. Pain. 2019;160(2):385-94.
8. Rubio-Beltrán E, Labastida-Ramírez A, Villalón CM, et al. Is selective 5-HT1F receptor agonism an entity apart from that of the triptans in antimigraine therapy? Pharmacol Ther. 2018;186:88-97.
9. Bouchelet I, Case B, Olivier A, et al. No contractile effect for 5-HT1D and 5- HT1F receptor agonists in human and bovine cerebral arteries: similarity with human coronary artery. Br J Pharmacol. 2000;129:501-8.
10. Nilsson T, Longmore J, Shaw D, et al. Characterisation of 5-HT receptors in human coronary arteries by molecular and pharmacological techniques. Eur J Pharmacol 1999;372:49-56.
11. Lamb YN. Lasmiditan: first approval. Drugs. 2019;79:1989-96.
12. Goadsby PJ, Wietecha LA, Dennehy EB, et al. Phase 3 randomized, placebo-controlled, double-blind study of lasmiditan for acute treatment of migraine. Brain. 2019;142(7):1894-904.
13. Kuca B, Silberstein SD, Wietecha L, et al.; COL MIG-301 Study Group. Lasmiditan is an effective acute treatment for migraine: A phase 3 randomized study. Neurology. 2018;91(24) 2222-32.
14. Brandes JL, Klise S, Krege JH, et al. Interim results of a prospective, randomized, open-label, phase 3 study of the long-term safety and efficacy of lasmiditan for acute treatment of migraine (the GLADIATOR study). Cephalalgia. 2019;39:1343-57.
15. Lipton RB, Lombard L, Ruff DD, et al. Trajectory of migraine-related disability following long-term treatment with lasmiditan: results of the GLADIATOR study. J Headache Pain. 2020;21:20.
16. ClinicalTrials.gov. (2019). Lasmiditan compared to placebo in the acute treatment of migraine: (SAMURAI), NCT02439320. [online] Available from https://classic.clinicaltrials.gov/ct2/show/NCT02439320 [Last accessed July, 2023].
17. ClinicalTrials.gov. (2019). Three doses of lasmiditan (50 mg, 100 mg and 200 mg) compared to placebo in the acute treatment of migraine (SPARTAN), NCT02605174. [online] Available from

https://classic.clinicaltrials.gov/ct2/show/NCT02605174 [Last accessed July, 2023].

18. Ashina M, Reuter U, Smith T, et al. Randomized, controlled trial of lasmiditan over four migraine attacks: findings from the CENTURION study. Cephalalgia. 2021;41:294-304.
19. Shapiro RE, Hochstetler HM, Dennehy EB, et al. Lasmiditan for acute treatment of migraine in patients with cardiovascular risk factors: Post-hoc analysis of pooled results from 2 randomized, double-blind, placebo-controlled, phase 3 trials. J Headache Pain. 2019;20(1):90.
20. Loo LS, Plato BM, Turner IM, et al. Effect of a rescue or recurrence dose of lasmiditan on efficacy and safety in the acute treatment of migraine: findings from the phase 3 trials (SAMURAI and SPARTAN). BMC Neurol. 2019;19:191.
21. Yang CP, Liang CS, Chang CM, et al. Comparison of new pharmacologic agents with triptans for treatment of migraine: a systematic review and meta-analysis. JAMA Netw Open. 2020;4:e2128544.
22. Doods H, Hallermayer G, Wu D, et al. Pharmacological profile of BIBN4096BS, the first selective small molecule CGRP antagonist. Br J Pharmacol. 2000;129:420-3.
23. Olesen J, Diener H, Husstedt IW, et al. Calcitonin gene–related peptide receptor antagonist BIBN 4096 BS for the acute treatment of migraine. Society. 2004;350(11):1104-10.
24. Bigal ME, Walter S, Rapoport AM. Calcitonin gene-related peptide (CGRP) and migraine current understanding and state of development. Headache. 2013;53:1230-44.
25. Moreno-Ajona D, Villar-Martinez MD, Goadsby PJ. New Generation Gepants: Migraine Acute and Preventive Medications. J Clin Med. 2022;11(6):1656.
26. ClinicalTrials.gov. (2017). Efficacy, Safety, and Tolerability Study of Oral Ubrogepant in the Acute Treatment of Migraine (ACHIEVE I), NCT02828020. [online] Available from https://clinicaltrials.gov/ct2/show/NCT02828020?cond=NCT02828020&draw=2&rank=1 [Last accessed July, 2023].
27. Lipton RB, Dodick DW, Ailani J, et al. Effect of ubrogepant vs placebo on pain and the most bothersome associated symptom in the acute treatment of migraine: the ACHIEVE II randomized clinical trial. JAMA. 2019;322(19):1887-98.
28. ClinicalTrials.gov. (2018). An Extension Study to Evaluate the Long-Term Safety and Tolerability of Ubrogepant in the Treatment of Migraine, NCT02873221. [online] Available from https://clinicaltrials.gov/ct2/show/study/NCT02873221?cond=NCT02873221&draw=2&rank=1 [Last accessed July, 2023].
29. Scott LJ. Ubrogepant: First Approval. Drugs. 2020;80:323-8.
30. Ailani J, Lipton RB, Goadsby PJ, et al. Atogepant for the preventive treatment of migraine. N Engl J Med. 2021;385:695-706.
31. Lipton R, Coric V, Stock E, et al. Rimegepant 75 mg, an oral calcitonin gene-related peptide antagonist, for the acute treatment of migraine: Two phase 3, double-blind, randomized, placebo-controlled trials. Cephalalgia. 2018;38:140-1.
32. Lipton RB, Croop R, Stock EG, et al. Rimegepant, an Oral Calcitonin Gene-Related Peptide Receptor Antagonist, for Migraine. N Engl J Med. 2019;381:142-9.
33. Croop R, Goadsby PJ, Stock DA, et al. Efficacy, safety, and tolerability of rimegepant orally disintegrating tablet for the acute treatment of migraine: A randomised, phase 3, double-blind, placebo-controlled trial. Lancet. 2019;394:737-45.
34. ClinicalTrials.gov. (2019). Open Label Safety Study in Acute Treatment of Migraine, NCT03266588. [online] Available from https://clinicaltrials.gov/ct2/show/NCT03266588?cond=NCT03266588&draw=2&rank=1 [Last accessed July, 2023].
35. ClinicalTrials.gov. (2018). Safety and Efficacy in Adult Subjects with Acute Migraines, NCT03237845. [online] Available from https://clinicaltrials.gov/ct2/show/NCT03237845?cond=NCT03237845&draw=2&rank=1 [Last accessed July, 2023].
36. ClinicalTrials.gov. (2018). Trial in Adult Subjects with Acute Migraines, NCT03461757. [online] Available from https://clinicaltrials.gov/ct2/show/NCT03461757?cond=NCT03461757&draw=2&rank=1 [Last accessed July, 2023].
37. Powell LC, L'Italien G, Popoff E, et al. Health State Utility Mapping of Rimegepant for the Preventive Treatment of Migraine: Double-Blind Treatment Phase and Open Label Extension (BHV3000-305). Adv Ther. 2023;40:585-600.
38. Croop R, Madonia J, Conway C, et al. Intranasal Zavegepant is Effective and Well Tolerated for the Acute Treatment of Migraine: A Phase 2/3 Dose-Ranging Clinical trial. Neurology. 2021;96:4976.
39. Croop R, Lipton RB, Kudrow D, et al. Oral rimegepant for preventive treatment of migraine: A phase 2/3, randomised, double-blind, placebo-controlled trial. Lancet. 2021;397:51-60.
40. Goadsby PJ, Dodick DW, Ailani J, et al. Safety, tolerability, and efficacy of orally administered atogepant for the prevention of episodic migraine in adults: A double-blind, randomised phase 2b/3 trial. Lancet Neurol. 2020;19:727-37.

CHAPTER 11

Non-headache Symptoms in Migraine: What do They Mean?

Farsana MK, Thomas Mathew, Girish Baburao Kulkarni

ABSTRACT

Migraine is one of the most common primary headache disorders, characterized by recurrent episodes of disabling headaches, which are the defining features of this disease. Apart from headache other symptoms and associated comorbidities have a bearing in diagnosis disability and management of migraine, and frequently make migraine patients more incapacitated. Despite reports of fatigue associated with migraine dating back to the 19th century, the broader phenotype of an adult migraine attack has only recently been described non-headache symptoms may precede the headache phase by up to 72 hours and persist for a day after the headache resolution in the postdrome. The highest occurrence of non-headache symptoms is during the headache phase compared to the prodrome and postdrome. The most commonly reported non-headache symptom in the prodromal phase is neck stiffness, as compared to the difficulty in concentration during the headache phase and fatigue during the postdrome. The highest co-occurring symptoms were neck stiffness, thirst, and abdominal pain. Another important aspect of migraine heterogeneity is comorbidity with other neurological diseases (stroke or seizures), cardiovascular disorders, and psychiatric illnesses (anxiety and depression). The potential effect of acute and preventive treatments on non-headache symptoms has been poorly investigated. Given the clinical consequences, further research must be directed to specifically study these issues from a therapeutic point of view, to improve the quality of migraine patient care.

Keywords: Migraine, Non-headache symptoms, Variants, Comorbidities, Treatment.

INTRODUCTION

Migraine is one of the most common primary headache disorders characterized by recurrent episodes of disabling headaches.[1] Many epidemiological studies have demonstrated its higher incidence and the effects on socioeconomic and personal aspects of life. Migraine was listed one among the highest global causes of disability under 50 years of age in the Global Burden of Disease (GBD) 2019, and affects around 1 billion people worldwide.[2] A migraine attack classically has four phases, namely the prodromal (premonitory), aura, headache, and postdrome, which often overlap.[3] Along with severe headaches, non-headache symptoms associated with migraine attacks and comorbid diseases frequently make migraine patients more incapacitated.[4] Better recognition of the evolution of non-headache symptoms through the different phases of migraine can improve our understanding of migraine pathophysiology and help in the management of the disease.[5,6]

NON-HEADACHE SYMPTOMS IN MIGRAINE

Although the cardinal symptom of migraine is recurrent episodes of disabling headaches, it may not necessarily be always the most bothersome for all patients.[7] Non-headache symptoms may precede the headache phase by up to 72 hours and persist for a day after the headache resolution in the postdrome phase.[8-10] Despite reports of fatigue linked to migraine dating back to the 19th century, the broader phenotype of an adult migraine attack has only recently emerged in the past 30–40 years through several prevalence and phenotypic studies in which these symptoms were assessed.[11,12] Non-headache symptoms such as nausea, vomiting, photophobia, and phonophobia are an established part of the International Headache Society (IHS) criteria for migraine, and the recent International Classification of Headache Disorders-3 (ICHD-3) **(Box 1)** lists variants of migraine with non-headache symptomatology as well.[13]

According to a recent study by Messina et al., 99% of patients reported at least one non-headache symptom in one phase of the migraine attack, and 54% had at least one non-headache symptom occurring across the phases of the migraine.[6] Non-headache symptoms were higher during the headache phase compared to the prodrome and postdrome. Most symptoms occurred throughout all three phases, implying ongoing brain events with headache as just one feature of the attack. The highest co-occurring symptoms were neck stiffness, thirst, and abdominal pain. Patients with non-headache symptoms during all three phases of migraine were more likely to be female, had chronic migraine with higher levels of disability, and experienced drug overuse headaches more frequently. In addition, there were no discernible differences in the frequency of non-headache symptoms between patients with and without aura, those on prophylactic medication, or those with episodic and chronic headaches.[6] **Table 1** lists the various non-headache symptoms across the four phases of migraine.

PATHOPHYSIOLOGY OF NON-HEADACHE SYMPTOMS

Susceptibility for migraine is genetically inherited, but several additional factors also influence symptomatology and disease activity. The complex biology of migraine remains unsolved and involves a series of central and peripheral nervous system areas and networks. More recently, migraine was considered a disorder of sensory brain processing, where impairment of the filtering of sensory and nociceptive inputs causes ordinarily unbothersome sensations to be perceived as disturbing.[14]

Functional neuroimaging of non-headache symptoms across migraine phases reveals a substantial involvement in numerous subcortical and cortical areas. Sensory afferents from the head and neck region, along with the nociceptive input from the cranial vasculature and dura, converge in the trigeminocervical complex (TCC) located in the brainstem through the trigeminal (TG) and cervical ganglia (CG). Numerous ascending and descending connections project to the rostroventral medulla (RVM), locus coeruleus (LC), periaqueductal grey (PAG), hypothalamus, thalamus, and cerebral cortex.[14]

Cortical spreading depression (CSD) is thought to be the neurophysiological correlate of migraine, characterized by a slow (2–6 mm/min) propagating depolarization wave in neuronal and glial cell membranes followed by cortical suppression lasting up to 30 minutes. This pattern of activity coincides with the initiation and progression of aura symptoms and is associated with a wave of hyperemia, followed by a prolonged phase of cortical oligemia.[3] **Table 2** and **Figure 1** summarize the brain areas and neurochemical systems implicated in non-headache symptoms of migraine.

■ Symptoms during the Prodromal Phase

The migraine prodrome is defined in ICHD-3 beta as symptoms preceding and forewarning a migraine attack by 2–48 hours, occurring before the aura in migraine with

> **BOX 1: The International Classification of Headache Disorders (ICHD-3) classification of migraine.**
>
> 1. Migraine
>   1.1 Migraine without aura
>   1.2 Migraine with aura
>   1.2.1 Migraine with typical aura
>   1.2.1.1 Typical aura with headache
>   1.2.1.2 Typical aura without headache
>   1.2.2 Migraine with brainstem aura
>   1.2.3 Hemiplegic migraine
>   1.2.3.1 Familial hemiplegic migraine (FHM)
>   1.2.3.1.1 Familial hemiplegic migraine type 1 (FHM1)
>   1.2.3.1.2 Familial hemiplegic migraine type 2 (FHM2)
>   1.2.3.1.3 Familial hemiplegic migraine type 3 (FHM3)
>   1.2.3.1.4 Familial hemiplegic migraine, other loci
>   1.2.3.2 Sporadic hemiplegic migraine (SHM)
>   1.2.4 Retinal migraine
>   1.3 Chronic migraine
>   1.4 Complications of migraine
>   1.4.1 Status migrainosus
>   1.4.2 Persistent aura without infarction
>   1.4.3 Migrainous infarction
>   1.4.4 Migraine aura-triggered seizure
>   1.5 Probable migraine
>   1.5.1 Probable migraine without aura
>   1.5.2 Probable migraine with aura
>   1.6 Episodic syndromes that may be associated with migraine
>   1.6.1 Recurrent gastrointestinal disturbance
>   1.6.1.1 Cyclical vomiting syndrome
>   1.6.1.2 Abdominal migraine
>   1.6.2 Benign paroxysmal vertigo
>   1.6.3 Benign paroxysmal torticollis

Non-headache Symptoms in Migraine: What do They Mean?

TABLE 1: Non-headache symptoms across various phases of migraine.

Prodromal phase			
Increased sensitivity to external stimuli: • Photophobia • Phonophobia • Osmophobia • Allodynia • Neck stiffness	*Cognitive/Behavioral symptoms*: • Fatigue/Lethargy • Difficulty in concentration • Mood changes • Irritability • Confusion • Disorientation • Speech difficulty	*Homeostatic and hormonal alterations*: • Yawning • Food craving/aversion • Thirst • Polyuria • Altered sleep–wake cycle	*Cranial autonomic symptoms*: • Lacrimation • Nasal stuffiness • Rhinorrhea • Aural fullness • Abnormal taste • Sensation of throat swelling
Aura phase			
Visual aura: • Flashes of light • Brightly colored spots • Zigzag lines • Foggy vision • Blind spots	*Brainstem aura*: • Dysarthria • Vertigo • Tinnitus • Hypoacusis • Diplopia • Ataxia • Decreased level of consciousness	*Sensory-motor aura*: • Tingling • Numbness • Paresthesia • Weakness	*Speech and language*: • Word-finding difficulty *Retinal*: • Monocular positive, or negative visual symptoms
Headache phase			
Gastrointestinal symptoms: • Nausea • Vomiting • Abdominal pain	*Sensory hypersensitivity*: • Phonophobia • Photophobia • Osmophobia • Allodynia • Neck stiffness	*Vestibular symptoms*: • Vertigo • Dizziness • Imbalance	*Cranial autonomic symptoms*: • Dizziness • Visual blurring • Conjunctival injection • Conjunctival tearing • Ptosis • Eyelid swelling • Nasal stuffiness • Rhinorrhea • Aural fullness • Pupillary change • Facial flushing • Facial sweating • Taste disturbance
Postdromal phase			
Cognitive/Mood/Energy: • Fatigue • Intolerant/Irritable • Yawning • Emotional • Difficulty with thoughts • Difficulty reading or writing • Difficulty with speech • Concentration difficulties • Mood changes	*Autonomic*: • Dizziness • Pale face • Constipation/Diarrhea • Frequent urination • Hunger/Food craving • Thirst	*Gastrointestinal symptoms*: • Nausea/Vomiting • Flatulence • Abdominal pain • Anorexia	*Sensory hypersensitivity*: • Neck stiffness • Phonophobia • Photophobia • Head discomfort • Movement sensitivity

aura and before the onset of pain in migraine without aura. Previous studies report its occurrence in 8–87% of adults and 67% of pediatric patients with migraine.[15]

Prodromal symptoms can be broadly divided into increased sensitivity to sensory stimuli, cognitive and behavioral changes, homeostatic and hormonal alterations, and cranial autonomic symptoms.[14] Neck discomfort was the most commonly reported symptom in a recent study by Messina et al., and 39% of patients experienced the neck discomfort early in the premonitory stage. Early activation of

TABLE 2: Brain areas and neurochemical systems implicated in non-headache symptoms of migraine.		
Non-headache symptoms	**Brain areas implicated**	**Neurochemicals implicated**
Fatigue	Several cortical regions, hypothalamus, and LC	NA, orexins, and DA
Neck discomfort	PAG, TCC, hypothalamus, and thalamus	CGRP, neuronal NOS, NA, DA, and glutamate
Photophobia	Occipital cortex and thalamus	CGRP, neuronal NOS, NA, DA, and glutamate
Nausea	Rostral dorsal medulla and PAG	DA, serotonin, Ach, histamine, and substance P
Yawning	Hypothalamus	DA
Thirst, polyuria	Hypothalamus	ADH and orexins
Food cravings	Hypothalamus, BG, and limbic system	NPY, orexins, and CCK
Cranial autonomic symptoms	Superior salivatory nucleus	VIP and PACAP
Mood change	Limbic system (CC, insula, amygdala) and caudate nucleus	Serotonin, DA, and NA
Difficulty in concentration and memory disturbances	Frontal cortex, caudate nucleus, anterior temporal lobe, and hippocampus	DA, NA, and serotonin

(Ach: acetylcholine; ADH: antidiuretic hormone; BG: basal ganglia; CGRP: calcitonin gene-related peptide; CC: cingulate cortex; CCK: cholecystokinin; DA: dopamine; LC: locus coeruleus; NA: noradrenaline; NOS: nitric oxide synthase; NPY: neuropeptide Y; PAG: periaqueductal grey; PACAP: pituitary adenylate cyclase-activating peptide; TCC: trigeminocervical complex; VIP: vasoactive intestinal peptide)

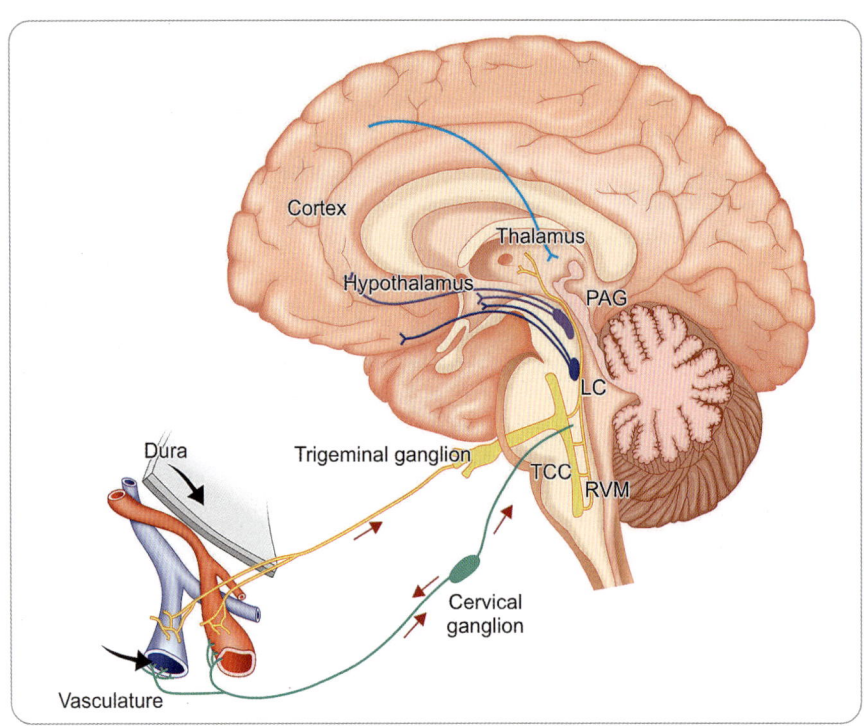

FIG. 1: Pathophysiology of migraine symptomatology. Sensory afferents from the head and neck region, along with the nociceptive input from the cranial vasculature and dura, converge in the trigeminocervical complex (TCC) located in the brainstem through the trigeminal and cervical ganglia. Numerous ascending and descending connections project to the rostroventral medulla (RVM), locus coeruleus (LC), periaqueductal grey (PAG), hypothalamus, thalamus, and cerebral cortex.

the TCC before the ascending input to the thalamus, where the headache presumably arises, explains its occurrence before the headache.[6] Previous studies also reported yawning, mood changes, lethargy, and light sensitivity in the order of decreasing frequency.[15] According to Giffin et al., tiredness or fatigue was the most common, reported in 72% of patients, followed by difficulty with concentration (51%) and stiff neck (50%). A high number of patients experience photophobia (49%), phonophobia (38%), and nausea (24%) as well, in the premonitory period continuing through the headache phase to the postdrome.[11]

Photo- and phonophobia showed the highest co-occurrence, which might represent their common origin, whereas yawning had a high co-occurrence with many other symptoms such as lethargy, craving, and mood changes. Prodrome was more common in females. 72% of the patients could correctly predict headache onset within 72 hours based on premonitory symptoms; yawning had the highest predictability.[11,15]

Symptoms during the Aura Phase

A migraine aura is a transient and reversible visual, sensory, or other neurological symptom that classically precedes a migraine headache, occurring in about 30% of patients. Aura can be visual, sensory, speech/language, motor, brainstem, or retinal. Individual symptoms can last 5-60 minutes and >60 minutes if there is more than one aura symptom.[16]

Visual aura accounts for 98–99% of all migraine auras, whereas sensory and language disturbances occur respectively in 36% and 10% of cases. Visual auras are usually seen in isolation, whereas the other symptoms co-occur.[17]

In a systematic review of clinical features of visual aura by Michele Viana et al., commonly reported visual aura included foggy, blurred vision or dimness (25–54%), zigzag or jagged lines (24–81%), scotoma (23–77%), phosphenes (small bright dots 19–70%), flashes of bright light or star-shaped figures (16–38%), flickering light (12–91%), hemianopia (7–22%), black dots (3–17%), and visual snow (7%).[18]

A Brazilian study on 122 migraines with aura patients showed blurred vision (54.1%) and small bright dots (47.5%) more common, whereas the frequencies of classic zigzag or jagged lines (41.8%) and the typical "C" crescentic shape were low (16.4%).[19]

Visual snow is a rare phenomenon characterized by alterations in the visual field, which persists even when the eyes are closed. Hypermetabolism of the right lingual gyrus and the anterior lobe of the left cerebellum was found in patients with visual snow in a [18F]-fluorodeoxyglucose positron emission tomography (PET) study.[20]

An auditory aura includes tinnitus, music, or noises; a sensory aura as tingling, numbness, or paresthesias; and a motor aura can present as hemiparesis. Language aura is rare and can occur as word-finding difficulty or trouble understanding words. The prevalence of these less common auras varies widely in different studies.

Most frequently reported brainstem aura includes dysarthria, vertigo, tinnitus, hyperacusis, diplopia, ataxia, and decreased level of consciousness. A recent review has suggested cortical localization of brainstem aura to vestibular cortex, temporo-parieto-occipital junction, posterior and superior parietal lobe, and temporal-insular regions. Retinal aura can be repeated, with monocular, positive, or negative visual symptoms, and is considered rare. The pathophysiology is reversible retinal vasospasm, retinal spreading depression, or both. Recent reports include alien hand syndrome, gelastic aura, and auditory or olfactory hallucinations.[16]

SYMPTOMS DURING THE HEADACHE PHASE

In 99% of cases, the headache phase coexists with non-headache symptoms. Most premonitory symptoms became more prevalent during the headache phase, except yawning, hunger or food cravings, and increased energy. In a recent study by Messina et al., difficulty concentrating was the most frequently reported non-headache symptom during the headache phase (87%).[6]

About 70–80% of migraine sufferers have nausea, and 30% experience vomiting, followed by anorexia and delayed gastric emptying.[21] Patients with gastrointestinal symptoms from migraines may have autonomic nervous system dysfunction. Patients with frequent nausea during migraines are twice as likely to develop chronic migraines than those with less frequent nausea.[22,23]

Around 70–90% of migrants have sensory hypersensitivity, including photophobia, phonophobia, osmophobia, and allodynia, in conjunction with the headache phase. At least one cranial autonomic symptom may be present in 74% of the population, with 70% having two or more. Lacrimation (45.5%), conjunctival injection (34.5%), eyelid edema (34%), aural fullness (27.5%), facial sweating (25%), facial flushing (17.5%), nasal congestion (9%), rhinorrhea (5%), and ptosis (4%) were the symptoms most frequently observed. About 30–50% of migraine patients report associated vertigo, dizziness, or imbalance. The vertigo can be spontaneous or positional.[24,25]

Symptoms during the Postdrome

The migraine postdrome is a constellation of symptoms occurring after the acute headache has subsided. This entity is yet to be defined in the ICHD. In a cohort of 827 individuals, studied by Kelman, 68% of the patients reported postdrome symptoms. The average duration of the postdrome was 25.2 hours. Tiredness (71.8%), headache (33.1%), cognitive difficulties (11.7%), hangover (10.7%), gastrointestinal symptoms (8.4%), mood changes (6.8%), and weakness (6.2%) were the most prevalent symptoms.[26]

The most prevalent individual postdrome symptoms were asthenia (55%), tiredness (46%), somnolence (29%), concentration difficulties (28%), phonophobia (27%), photophobia (26%), unhappiness (26%), and yawning (24%). Giffin et al., in a recent study, found that 97 individuals (81%) had at least one non-headache symptom during the postdrome, including fatigue/weariness (88%) and difficulty concentrating (56%) in that order, as well as stiff neck

(42%).⁹ Postdrome effects disappear in 93% of attacks within 24 hours following headache relief. There was no connection between the duration of the postdrome and the intensity of the migraine or the use of medication.[27]

MIGRAINE VARIANTS

Episodic syndromes that may be associated with migraine, also called migraine variants, are recurrent, periodic, paroxysmal disorders in children and adolescents. These episodic syndromes are diagnosed after excluding other conditions and are characterized by sudden onset, spontaneous resolution without permanent sequel, and may or may not be associated with headaches. In a pediatric migraine cohort, 9.8% had migraine variants, of which 10–70% had coexisting migraine. The most common types were benign paroxysmal vertigo (BPV) (38%), acephalgic migraine (29%), abdominal migraine/cyclic vomiting syndrome (CVS) (19%), benign paroxysmal torticollis (BPT) (10%), and confusional migraine (5%).[28,29] **Table 3** summarizes the salient features of important migraine variants.

COMORBIDITIES IN MIGRAINE

An important aspect of migraine heterogeneity is comorbidity with other neurological diseases, cardiovascular disorders, and psychiatric illnesses.

■ Psychiatric Illness

Psychiatric comorbidities are more common in migraine with aura than without aura, depressive disorders being the most common. Patients with psychiatric comorbidities are at high risk of transformation into chronic migraine. Identification of comorbidity will help in improved patient management. Migraineurs are two to four times more likely to experience severe depression in their lifetime. The pathophysiology of this comorbid association remains unknown, but genetic factors, serotonergic dysfunction, ovarian hormone influences, and hypothalamic–pituitary–adrenal axis dysregulation are implicated.[30]

Migraine patients are reported to have a higher risk of comorbid bipolar disorder and seem to more likely to have a rapid cycling illness course. Anxiety is more prevalent in chronic migraine patients than in those with episodic migraine, and it is two to five times as common in migraine patients overall. The risk of developing generalized anxiety disorder was higher in migraine patients, increased with headache frequency.[4]

■ Other Neurological and Cardiovascular Diseases

Sleep disruptions are linked to migraine type and intensity, indicating their strong and significant association.

TABLE 3: Salient features of important migraine variants.

Migraine variant	Important clinical characteristics
Benign paroxysmal vertigo	• Less than 4 years, equal in boys and girls • Disabling vertigo without provocation or prodrome • Lasts for seconds to minutes • Pallor and sweating, vomiting, and nystagmus • Electroencephalography shows no epileptiform activity
Benign paroxysmal torticollis	• Without premonitory symptoms • Head tilt with rotation • Pallor, agitation, irritability, and vomiting • Lasts hours to days, 2–3 times/month • Spontaneous and stereotypic • Attacks may remain one sided or alternate sides • The attacks frequently cease by age 3 or 4
Cyclic vomiting syndrome	• Age of onset is 5 years. Male–female ratio is equal • Recurrent episodes of severe vomiting usually beginning in the early morning, stereotypical recurring intervals • Self-limited and often ends at puberty • Premonitory abdominal pain, anorexia, or nausea the night before • Episodes may last hours to days (24–40 hours), average 12 episodes/year • Characteristic for each patient nausea, anorexia, abdominal pain, headache, phonophobia, photophobia, lethargy, pallor, and less frequently, diarrhea, and fever
Abdominal migraine	• Children with a positive family history of migraine • Stereotypical recurrent paroxysmal bouts of abdominal pain, separated by periods of wellness • Pain is sore, dull, and periumbilical in location • Severe enough to interfere with normal activity, lasts at least an hour • Associated pallor, anorexia, and nausea and vomiting
Hemiplegic migraine	• Familial or sporadic • Fully reversible motor weakness or fully reversible visual, sensory and/or speech/language symptoms • Associated other neurological features such as ataxia, epilepsy, periodic paralysis, retinitis pigmentosa, sensorineural deafness, essential tremor, and nystagmus • History of the more usual forms of migraine • Family history of migraine

Insomnia, sleep-related breathing disorders (such as obstructive sleep apnea), sleep-related movement disorders (such as restless leg syndrome), central disorders of hypersomnolence (such as narcolepsy), circadian rhythm-related sleep-wake disorders, and parasomnia are all linked to migraine.

Both migraines and epilepsy share several systemic symptoms, including olfactory dysfunction, nausea, vomiting, and visual and other sensory problems. CSD, the pathophysiological hallmark of aura, further suggests that excessive neuronal activity causes the recruitment of larger populations of rhythmically firing neurons, which in turn causes epileptic seizures.

Migraine is thought to increase the risk of cardiovascular disease as well. People with migraine with aura are more likely to experience ischemic, hemorrhagic, and subclinical ischemic strokes. Oral contraceptive use, smoking, female, and older age are all possible risk factors for ischemic stroke among migraineurs.[31]

DIFFERENTIAL DIAGNOSIS

Non-headache symptoms of migraine, especially aura, should be differentiated from other causes of transient neurological symptoms such as transient ischemic attack (TIA), seizures, and syncope. The main differentiating features are listed in **Table 4**.

MANAGEMENT OF NON-HEADACHE SYMPTOMS IN MIGRAINE

Patients with vascular risk factors should be evaluated along the lines of TIA, including MRI of the brain with angiography, when non-headache symptoms in form of aura occur abruptly. If there is a seizure suspicion, electroencephalography (EEG) can be performed and a thorough cardiac workup for syncope.

Non-headache symptoms can be challenging to treat since they resolve spontaneously before the drugs have a chance to start working. Many patients may not require treatment if their symptoms are short-lasting. The potential effect of acute and preventive treatments on non-headache symptoms has been poorly investigated. The adverse effects of several acute migraine treatments, such as acetaminophen, nonsteroidal anti-inflammatory drugs, and triptans, might be similar to the non-headache symptoms such as nausea, dizziness, paresthesia, and somnolence. Only one study looked at whether acute migraine treatments could reduce non-headache symptoms, it found that triptans had no effects on such symptomatology during the postdromal phase.[9] Another recent study found that patients who received treatment with monoclonal antibodies targeting the calcitonin gene-related peptide (CGRP) pathway experienced relief in non-headache symptoms, like irritability and mood swings as well. Additionally, this study

TABLE 4: Differential diagnosis of non-headache symptoms in migraine.				
Characteristics	Non-headache aura symptoms of migraine	Transient ischemic attack	Seizure	Syncope
Age and gender	More common in younger age and females	More common in older age and males	No age or gender predilection	Any age
Clinical presentation	<ul><li>Both positive and negative symptoms</li><li>Visual the most common</li><li>May evolve into other modality (spreading character) visual to somatosensory</li><li>No complete loss of consciousness</li><li>Mental slowing and confusion</li></ul>	<ul><li>Predominantly negative symptoms</li><li>Maximum at onset</li><li>No spreading character</li><li>Loss of consciousness is rare</li></ul>	<ul><li>Predominantly positive symptoms</li><li>Loss of consciousness and amnesia for event common</li><li>Postictal negative symptoms may persist for hours to days</li></ul>	<ul><li>Light-headedness, darkening of vision, or muffled hearing</li><li>Brief period of impaired awareness</li></ul>
Onset and duration	<ul><li>Gradual on set progressive over 5 minutes</li><li>Last for 20–60 minutes</li><li>Can be prolonged and recur anytime</li></ul>	<ul><li>Abrupt onset and gradual recovery (minutes)</li><li>Last for minutes to <1 hour</li><li>Recur over days or weeks</li></ul>	<ul><li>Brief <2 minutes</li><li>Can recur anytime</li></ul>	<ul><li>Brief seconds to less than a minute</li><li>Can recur anytime</li></ul>
Other features	Headache can precede, co-occur, or follow the non-headache symptoms	Headaches may occur, usually during the attacks	<ul><li>Tongue bite, incontinence</li><li>Postictal-myalgia, confusion, and headache</li></ul>	Sweating, pallor, nausea, and rapid and complete recovery

demonstrated that anti-CGRP monoclonal antibodies could delay the onset of non-headache symptoms in addition to pain.[32] The use of acute and prophylactic medications for migraine management can be planned so as to help treating the non-headache symptoms and comorbidities. For example, use of antiemetics for nausea and vomiting, avoiding ergots in patients with aura, and use of parenteral medications when patient has vomiting. With respect to prophylactic drugs presence of comorbidities in a given patient can be considered for appropriate selection of drugs (e.g., depression, obesity, asthma, etc.).

CONCLUSION

Many non-headache symptoms and comorbidities of migraine have a significant negative impact on the quality of life. Early recognition and management of non-headache symptoms is important. Given the clinical consequences, further research must be done to specifically study these issues from a therapeutic point of view, to improve the quality of migraine patient care.

REFERENCES

1. Ferrari MD, Goadsby PJ, Burstein R, et al. Migraine. Nat Rev Dis Primer. 2022;8(1):1-20.
2. Vos T, Lim SS, Abbafati C, et al. Global burden of 369 diseases and injuries in 204 countries and territories, 1990–2019: a systematic analysis for the Global Burden of Disease Study 2019. The Lancet. 2020;396(10258):1204-22.
3. Dodick DW. A Phase-by-Phase Review of Migraine Pathophysiology. Headache. 2018;58 Suppl 1:4-16.
4. Chen PK, Wang SJ. Non-headache symptoms in migraine patients. F1000Research. 2018;7:188.
5. Charles A. Migraine: a brain state. Curr Opin Neurol. 2013;26(3):235-9.
6. Messina R, Cetta I, Colombo B, et al. Tracking the evolution of non-headache symptoms through the migraine attack. J Headache Pain. 2022;23(1):149.
7. Lampl C, Thomas H, Stovner LJ, et al. Interictal burden attributable to episodic headache: findings from the Eurolight project. J Headache Pain. 2016;17:9.
8. Bose P, Goadsby PJ. The migraine postdrome. Curr Opin Neurol. 2016;29(3):299-301.
9. Giffin NJ, Lipton RB, Silberstein SD, et al. The migraine postdrome: An electronic diary study. Neurology. 2016;87(3):309-13.
10. Karsan N, Peréz-Rodríguez A, Nagaraj K, et al. The migraine postdrome: Spontaneous and triggered phenotypes. Cephalalgia. 2021;41(6):721-30.
11. Giffin NJ, Ruggiero L, Lipton RB, et al. Premonitory symptoms in migraine: An electronic diary study. Neurology. 2003;60(6):935-40.
12. Karsan N, Bose PR, Thompson C, et al. Headache and non-headache symptoms provoked by nitroglycerin in migraineurs: A human pharmacological triggering study. Cephalalgia. 2020;40(8):828-41.
13. Headache Classification Committee of the International Headache Society (IHS) The International Classification of Headache Disorders, 3rd edition. Cephalalgia. 2018;38(1):1-211.
14. Karsan N, Goadsby PJ. Biological insights from the premonitory symptoms of migraine. Nat Rev Neurol. 2018;14(12):699-710.
15. Laurell K, Artto V, Bendtsen L, et al. Premonitory symptoms in migraine: A cross-sectional study in 2714 persons. Cephalalgia. 2016;36(10):951-9.
16. Lai J, Dilli E. Migraine Aura: Updates in Pathophysiology and Management. Curr Neurol Neurosci Rep. 2020;20(6):17.
17. Russell MB, Olesen J. A nosographic analysis of the migraine aura in a general population. Brain J Neurol. 1996;119 (Pt 2):355-61.
18. Viana M, Tronvik EA, Do TP, et al. Clinical features of visual migraine aura: a systematic review. J Headache Pain. 2019;20(1):64.
19. Queiroz LP, Friedman DI, Rapoport AM, et al. Characteristics of migraine visual aura in Southern Brazil and Northern USA. Cephalalgia. 2011;31(16):1652-8.
20. Schankin CJ, Maniyar FH, Sprenger T, et al. The relation between migraine, typical migraine aura and "visual snow." Headache. 2014;54(6):957-66.
21. Choi JY, Oh K, Kim BJ, et al. Usefulness of a photophobia questionnaire in patients with migraine. Cephalalgia. 2009;29(9):953-9.
22. Chelimsky TC, Chelimsky GG. Autonomic abnormalities in cyclic vomiting syndrome. J Pediatr Gastroenterol Nutr. 2007;44(3):326-30.
23. Reed ML, Fanning KM, Serrano D, et al. Persistent frequent nausea is associated with progression to chronic migraine: AMPP study results. Headache. 2015;55(1):76-87.
24. Vuković V, Plavec D, Galinović I, et al. Prevalence of vertigo, dizziness, and migrainous vertigo in patients with migraine. Headache. 2007;47(10):1427-35.
25. Tiwari A, Maurya PK, Qavi A, et al. Cranial Autonomic Symptoms in Migraine: An Observational Study. Ann Indian Acad Neurol. 2022;25(4):654-9.
26. Kelman L. The postdrome of the acute migraine attack. Cephalalgia. 2006;26(2):214-20.
27. Quintela E, Castillo J, Muñoz P, et al. Premonitory and resolution symptoms in migraine: a prospective study in 100 unselected patients. Cephalalgia. 2006;26(9):1051-60.
28. Rothner AD, Parikh S. Migraine Variants or Episodic Syndromes That May Be Associated With Migraine and Other Unusual Pediatric Headache Syndromes. J Head Face Pain. 2016;56(1):206-14.
29. Rothner AD. Migraine Variants in Children. Pediatr Ann. 2018;47(2):e50-4.
30. Antonaci F, Nappi G, Galli F, et al. Migraine and psychiatric comorbidity: a review of clinical findings. J Headache Pain. 2011;12(2):115-25.
31. Amiri P, Kazeminasab S, Nejadghaderi SA, et al. Migraine: A Review on Its History, Global Epidemiology, Risk Factors, and Comorbidities. Front Neurol. 2022;12:800605.
32. Iannone LF, De Cesaris F, Ferrari A, et al. Effectiveness of anti-CGRP monoclonal antibodies on central symptoms of migraine. Cephalalgia. 2022;42(13):1323-30.

CHAPTER 12

Managing Chronic Migraine: An Update

Kamakshi Dhamija, Tanushree Chawla

ABSTRACT

With a prevalence of 1.4–2.2% worldwide, chronic migraine (CM) is a disabling condition that places a heavy financial burden. About 2–3% of people annually develop chronic migraine from episodic migraine. Although central sensitization and increased excitability of the trigeminal nociceptive pathway are thought to be the most significant factors, pathophysiology is still not fully understood. Certain modifiable and nonmodifiable risk factors predispose patients for chronification of migraine. Management of chronic migraine can be divided into pharmacological (oral and injectable medications) and nonpharmacological (neuromodulation and behavioural therapy) therapies. Patient education is an integral part of chronic migraine management and should be done at all potential points of patient contact. In this chapter, we have discussed the evidence available for the commonly used drugs in chronic migraine and the potential emerging therapies.

Keywords: Chronic migraine, Pathophysiology, Management, Topiramate, Onabotulinum toxin, Greater occipital nerve block, CGRP-related therapies, Neuromodulation.

INTRODUCTION

Migraine, a primary headache disorder, is one of the most common conditions that we encounter on daily basis in our outpatient clinics. It can be classified into episodic migraine (EM) and chronic migraine (CM) based on the frequency of the attacks. CM is diagnosed when a patient experiences >15 days of headache in a month for 3 months and out of which 8 attacks are migrainous in character. Prevalence of CM ranges between 1.4 and 2.2% globally, and is directly proportional to the age, also being more common in females. The impact and the disability cost attributable to migraine are often underestimated by the treating physicians. According to global disease burden analysis (2016), migraine was associated with 42.1 million years lived with disability (YDLs), was highest in women between 15 and 49 years of age group, when the productivity is at the peak.[1] The economic burden of CM can be gauged by the fact that approximately $9,000/year higher costs are bared by people living with migraine compared to those without.[2] Hence, it can be inferred that it is utmost important to promptly diagnose and treat patients with CM in order to improve their health-related quality of life.

DIAGNOSTIC CRITERIA OF CHRONIC MIGRAINE

The term CM was first introduced by Manzoni et al. in 1995. The diagnostic criteria for CM were first introduced in the International Classification of Headache Disorders, 2nd edition (ICHD-2) in 2005, revised in ICHD-2R in 2006, and established in 2018 with the ICHD-3. ICHD-3 allows diagnosis of both CM and medication overuse headache (MOH) in the same patient, as few patients might not revert to EM on withdrawal of analgesics. A few issues around the diagnosis of CM remain unresolved, including the observation that patients with chronic daily headache may lose the migrainous character over time, variability of headache frequency over time, and whether MOH is a risk factor for transformation or an entirely separate disorder. Lack of a uniform inclusive standardized definition of CM over the years has led to exclusion of these patients from the drug trials, consequently leading to limitation of evidence-based data for its management. The current ICHD-3 diagnostic criteria for CM are as follows:[3]

A. Headache (migraine-like or tension-type-like) on ≥15 days/month for >3 months
B. Occurring in a patient who has had at least five attacks fulfilling criteria for migraine with or without aura
C. On ≥8 days/month for >3 months, fulfilling any of the following:
   1. Criteria for migraine with or without aura or
   2. Believed by the patient to be migraine at onset and relieved by a triptan or ergot derivative

PATHOPHYSIOLOGY

Chronic migraine most often develops from EM. While the mechanisms behind this transformation are complex, the pathophysiology is still not completely understood. Less than 5% of patients with CM are able to traverse the three barriers of "consultation, diagnosis, and treatment", emphasizing the large unmet need for appropriate management of patients with CM.[4] It is a multifactorial disorder with a presumed interplay of both genetic and environmental factors. Genomic susceptibility has been evidenced to exist for migraine in general, but data for migraine subphenotypes as CM is scarce. Prospective studies such as the Frequent Headache Epidemiology Study, American Migraine Prevalence and Prevention study, and the CaMEO study have attempted to address the rates and risk factors for transition.[5] Around 2–3% of patients experience this transformation over time. The transformation often occurs gradually, and patients have been reported to oscillate to and fro among these two categories. The risk factors for transformation are:

- *Modifiable risk factors*:
  o Higher baseline EM frequency
  o Obesity
  o Higher use of abortive medications
  o Caffeine overuse
  o Overuse of certain medications as barbiturates and opioids
- *Nonmodifiable risk factors*:
  o Increasing age
  o Female gender
  o Low socioeconomic status
  o Low educational status
  o A past history of mild head injury
  o Past history of stressful life events

Hence, it is of utmost importance to address the modifiable risk factors in order to mitigate the chances of transformation. In corollary, CM can revert to EM. *Thus, CM is a preventable disorder*, amongst a subset of "at risk" population. Development of central sensitization and heightened excitability of trigeminal nociceptive pathways is a central pathophysiological link in migraine chronification. There are more marked, structural, physiological, and biochemical changes in brains of chronic migraineurs as compared to those in patients with EM. Neurogenic inflammation is the key biochemical substrate for development of central sensitization in CM. Studies have shown that chronic migraineurs express increased levels of vanilloid-type 1 receptor along the scalp arteries and smaller sensory neurons, which augments the release of calcitonin gene-related peptide (CGRP) and substance P. The role of CGRP needs a separate mention here as we have now entered into an era of monoclonal antibodies targeting this pathway specifically. CGRPergic nociceptive neurons interact with receptors in trigeminal ganglion to release nitrous oxide which in turns creates a vicious cycle for additional CGRP release, resulting in heightened sensitization of trigeminal ganglion. Nearly 30% of trigeminal ganglion neurons express CGRP. CGRP expressing neurons are either Aδ or C-fibers. Peripheral projection of CGRP also results in vasodilatation of meningeal vessels, augmenting neurogenic inflammation further. The heightened sensitization also spreads to spinal nucleus of trigeminal ganglion as well as thalamus upstream, which are the substrates for orofacial pain and allodynic body symptoms in CM.[6] Thus, CGRP is a very potent vasodilator and considered to have a sentinel role in inflammatory and nociceptive processes. Levels of other vasoactive neuropeptides as vasoactive intestinal peptide (VIP) and pituitary adenylate cyclase-activating polypeptide-38 (PACAP-38) are also higher in chronic migraineurs than in controls or in patients with EM. There is apparently widespread expression of PACAP-38 in headache-implicated areas as hypothalamus, brainstem, pituitary, and cortex. Thus, the atypical pain processing mechanisms of subcortical structures resulting in cortical hyperexcitability due to an inflammatory milieu serve as substrate for migraine chronification.

MANAGEMENT OF CHRONIC MIGRAINE

Goals of Treatment in Chronic Migraine

The goals of treatment of CM are prevention of headache attacks; prevention of conversion of frequent EM to CM, and lastly to prevent MOH. Parameters used for assessment of efficacy of treatment are reduction in monthly migraine or headache days; reduction in duration, frequency or severity of attacks; reduction in analgesic use; improvement of response to analgesics; and improvement in quality of life.

Management of CM can be subdivided into:
- Pharmacological treatment
- Nonpharmacological treatment

Pharmacological Treatment

Pharmacological treatment of CM includes management of acute migraine attacks and prophylactic treatment. Acute migraine treatment is similar to the management of acute attacks in EM, hence is not included for the purpose of this review. The prophylactic CM treatment includes oral drugs and injectables. The evidence for the most pharmacological agents in CM is largely extrapolated from the trials for the drugs used for prophylaxis in EM. Robust evidence for efficacy in CM is available only for topiramate (TOP) and onabotulinum toxin A (Ona-BT A), and thus they are recommended as first-line medications by Latin American guidelines.[7] Initial pharmacological agent shall not only be chosen based on the recommendation but comorbidities should also be taken into account. One must start with the lowest dose and gradually titrate upward every 2 weeks till the maximum dose is reached or unacceptable side-effects appear. Patients shall always be advised to maintain a headache diary, where they should record the frequency, severity, intensity of the headache, and analgesic usage. In addition, functional impairment should be assessed at the first visit using scales like Headache Impact Test-6 (HIT-6) and Migraine Disability Assessment (MIDAS), and patients must be advised to keep a record of the same as well. Evaluation should be done every 2–3 months focusing on the reduction in frequency, intensity, and improvement in functional impairment. 50% improvement in the parameters reflects efficacy. The effective dose of medication should be continued for 6 months to 1 year and then gradually tapered. Patient education plays a vital role. The role of behavioral therapies must be emphasized from the very first encounter. Avoidance of triggers should be emphasized and indiscriminate use of over-the-counter analgesics should be discouraged. The treatment expectations must be discussed openly. Patient should always be educated about the chances of recurrence on stopping the medications.

Oral Medications

Anticonvulsants

Topiramate: It has consistently displayed benefit over the placebo in terms of reduction in headache frequency, mean number of monthly headache days, thus establishing its efficacy in CM. It has also shown improvement in the patient-reported outcomes and quality of health-related outcomes across various studies.[8-10] Although TOP is quite effective in CM, there are substantial adverse effects such as paresthesias, renal stones, glaucoma, etc., that can interfere with the compliance. In a few trials that compared TOP to other drugs, it was shown that TOP produced superior results to valproate and propranolol, while Ona-BT A and flunarizine appear to perform better in terms of migraine control, patient-reported outcomes, and side effect profiles. **Table 1** gives a summary of the randomized controlled trials (RCTs) of TOP in CM.

TABLE 1: Summary of the trials of topiramate and propranolol.				
Drug	**Number of trials**	**Primary outcomes**	**Results**	**Adverse effects**
Topiramate	• Total 13 randomized trials • Placebo-controlled—6 • TOP vs. Botox—4 (2 blinded, 2 open-labeled) • TOP vs. VA—1 • TOP vs. FLU—1 • TOP vs. Propranolol—1	• Reduction in headache frequency • Monthly migraine days • Efficacy of acute medications • Quality of life and patient-reported outcomes • Physician global assessment scale • Headache days and migraine days • >50% reduction in headache days	• TOP was better than placebo in all six placebo-controlled RCTs • TOP was more effective than VA at month 9 • FLU was found to be more effective than TOP • Onabotulinum toxin was better in both in efficacy and quality of life parameters • TOP was better than propranolol	• 35.7–75% minor adverse effects reported across the studies • On comparison to botox—TOP group reported 24.1% AEs vs. 2.1% in onabotulinum toxin group • The discontinuation rate was also higher in TOP (42%) group vs. botox group (1%) • Paresthesias was the most common SE
Propranolol	• RCT—4 • Propranolol vs. divalproex—1 • Propranolol vs. NT vs. combination—1 • Propranolol vs. TOP—1 • Propranolol as add-on therapy with TOP—1	• Frequency of migraine attacks • Number of migraine days • Proportion of patients with 50% reduction in number of headache days • Moderate-to-severe headache days/28 days	• All trials showed that propranolol was efficacious in CM • No significant difference was seen in propranolol vs. divalproex, nortriptyline or TOP	• TEAE seen in 36% in one study • Dizziness, fatigue, and hypotension were the commonly reported SEs

(CM: chronic migraine; FLU: flunarizine; NT: nortryptyline; RCT: randomized controlled trial; SE: side effect; TEAE: treatment-emergent adverse event; TOP: topiramate; VA: valproic acid)

Valproic acid or divalproex sodium: It primarily works by inhibition of gamma-aminobutyric acid (GABA) transaminase. Valproic acid (VA) has high metabolism, needs to be given at frequent intervals, whereas divalproex sodium is an enteric-coated tablet with sustained-release formulations, which may be given once daily. Efficacy of both the compounds has been proven in RCTs for EM but again no data exist for its use in CM. Meta-analysis of three trials of 510 patients of migraine (unspecified) showed an odds ratio of 2.74 for having a reduction of >50% in migraine frequency compared with placebo.[11] One study where VA was studied in chronic daily headaches [CM 29, chronic tension-type headache (CTTH) 41], VA decreased the maximum pain visual analog scale (VAS) level, general pain VAS levels, and pain frequency (PF) significantly in CM ($p = 0.006$, $p = 0.03$, and $p = 0.000$, respectively) and PF was reduced significantly in CTTH, indicating valproate is an effective agent in chronic daily headache more so in patients with CM compared to CTTH.[12] One of the major complications associated with VA is teratogenicity. Thus, one should be extremely careful in childbearing age group. It has significant side effects such as weight gain, hair loss, tremors, and hepatic failure.

Antihypertensives

Propranolol: There is no dearth of data for efficacy of propranolol in prevention of EM, but there are only four RCT on its use in CM.[13-16] None of the trial were placebo controlled, it was compared with valproate, nortriptyline, TOP, whereas in one clinical trial propranolol was tested as an add-on therapy to TOP. All these trials suggested propranolol was effective in CM, but add-on treatment was not useful. It was noted that propranolol leads to significant reduction in frequency of migraine attacks by 63% and monthly migraine days were reduced by 4.5–4.6 days. Comparative analysis suggested no significant difference in the efficacy of propranolol compared to valproate or TOP or nortriptyline. In the most recent RCT conducted by Chowdhury et al. (2022) comparing TOP ($n = 93$) to propranolol ($n = 82$), propranolol was found to be noninferior to TOP with a comparable tolerability (change in migraine days in TOP group was -5.3 ± 1.2 vs. -7.3 ± 1.1 days in the propranolol group, $p = 0.226$).[16] Most common side effects observed in the trials were fatigue, dizziness, and hypotension. **Table 1** summarizes the major trials of propranolol in CM.

Candesartan: An RCT of candesartan in EM in 2003 found that candesartan significantly reduced the mean number of headache days compared to placebo with comparable tolerability.[17] The other placebo-controlled RCT comprising both EM and CM patients, comparing efficacy with placebo and propranolol, found that candesartan was noninferior to propranolol and superior to placebo.[18]

Antidepressants

Tricyclic antidepressants (TCAs), serotonin norepinephrine reuptake inhibitors (SNRIs), and selective serotonin reuptake inhibitors (SSRIs) are all used for migraine prophylaxis. However, there are no systematically conducted trials for antidepressants in patients with CM.

A Cochrane review by Xu et al. 2017 analyzed 16 randomized clinical trials of antidepressants in migraine prophylaxis (unspecified population—EM/CM). They found a significant improvement in the headache frequency and headache index with antidepressants compared to placebo (standard mean difference of -0.79; CI -1.13 to -0.45; $p < 0.00001$), although there was significant heterogeneity in the trial design. TCAs are a commonly accepted treatment for migraine, but the data in relation to SNRI and SSRI is limited and conflicting. In the meta-analysis, the SNRI and SSRI benefitted the migraineurs but the level of evidence was low due to underpowered study and limited sample size.[19]

Calcium Channel Blockers

Common calcium channel blockers (CCBs) used in migraine prophylaxis are flunarizine, cinnarizine, and verapamil. There are no placebo-controlled trials of CCBs in CM. There are a handful of comparative trial of CCBs with other drugs in CM. Nifedipine has been tried previously in EM. It was comparable in efficacy to flunarizine but was observed to be inferior to propranolol in migraine prophylaxis with significant side effects.[20] Cinnarizine was found to be as effective in migraine prophylaxis of refractory migraine as sodium valproate. However, cinnarizine is commonly associated with extrapyramidal adverse effects, which could be quite disabling. TOP and flunarizine were comparable in the efficacy parameters in another study but the combination therapy lead to significantly better results compared to either alone.[21] Based on the above results, flunarizine may be used as an alternative or as an add-on agent in refractory migraine.

Injectables

The difficulty of treating migraines is made worse by the high rate of drug discontinuation due to either side effects, inefficacy, or occasionally due to the inability to take oral medications due to nausea and vomiting. Alternative therapy methods to address this problem include Ona-BT A, nerve blocks, and CGRP antagonists.

Onabotulinum Toxin A

The pathogenesis behind transformation accounts for the resistance of CM to therapies currently effective for EM. Before the Food and Drug Administration (FDA) approval of Ona-BT A for CM, TOP was the only oral drug for which high-quality evidence existed in favor of its efficacy and safety in this patient group. In the era of emerging popularity of Ona-BT A, there was an accidental observation that when it was being given for the forehead rejuvenation, the patients reported elimination of their concurrently existing migraine headaches. Subsequently, two robust phase 3 randomized placebo-controlled trials [PREEMPT (Phase 3

REsearch Evaluating Migraine Prophylaxis Therapy) 1 and 2] established the efficacy of Ona-BT A for CM treatment. Currently, Ona-BT A has level A evidence for its usage in CM. The treatment is usually offered to CM patients who have failed two to three migraine prophylactics (European Headache Federation 2018 guidelines) unless it is contraindicated by comorbid disorders.[22] The mechanisms for action of Ona-BT A in CM are diverse. The potential mechanisms go beyond its action of local "muscle tension" release. Apart from the decrease in peripheral muscle overactivity, which results in reduced nociceptive signaling centrally, there is sufficient evidence to believe that the toxin reduces the proinflammatory cytokine release at the nerve terminals such as substance P, ATP, CGRP, enkephalin, and other similar transmitters resulting in decrease in "inflammatory signaling" in the local milieu. Changes in surface expression of receptors and cytokines as well as enhancement of opioidergic transmission have also been postulated as valid mechanisms.[23] **Table 2** summarizes major trials for Ona-BT A use in CM. The considerations for Ona-BT A use in CM are:

- The dosages of Ona-BT A are usually given as per the PREEMPT protocol. Dose ranges from 155 to 195 U given in 31 fixed sites and fixed doses (5 U each) across seven specific head/neck muscle areas. The physician can, hence, additionally use 40 U into the temporalis,

TABLE 2: Key findings of landmark studies for botulinum toxin use in chronic migraine.			
Trial	Trial design	Duration of study	Key trial findings
PREEMPT 1 and 2[24,25] (pre-marketing trials)	• Phase 3 research trials conducted at 56 North American sites (PREEMPT 1), 66 North American and European sites (PREEMPT 2) • *Trial design*: A 24-week, 2-treatment cycle, double-blind, randomized, placebo-controlled, parallel-group phase, followed by a 32-week, 3-treatment cycle, open-label phase	• 56 weeks • *Protocol followed*: Fixed dose, fixed site with discretion of using additional 40 U according to "follow-the-pain" strategy	• ≥50% responder rate in terms of frequency of headache days—49% after first treatment cycle, additional 11% after second treatment cycle, further 10% in third treatment cycle • >50% patients benefitted in terms of moderate-to-severe headache days, total cumulative hours of headache, HIT-6 score after first treatment cycle • Adverse effects with >5% incidence—neck pain and muscle stiffness
COMPEL study[26] (post-marketing trial)	*Trial design*: Multicenter, open-label long-term prospective study conducted at 35 sites in US, Korea, and Australia	• 108 weeks • *Protocol followed*: Fixed dose, fixed site	• ≥50% responder rate in terms of frequency of headache days—39.5% at week 24, 61.1% at week 108 • Statistically significant improvement observed in terms of moderate-to-severe headache days, starting at week 24, maintained till week 108 • Treatment effects seem to cumulate over time • TRAEs—18.3% • Most common adverse events—neck pain followed by eyelid ptosis • Recommended to continue treatment for at least 12 months of good headache control
REPOSE[27] (post-marketing trial)	Multicenter, prospective, observational, noninterventional study conducted at 78 centers in Germany, Italy, Norway, Russia, Sweden, Spain, and the United Kingdom	• 24 months • *Protocol studied*: Both fixed dose and follow-the-pain strategies	• Statistically significant reductions from baseline observed in headache-day frequency at all postbaseline visits • Statistically significant changes from baseline observed in all three migraine-specific quality of life questionnaire domains at all administration visits (visit 2–8) • Adverse drug events—18.3% • Most commonly noticed adverse events: Eyelid ptosis, neck pain, and musculoskeletal stiffness • Most frequent interinjection interval employed is >13 weeks
CM-PASS[28]	Multicenter, prospective, observational, noninterventional study conducted at 58 centers in Germany, Sweden, Spain, and the United Kingdom	64 weeks	• 74.4% patients were satisfied/extremely satisfied with Ona-BT A therapy. This included 83% and 65% of patients who had and had not previously received Ona-BT A, respectively • ≥1 TRAE seen in 25.1% patients, most common being neck pain and eyelid ptosis
(HIT: Headache Impact Test; TRAE: treatment-related adverse event)			

occipitalis, and/or trapezius muscles using a follow-the-pain strategy.[29]
- Abbreviated Ona-BT A regimen tailored to individual myofascial trigger points in head, neck, and shoulder instead of a fixed site/fixed dose protocol is also reported to be reasonably effective. Such regimens can be especially employed where financial constraints preclude standard injection protocols.
- "Follow-the-suture" protocol wherein 90 U of Ona-BT A is injected at 18 sites over the area of cranial sutures (postulating the zones where collaterals from meninges penetrate the skull) can also be employed.
- Ona-BT A therapy should be repeated every 3 months; treatment effect is seen to cumulate over time.
- Predictors of Ona-BT A response include ocular or imploding character of headache, unilaterality of pain, presence of allodynia, pericranial tenderness, previous response to triptans, and a shorter disease duration.
- The adverse reactions with Ona-BT A are usually mild or moderate in severity and resolve without sequelae. Majorly they include neck pain and muscular weakness as eyelid ptosis. Minor side effects noticed are erythema, injection-site edema, and itching. Treatment discontinuations attributable by adverse reactions to the drug are rare.
- Wearing off response may be seen with Ona-BT A use 2–4 weeks prior to next scheduled dose. This can usually be managed with greater occipital nerve (GON) blocks, a higher next dose of Ona-BT A, adding a prophylactic and abbreviating the interinjection period to 8–10 weeks.
- It is recommended that when CM reverts to EM and the frequency of headache remains stable in the EM range for consecutive 3 months, the Ona-BT A treatment can be stopped according to National Institute for Health and Care Excellence (NICE) guidelines.[30] Another strategy that has been recommended is that in those subjects who are stable responders to Ona-BT A for at least 1 year, interinjection period may be extended to verify durability of Ona-BT A treatment. Patients should be evaluated after 4–5 months of stopping treatment in order to ensure nonreversion to CM.
- On the other hand, treatment unresponsiveness is defined by NICE guidelines as a <30% reduction in headache days per month after two adequate treatment cycles, following which the treatment can be stopped assuming to its nonbenefit.

Nerve Blocks (Table 3)

Local nerve blocks using local anesthetics (LA)/steroids in the GON, supraorbital nerve (SON), or sphenopalatine ganglion (SPG) have been used in migraine and other headaches. These blocks take the advantage of functional and anatomical convergence of branches of trigeminal and cervical nerves at the trigeminal cervical complex. The afferent stimuli from the area supplied by cutaneous nerve are blocked thus inhibiting anesthetic sensitization of the C2 dorsal horn convergent neurons by decreasing their input.

Greater Occipital Nerve Block

Use of GON block has been studied in a few ($n = 11$) RCTs, though the trial designs were significantly heterogeneous. The same was suggested by a recent critical review by Chowdhury et al. (2020). They identified nine open-label trials which reported a consistent reduction in frequency and that 35–68% reduction in frequency and severity of headaches in 38–68% cases.[31] Despite the significant heterogeneity, the following observations can be made:
- GON block lead to significant reduction in headache severity, monthly migraine days, and headache frequency.[32,33]
- The addition of steroids to the GON block did not show better outcome. The dose and type of LA/steroid used varied amongst the trials.
- Ultrasonography (USG)-guided approach to administer GON block was found to be effective, though the utility appears to be limited to the patients with anatomical variations, as GON can be easily localized by palpating the occipital artery. There are yet no RCTs comparing blind technique to USG-guided approach.
- A USG-guided proximal approach was introduced in 2010, considering it might provide better results, because of ease of visualization sonographically and on the presumption that smaller divided branches distally may reduce the efficacy of the block. The study by Flamer et al. compared the proximal to distal approach and found no significant difference in the reduction of numerical rating scale (NRS) scores in the two groups although the proximal group showed a sustained effect up to 3 months after single block. However, the proximal approach is technically more demanding because of its close relation with vital structure such as spinal cord and vertebral artery and may be associated with more discomfort due to a deeper location.[34] Thus larger studies are required to compare the efficacy and safety of the two approaches.
- Palamar et al. detected that GON block is effective only on injected site.[35] Inan et al. did not find any significant different between unilateral or bilateral injections.[36] This may suggest that unilateral GON block can be used to minimize the side effects, one may consider bilateral blocks if unilateral block is ineffective.
- The GON tenderness did not affect the results according to the results of Kashipaza et al.,[37] whereas Cuadrado et al.[38] found that GON hypersensitive patients responded 50% less. A systematic study is required to assess the predictive factor for response to GON block.
- Consumption of prophylactic medications did not make any significant difference in the outcome, though study by Chowdhury et al. who systematically reviewed

TABLE 3: Summary of the trials on GON block and SPG block in chronic migraine.

Nerve block	No. of trials	Drugs and dosage used	Site of application	Frequency of application	Primary outcomes used	Results	Adverse effects

GON block	• RCTs—11
	• GON block vs. placebo—6
	• GON block with or without steroids—3
	• Proximal vs. distal block—1
	• TOP as add-on therapy with GON bock—1
		• *Lidocaine 2%:* 1–4.5 mL
		• *Bupivacaine 0.5%:* 1–4.5 mL
		• In combination with or without steroids
		  ○ Steroids used—triamcinolone (40 mg/1 mL) Or
		  ○ MPS 40 mg/1 mL
			• Medial third to distance from Po to mastoid process
			• 2 cm lateral and 2 cm inferior to Po
			• 3 cm below and 1.5 cm inferior to inion
			• USG-guided—distal block—just medial to occipital artery
			• Proximal block—at the level of C2 spinous process GON was identified as a honeycombed structure lying in the interfascial plane between the IOCM and the SSCM
				• Applied once
				• Once weekly for weeks
				• Once monthly for 3 months
					50% reduction in frequency/28 days, reduction in pain, frequency, and duration of headache, mean frequency of monthly headaches, number of headache days	• Significant difference between the GON block and placebo was seen in majority of the studies except one
						• No significant difference was seen between the group with or without steroids
						• Sustained relief was observed in the proximal block group in the USG-guided distal vs. proximal block
							Transient and minor adverse effects were noted

SPG block	• RCT-2 • Both were placebo controlled • Second was extension of the first trial to assess the sustains effects of SPG	0.3 mL of 0.5% bupivacaine	Transnasal approach	12 SPG blocks over a 6-week period (2/week)	• NRS scores at pretreatment baseline vs. 15 minutes, 30 minutes, and 24 hours postprocedure for all 12 treatments • Change in the number of headache days and acute medications usage from treatment to last 28 days of treatment and 1 month post-treatment	NRS scores at 15 minutes, 30 minutes, and 24 hours were significantly reduced but did not achieve statistical significance in headache days over 1 month or 6 months post-treatment	

(GON: greater occipital nerve; IOCM: inferior obliquus capitis muscle; MPS: methylprednisolone; NRS: numerical rating scale; RCT: randomized controlled trial; SSCM: splenius semicapitis muscle; SPG: sphenopalatine ganglion; TOP: topiramate; USG: ultrasonography) addition of GON to usual TOP therapy observed a significant difference in the outcome in the steroid and lidocaine group added on to TOP therapy.[39]

- Studies where single dose of GON block was administered, benefits lasted up to 4–8 weeks,[35,37] whereas in a study by Gul et al. where weekly blocks were given weekly for 4 weeks, a sustained benefit was seen even up to 3 months.[33] This suggested that single injection may show sustained effects but in patients not showing adequate response repeated weekly or monthly injections may be tried.
- A recent, methodologically robust, placebo-controlled RCT by Chowdhury et al. ($n = 44$) showed positive results favoring GON block in CM {mean reduction in the number of headache and migraine days was 4.2 days [95% confidence interval (CI) 7.5–0.8; $p = 0.018$] and 4.7 days [95% CI 7.7 to 1.7; $p = 0.003$], respectively}, in addition their results suggested that the effect accumulated over the time and reported clinically meaningful improvement in patient-reported improvements.[32]
- Chowdhury et al. (2022) conducted a parallel group, RCT comparing TOP alone ($n = 41$) to combination of TOP plus GON block with steroid and lidocaine ($n = 44$) or GON block with only lidocaine ($n = 40$). In conclusion, combination therapies showed greater reduction in monthly migraine days at month 3 compared to TOP alone and were well tolerated.[39]
- None of the study showed any serious adverse effects establishing the safety of the technique.

Sphenopalatine Block in Migraine

Sphenopalatine ganglion has a sensory, parasympathetic, and sympathetic root. The sensory root is connected with the maxillary division of trigeminal nerve and parasympathetic root also has trigeminal innervation. This physiological relationship with trigeminal innervation is the rational for its use in migraine. SPG blockade can be done using transnasal approach, where a cotton pledget soaked with LA is passed just below the middle turbinate through a nasal cannula or blindly to the nasopharynx or transoral approach or infrazygomatic approach under fluoroscopic guidance through pterygomaxillary fissure. Two pilot studies for immediate and sustained effects of SPG block in CM were conducted by Cady et al. They showed a significant effect in the NRS score at 15 minutes, 30 minutes, and 24 hours posttreatment in acute attack of migraine but did not find a sustained effect over 1 month and 6 month though a trend toward long-term benefit was seen. They did not report any serious adverse events. The studies were not adequately powered, and the treatment plan was randomly constructed. These results may give an impetus to conduct efficacy studies first to find an appropriate dosage of SPG block in CM.

Targeted Calcitonin Gene-related Peptide Therapies in Chronic Migraine

As discussed previously, CGRP is a neuropeptide having a key role in migraine pathophysiology. Hence, targeted CGRP molecules have been explored for their potential role in CM treatment. They can be classified into nonpeptide small molecules of oral CGRP antagonists (gepants) and monoclonal antibodies against CGRP (CGRP m-Abs). Gepants have been approved for acute and preventive migraine treatment.[40] However, they are yet to find their role in CM treatment. While being structurally very different to gepants, the CGRP m-Abs have a longer half-life allowing feasible and patient-friendly administration. To date, four agents have been studied for their use in EM and CM, in the pivotal trials, which are summarized in **Table 4**. These drugs are immunoglobulin G (IgG) molecules against either the CGRP ligand (fremanezumab, galcanezumab, and eptinezumab) or its receptor (erenumab). All these molecules showed a significant reduction in their primary study endpoints, which were either a mean reduction in their monthly migraine days or average duration of headache hours. The secondary outcomes as a mean reduction in monthly headache days, days with acute medication use, or migraine-related quality of life scores also showed a favorable trend for their efficacy. Given the robust evidence, fremanezumab, galcanezumab, and erenumab received FDA approval for preventive treatment of migraine in 2018, and eptinezumab in 2020. The key facts for these drugs are illustrated in **Table 5**. Given their favorable tolerability profile and infrequent administration schedule, they represent a convenient treatment option in CM. Patients who either fail to respond to an adequate trial of two appropriately chosen and well-tolerated prophylactics or to at least two sessions of Ona-BT A can be offered anti-CGRP therapies.[53] FOCUS trial was a phase 2b randomized, double-blind, placebo-controlled trial, which evaluated the efficacy of fremanezumab in patients with documented failure to 2–4 prophylactics in EM and CM. The trial reported a significant reduction in monthly migraine days over 12 weeks with quarterly or monthly fremanezumab versus placebo.[54] The drug had a good tolerability and safety profile as well. CONQUER trial similarly reported efficacy of galcanezumab in patients with previous failures to two or more drugs in EM and CM. Studies have also attempted to answer the question regarding the most efficacious CGRP m-Ab in CM.[55] In a recently reported network meta-analysis of RCTs, the data for CM favors erenumab over others at the end of 12 weeks.[56] Head-to-head trials for comparison with the conventional prophylactics in CM are lacking. A recent systematic review concluded that CGRP m-ABS might be slightly better in terms of safety and efficacy than Ona-BT A therapy in CM; however, this needs

TABLE 4: Key findings of landmark studies for CGRP monoclonal antibody use in chronic migraine.		
CGRP m-Ab molecule	Nature of trial	Results
Eptinezumab	Phase 2b randomized, double-blind, parallel group, placebo-controlled, dose-ranging trial[41]	• Significant reduction as compared to placebo in terms of migraine days and headache days in 300 mg, 100 mg, and 30 mg drug group • Most frequent adverse events—upper respiratory tract infections and dizziness; most adverse effects—mild to moderate
	Phase 3 multicentric, randomized, double-blind, placebo-controlled, parallel group trial (PROMISE-2)[42]	• Significant reduction in mean migraine days for both 100 mg and 300 mg doses compared to placebo • Significantly greater 75% migraine responder rate across week 1–4 and week 1–12 for both the doses compared to placebo • Significant reduction in acute medication days for both the doses compared to placebo • Significant reduction in mean HIT-6 score for both the doses compared to placebo • Only adverse event with >2% incidence over placebo-nasopharyngitis (in 300 mg group) • Follow-up study over 24-week period reported sustained benefit[43]
	2 year, open-label phase 3 trial, 48 week treatment phase followed by a second 48-week treatment phase (PREVAIL)[44]	• Drug has favorable safety and tolerability profile, 95.6% of adverse events are mild to moderate in nature • Early and sustained reduction in migraine-related disability and improvement in quality of life • No discernible clinical impact of neutralizing antidrug antibodies
Galcanezumab	Phase 3 randomized, double-blind, placebo-controlled study (REGAIN)[45]	• Significant reduction in monthly migraine headache days, monthly headache days, monthly migraine headache days with acute medication overuse, monthly migraine hours and monthly headache hours as compared to placebo • Significant improvement in migraine-specific quality of life scores across both dosages of drug tested as compared to placebo • Most common adverse event—injection site reaction • Open-label extension of REGAIN study reported high adherence for up to 12 months without any new adverse events[46]
Fremanezumab	Phase 2b multicentric, double-blind, randomized placebo-controlled trial[47]	• Significant reduction in headache hours, headache days, migraine days, moderate-to-severe headache days, and days with acute medication use for both the doses compared with placebo • Most common adverse effects—mild injection site pain and pruritis • A subsequent post hoc analysis demonstrated that the onset of therapeutic effect occurs as early as 1 week of initiation of therapy[48]
	Phase 3 double-blind, parallel group, placebo-controlled trial[49]	• Significant reduction in average number of headache days, migraine days, and headache disability compared to placebo • No direct comparisons between drug dosage group were made • Mild injection site reactions and transient transaminitis
	Multicentric, double-blind, randomized, placebo-controlled, parallel group trial in Japanese and Korean patients[50]	• Significant reduction in average frequency of moderate-to-severe headache days, migraine days per month, number of days with acute medication use per month and HIT-6 score in both the drug groups compared to placebo • Most common side effects—nasopharyngitis and injection site reactions; not precluding treatment
Erenumab	Phase 2 double-blind, placebo-controlled, randomized, multicentric trial[51]	• Both doses significantly reduced monthly migraine days as compared to placebo • Most frequent adverse events—injection site pain, upper respiratory tract infection, and nausea • A subgroup analysis revealed significant reductions in migraine frequency and acute medication days in patients with chronic migraine and medication overuse[52]
(CGRP: calcitonin gene-related peptide)		

TABLE 5: Salient comparison points for four CGRP monoclonal antibodies.

	Erenumab	Fremanezumab	Galcanezumab	Eptinezumab
Studied for	EM, CM	EM, CM, eCH, cCH	EM, CM, eCH, cCH	EM, CM
FDA approval	Preventive migraine treatment	Preventive migraine treatment	• Preventive migraine treatment • Episodic cluster headache	Preventive migraine treatment
Target	CGRP receptor	CGRP peptide	CGRP peptide	CGRP peptide
Antibody type	IgG2	IgG2α	IgG4	IgG1
Human component	100% human	95% human, 5% murine	90% human, 10% murine	90% human, 10% murine
Dose	70 mg/140 mg	225 mg monthly/675 mg quarterly	240 mg loading followed by 120 mg	100 mg/300 mg
Half life	21–23 days	31 days	28 days	31 days
Dosing	Monthly	Monthly or quarterly	Monthly	Quarterly
Route of administration	SC	SC	SC	IV

(CGRP: calcitonin gene-related peptide; cCH: chronic cluster headache; CM: chronic migraine; EM: episodic migraine; eCH: episodic cluster headache; FDA: Food and Drug Administration; IgG: immunoglobulin-G; SC: subcutaneous)

further exploration.[57] Some predictors for positive response to CGRP m-Abs include older age, fewer past treatment failures, and lack of history of immune rheumatological disorders. Positive response to triptans is also a predictor for good therapeutic effect with CGRP m-Abs. As for other prophylactics, these medications should be given an adequate trial of 3–6 months before their benefits are assessed. Some preclinical evidence also suggests that addition of Ona-BT A therapy to CGRP m-Abs may exert synergistic effects in CM. Theoretically, the fact may be plausible as CGRP (fremanezumab) prevents activation of Aδ fibers, while Ona-BT A acts on C-fibers. The theory requires further substantiation as our experience with these novel molecules grows. The drugs are, in general, well tolerated. Nevertheless, their availability and cost concerns may preclude their rampant use in Indian setup. The major concern with erenumab is the occurrence of hypertension. Hence, it is recommended that regular BP measurements must be done in first month of erenumab initiation. Also, it is reasonable to expect that over due course of time these antibodies may be neutralized by development of antidrug antibodies; hence, they might lose their efficacy over time. Although, this has not translated into loss of clinical efficacy as reported by the pivotal trials. However, longer follow-up is required to answer this concern. Furthermore, since their half-life is long, the adverse effects may not immediately cease upon cessation of treatment.

Nonpharmacological Therapies

Neuromodulation

Pharmacological therapies used for treatment of CM are associated with drawbacks such as noncompliance and adverse drug reactions. Nonpharmacological therapies circumvent these inconveniences. Neuromodulation uses electrical, magnetic, or chemical agents for stimulation of central or peripheral pathways, which either modulate or restore the function of aberrant pain pathways.

Transcutaneous Supraorbital Nerve Stimulation

A handful of open-label prospective studies of Cefaly device [transcutaneous supraorbital nerve stimulation (tSNS) device] in CM have shown encouraging results. Di Fiore et al. 2017 ($n = 23$) reported that 34.8% of cases achieved 50% reduction in the headache days with Cefaly device in refractory migraine.[58] Subsequent studies by Danno et al. (both CM and EM, $n = 83$) and Ordas et al. (CM, $n = 25$) showed a significant reduction in headache days, mean number of headache days, migraine days, and reduction in mean number of headache days respectively.[59,60] It is easy to use with acceptability rate of up to 90%. Only mild adverse effects were seen in 7.2–40% of patients across the studies.

Transcutaneous Vagal Nerve Stimulation

Gammacore Sapphire™ is a handheld transcutaneous vagal nerve stimulation (tVNS) device approved for EM in 2017. EVENT study, an RCT, ($n = 59$), did not demonstrate a significant difference between the tVNS and sham treatment group. However, results suggested that more extended use may be beneficial, as 15 completers had a mean change of –7.9 (95% CI –11.9 to –3.8, $p < 0.01$) after 8 months of treatment.[61] PREMIUM II study ($n = 113$, CM and EM), terminated prematurely due to COVID-19, demonstrated a greater responder rate with tVNS (44.87%) compared to sham (26.8%) treatment after 12 weeks.[62]

Transcranial Magnetic Stimulation

Prefrontal lobe dysfunction is involved in the pathogenesis of CM, thus repetitive transcranial magnetic stimulation (rTMS)—dorsolateral prefrontal cortex (DLPFC) has been explored as a treatment strategy for CM. DLPFC stimulation decreases pain perception by modulating the supraspinal pain pathways. A pilot study conducted by Brighina et al. with 11 patients of CM demonstrated positive effect of rTMS in CM.[63] Further studies conducted and demonstrated conflicting results. Deep TMS as add-on therapy was studied by Rapiseni et al. in 2016 ($n = 14$)[64] and was found to be effective. Studies with a larger sample size following a standardized protocol for regular usage are required to establish its effectiveness in CM.

BIOBEHAVIOR THERAPY IN CHRONIC MIGRAINE

Biobehavioral therapy in the form of cognitive behavioral therapy, biofeedback, and relaxation therapies has grade A evidence for use as preventive treatment in migraine as per American Headache Society recommendations.[53] They are particularly suitable for patients who are either intolerant to other pharmacotherapies or have inadequate response to them or else have one/more contraindications to their use. There may be a patient population who might prefer to be on nonpharmacological management, especially the pregnant females or those planning conception. Patients with MOHs are also suitable candidates, as are the patients who are stressed or have poor stress coping skills. Patients with comorbidities or low health-related quality of life are also ideal candidates. These therapies can also be added to the usual standard of care plan, and individualized as per patient preference. The biobehavioral therapies are usually delivered in-person, although virtual platforms have been developed which offer the ease of administration. Mindfulness-based techniques and acceptance and commitment therapies are an active intriguing area of research. Other integrative methods such as acupuncture, yoga, and tai-chi serve as complimentary therapies in migraine management with acceptable measurable effects. Nevertheless, addressing modifiable risk factors to prevent migraine chronification is of utmost importance. The need to start prophylactic migraine treatment cannot be underemphasized. Managing obesity, avoidance of triggers, and exercising regularly should be a part of holistic treatment approach even in CM patients.

Guidelines (adapted from American Headache Society recommendations 2021)[53] for preventive treatment in migraine are as **(Flowchart 1)**:

- Lifestyle modification is an integral part of migraine management. Avoidance of triggers, maintaining hydration and proper nutrition, good sleep hygiene,

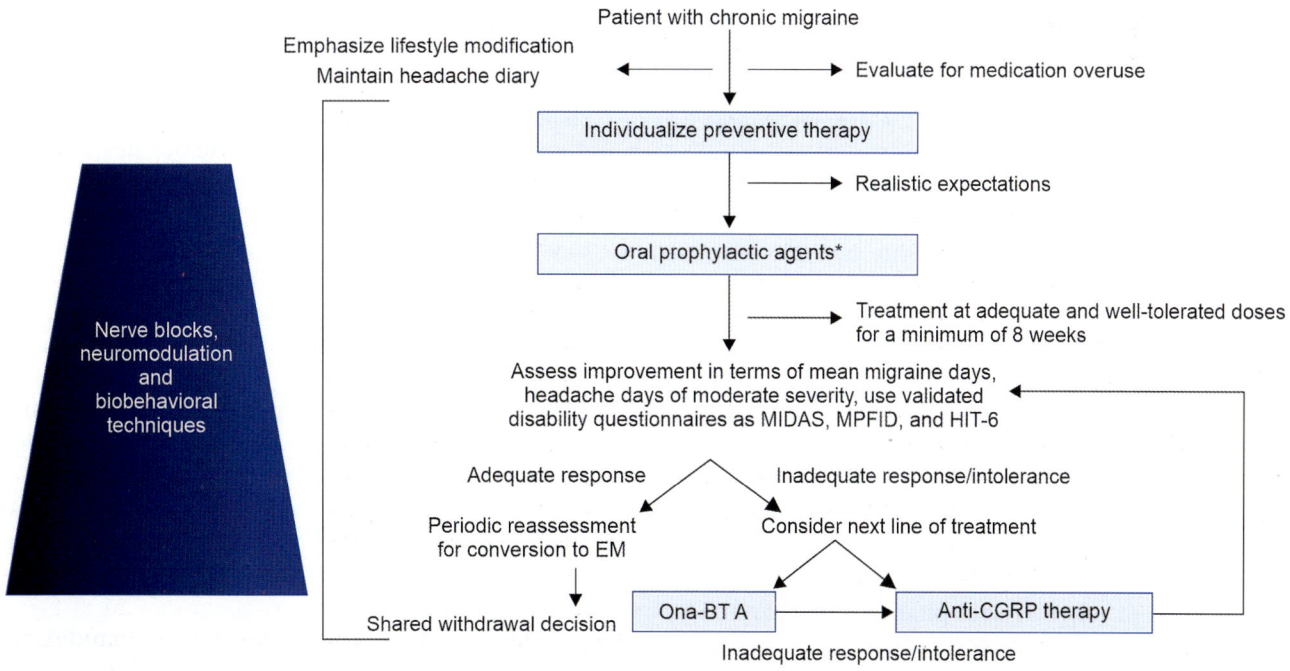

*Refer text for details.

FLOWCHART 1: Preventive treatment in migraine.
(CGRP: calcitonin gene-related peptide; EM: episodic migraine; HIT-6: Headache Impact Test-6; MIDAS: Migraine Disability Assessment; MPFID: Migraine Physical Function Impact Diary; Ona-BT A: onabotulinum toxin A)

- stress management, and regular exercise should be clearly emphasized alongside the pharmacological management.
- Preventive treatment must be individualized tailored to each patient's needs.
- Medication overuse should be actively sought and addressed.
- Guidelines for oral drugs in CM are challenged by the fact that most of the drugs have been studied for EM rather than CM. The best evidence for oral therapy exists for TOP. Oral treatment, in general, should be started at a low dose and titrated up slowly until the target response develops, the maximum or target dose is reached, or tolerability issues emerge. When there is a partial but suboptimal response or dose-limiting side-effects, combining preventive drugs from different classes may be useful.
- With oral treatments, prevention plans should be followed for a minimum of 8 weeks at a target therapeutic dose before lack of effectiveness can be determined. If there is no response to treatment after at least 8 weeks at a target or usual effective dose, switching preventive treatments is recommended. Patients with a partial response should be counseled that cumulative benefits may occur over 6–12 months of continued use.
- Ona-BT A has established efficacy in CM. The optimal initial dose of Ona-BT A is usually 155 units, while follow-the-pain protocol allowing higher doses is also approved in the European Union.
- Patients who fail to respond/tolerate an 8-week trial of two or more oral agents/minimum of 2-quarterly injections (6 months) of Ona-BT A are candidates for anti-CGRP therapy.
- Adequate response is usually defined in terms of reduction in mean migraine headache days or headache days of at least moderate severity by >50% relative to pretreatment baseline. Disability improvement is evaluated through any one of the following questionnaires—MIDAS, MPFID (Migraine Physical Function Impact Diary), or HIT-6.
- Combination of Ona-BT A and anti-CGRP therapy is probably effective for CM treatment.
- It is essential that all preventive pharmacotherapies be given an adequate trial (at least 3–6 months) before the benefits of treatment are assessed.
- Neuromodulation and biobehavioral therapies can be used alone or together with pharmacotherapy and/or other modalities in the acute and preventive treatment of appropriately selected patients.
- Once the control is established, as with the control of any chronic disease, the decision to discontinue or taper treatment should be a shared decision between patient and clinician.

Note: French Headache Society gives a strong recommendation for TOP, Ona-BT A, anti-CGRP therapy in CM, moderate strength of recommendation for valproate and amitriptyline, whereas weak recommendation in relation to propranolol, candesartan, and flunarizine.

BEST PRACTICE PEARLS IN CHRONIC MIGRAINE MANAGEMENT

- Chronic migraine is a disabling disorder, which causes a significant physical, social, and economic impact on the patients.
- There are more marked pathophysiological and neurochemical disturbances in brain of chronic migraineurs than in patients with EM, which accounts for the resistance of this entity to treatment with conventional prophylactics for EM.
- The presence of modifiable risk factors for migraine chronification entails that this is a preventable disorder.
- Patient education is an integral part of CM management.
- Indiscriminate use of analgesics must be condemned.
- Based on the strong evidence, both French and Latin American guidelines advocate TOP as the first line of treatment. However, depending on the patient's comorbidities, other medications such as propranolol, CCBs, VAs, and TCAs may also be tried. Each medication shall be titrated up to the maximally tolerated therapeutic dose and tried for 2–3 months before declaring it as ineffective.
- Patients having issues of noncompliance, intolerability to oral medication, or contraindication can be given a trial of injectables.
- Ona-BT A has level A evidence for usage in CM, being typically offered to patients failing/not tolerating oral agents.
- GON block is also emerging as a treatment option for CM, while further trials are required to standardize the dosing procedure.
- CGRP m-Abs have emerged as a lucrative option in CM treatment, with robust data on their clinical efficacy. However, the availability and cost concerns limit their use.
- Lifestyle modification and biobehavioral modification are supporting pillars in management of CM.

REFERENCES

1. Burch RC, Buse DC, Lipton RB. Migraine: Epidemiology, Burden, and Comorbidity. Neurol Clin. 2019;37(4):631-49.
2. Bonafede M, Sapra S, Shah N, et al. Direct and Indirect Healthcare Resource Utilization and Costs Among Migraine Patients in the United States. Headache. 2018;58(5):700-14.
3. IHS classification ICHD-3. 1.3 Chronic migraine. The International Classification of Headache Disorders, 3rd edition. [online] Available from https://ichd-3.org/1-migraine/1-3-chronic-migraine/ [Last accessed June, 2023].
4. Dodick DW, Loder EW, Manack Adams A, et al. Assessing Barriers to Chronic Migraine Consultation, Diagnosis, and Treatment: Results From the Chronic Migraine Epidemiology and Outcomes (CaMEO) Study. Headache. 2016;56(5):821-34.
5. Lipton RB. Tracing transformation: Chronic migraine classification, progression, and epidemiology. Neurology. 2009;72(5 Suppl):S3-7.
6. Mungoven TJ, Henderson LA, Meylakh N. Chronic Migraine Pathophysiology and Treatment: A Review of Current Perspectives. Front Pain Res. 2021;2:705276.
7. Giacomozzi ARE, Vindas AP, Junior AA da S, et al. Latin American consensus on guidelines for chronic migraine treatment. Arq Neuropsiquiatr. 2013;71:478-86.
8. Silberstein SD, Lipton RB, Dodick DW, et al. Efficacy and Safety of Topiramate for the Treatment of Chronic Migraine: A Randomized, Double-Blind, Placebo-Controlled Trial. Headache. 2007;47(2):170-80.
9. Diener HC, Bussone G, Oene JV, et al. Topiramate Reduces Headache Days in Chronic Migraine: A Randomized, Double-Blind, Placebo-Controlled Study. Cephalalgia. 2007;27(7):814-23.
10. Dodick DW, Silberstein S, Saper J, et al. The Impact of Topiramate on Health-Related Quality of Life Indicators in Chronic Migraine. Headache J Head Face Pain. 2007;47(10):1398-408.
11. Pringsheim T, Davenport WJ, Becker WJ. Prophylaxis of migraine headache. CMAJ Can Med Assoc J. 2010;182(7):E269-76.
12. Yurekli VA, Akhan G, Kutluhan S, et al. The effect of sodium valproate on chronic daily headache and its subgroups. J Headache Pain. 2008;9(1):37-41.
13. Kaniecki RG. A Comparison of Divalproex With Propranolol and Placebo for the Prophylaxis of Migraine Without Aura. Arch Neurol. 1997;54(9):1141-5.
14. Domingues RB, Silva ALP da, Domingues SA, et al. A double-blind randomized controlled trial of low doses of propranolol, nortriptyline, and the combination of propranolol and nortriptyline for the preventive treatment of migraine. Arq Neuropsiquiatr. 2009;67(4):973-7.
15. Silberstein SD, Dodick DW, Lindblad AS, et al. Randomized, placebo-controlled trial of propranolol added to topiramate in chronic migraine. Neurology. 2012;78(13):976-84.
16. Chowdhury D, Bansal L, Duggal A, et al. TOP-PRO study: A randomized double-blind controlled trial of topiramate versus propranolol for prevention of chronic migraine. Cephalalgia Int J Headache. 2022;42(4-5):396-408.
17. Tronvik E, Stovner LJ, Helde G, et al. Prophylactic Treatment of Migraine With an Angiotensin II Receptor Blocker: A Randomized Controlled Trial. JAMA. 2003;289(1):65.
18. Stovner LJ, Linde M, Gravdahl GB, et al. A comparative study of candesartan versus propranolol for migraine prophylaxis: A randomised, triple-blind, placebo-controlled, double cross-over study. Cephalalgia. 2014;34(7):523-32.
19. Xu XM, Yang C, Liu Y, et al. Efficacy and feasibility of antidepressants for the prevention of migraine in adults: a meta-analysis. Eur J Neurol. 2017;24(8):1022-31.
20. Lamsudin R, Sadjimin T. Comparison of the efficacy between flunarizine and nifedipine in the prophylaxis of migraine. Headache. 1993;33(6):335-8.
21. Luo N, Di W, Zhang A, et al. A randomized, one-year clinical trial comparing the efficacy of topiramate, flunarizine, and a combination of flunarizine and topiramate in migraine prophylaxis. Pain Med Malden Mass. 2012;13(1):80-6.
22. Lacković Z, Filipović B, Matak I, et al. Activity of botulinum toxin type A in cranial dura: implications for treatment of migraine and other headaches. Br J Pharmacol. 2016;173(2):279-91.
23. Do TP, Hvedstrup J, Schytz HW. Botulinum toxin: A review of the mode of action in migraine. Acta Neurol Scand. 2018;137(5):442-51.
24. Diener HC, Dodick DW, Aurora SK, et al. OnabotulinumtoxinA for treatment of chronic migraine: results from the double-blind, randomized, placebo-controlled phase of the PREEMPT 2 trial. Cephalalgia Int J Headache. 2010;30(7):804-14.
25. Aurora SK, Dodick DW, Turkel CC, et al. OnabotulinumtoxinA for treatment of chronic migraine: results from the double-blind, randomized, placebo-controlled phase of the PREEMPT 1 trial. Cephalalgia Int J Headache. 2010;30(7):793-803.
26. Blumenfeld AM, Stark RJ, Freeman MC, et al. Long-term study of the efficacy and safety of OnabotulinumtoxinA for the prevention of chronic migraine: COMPEL study. J Headache Pain. 2018;19(1):13.
27. Ahmed F, Gaul C, García-Moncó JC, et al.; on behalf of the REPOSE Principal Investigators. An open-label prospective study of the real-life use of onabotulinumtoxinA for the treatment of chronic migraine: the REPOSE study. J Headache Pain. 2019;20(1):26.
28. ClinicalTrials.gov. (2015). BOTOX® Prophylaxis in Patients with Chronic Migraine. [online] Available from https://clinicaltrials.gov/ct2/show/NCT01432379 [Last accessed June, 2023].
29. Silberstein SD, Dodick DW, Aurora SK, et al. Per cent of patients with chronic migraine who responded per onabotulinum toxin A treatment cycle: PREEMPT. J Neurol Neurosurg Psychiatry. 2015;86(9):996-1001.
30. NICE. (2012). Guidance. Botulinum toxin type A for the prevention of headaches in adults with chronic migraine. [online] Available from https://www.nice.org.uk/guidance/ta260/chapter/1-Guidance [Last accessed June, 2023].
31. Chowdhury D, Mundra A. (2020). Role of greater occipital nerve block for preventive treatment of chronic migraine: A critical review. [online] Available from https://journals.sagepub.com/doi/epub/10.1177/2515816320964401 [Last accessed June, 2023].
32. Chowdhury D, Tomar A, Deorari V, et al. Greater occipital nerve blockade for the preventive treatment of chronic migraine: A randomized double-blind placebo-controlled study. Cephalalgia Int J Headache. 2023;43(2):3331024221143541.
33. Gul HL, Ozon AO, Karadas O, et al. The efficacy of greater occipital nerve blockade in chronic migraine: A placebo-controlled study. Acta Neurol Scand. 2017;136(2):138-44.
34. Flamer D, Alakkad H, Soneji N, et al. Comparison of two ultrasound-guided techniques for greater occipital nerve injections in chronic migraine: a double-blind, randomized, controlled trial. Reg Anesth Pain Med. 2019;44(5):595-603.

35. Palamar D, Uluduz D, Saip S, et al. Ultrasound-guided greater occipital nerve block: an efficient technique in chronic refractory migraine without aura? Pain Physician. 2015;18(2):153-62.
36. Inan LE, Inan N, Karadaş Ö, et al. Greater occipital nerve blockade for the treatment of chronic migraine: a randomized, multicenter, double-blind, and placebo-controlled study. Acta Neurol Scand. 2015;132(4):270-7.
37. Kashipazha D, Nakhostin-Mortazavi A, Mohammadianinejad SE, et al. Preventive effect of greater occipital nerve block on severity and frequency of migraine headache. Glob J Health Sci. 2014;6(6):209-13.
38. Cuadrado ML, Aledo-Serrano Á, Navarro P, et al. Short-term effects of greater occipital nerve blocks in chronic migraine: A double-blind, randomised, placebo-controlled clinical trial. Cephalalgia Int J Headache. 2017;37(9):864-72.
39. Chowdhury D, Mundra A, Datta D, et al. Efficacy and tolerability of combination treatment of topiramate and greater occipital nerve block versus topiramate monotherapy for the preventive treatment of chronic migraine: A randomized controlled trial. Cephalalgia Int J Headache. 2022;42(9):859-71.
40. Moreno-Ajona D, Pérez-Rodríguez A, Goadsby PJ. Small-molecule CGRP receptor antagonists: A new approach to the acute and preventive treatment of migraine. Med Drug Discov. 2020;7:100053.
41. Dodick DW, Lipton RB, Silberstein S, et al. Eptinezumab for prevention of chronic migraine: A randomized phase 2b clinical trial. Cephalalgia Int J Headache. 2019;39(9):1075-85.
42. Lipton RB, Goadsby PJ, Smith J, et al. Efficacy and safety of eptinezumab in patients with chronic migraine: PROMISE-2. Neurology. 2020;94(13):e1365-77.
43. Silberstein S, Diamond M, Hindiyeh NA, et al. Eptinezumab for the prevention of chronic migraine: efficacy and safety through 24 weeks of treatment in the phase 3 PROMISE-2 (Prevention of migraine via intravenous ALD403 safety and efficacy–2) study. J Headache Pain. 2020;21(1):120.
44. Kudrow D, Cady RK, Allan B, et al. Long-term safety and tolerability of eptinezumab in patients with chronic migraine: a 2-year, open-label, phase 3 trial. BMC Neurol. 2021;21(1):126.
45. Detke HC, Goadsby PJ, Wang S, et al. Galcanezumab in chronic migraine. Neurology. 2018;91(24):e2211-21.
46. Pozo-Rosich P, Detke HC, Wang S, et al. Long-term treatment with galcanezumab in patients with chronic migraine: results from the open-label extension of the REGAIN study. Curr Med Res Opin. 2022;38(5):731-42.
47. Bigal ME, Edvinsson L, Rapoport AM, et al. Safety, tolerability, and efficacy of TEV-48125 for preventive treatment of chronic migraine: a multicentre, randomised, double-blind, placebo-controlled, phase 2b study. Lancet Neurol. 2015;14(11):1091-100.
48. Bigal ME, Dodick DW, Krymchantowski AV, et al. TEV-48125 for the preventive treatment of chronic migraine: Efficacy at early time points. Neurology. 2016;87(1):41-8.
49. Silberstein SD, Dodick DW, Bigal ME, et al. Fremanezumab for the Preventive Treatment of Chronic Migraine. N Engl J Med. 2017;377(22):2113-22.
50. Sakai F, Suzuki N, Kim BK, et al. Efficacy and safety of fremanezumab for chronic migraine prevention: Multicenter, randomized, double-blind, placebo-controlled, parallel-group trial in Japanese and Korean patients. Headache. 2021;61(7):1092-101.
51. Tepper S, Ashina M, Reuter U, et al. Safety and efficacy of erenumab for preventive treatment of chronic migraine: a randomised, double-blind, placebo-controlled phase 2 trial. Lancet Neurol. 2017;16(6):425-34.
52. Tepper SJ, Diener HC, Ashina M, et al. Erenumab in chronic migraine with medication overuse. Neurology. 2019;92(20):e2309-20.
53. Ailani J, Burch RC, Robbins MS; Board of Directors of the American Headache Society. The American Headache Society Consensus Statement: Update on integrating new migraine treatments into clinical practice. Headache. 2021;61(7):1021-39.
54. Ferrari MD, Diener HC, Ning X, et al. Fremanezumab versus placebo for migraine prevention in patients with documented failure to up to four migraine preventive medication classes (FOCUS): a randomised, double-blind, placebo-controlled, phase 3b trial. The Lancet. 2019;394(10203):1030-40.
55. Mulleners WM, Kim BK, Láinez MJA, et al. Safety and efficacy of galcanezumab in patients for whom previous migraine preventive medication from two to four categories had failed (CONQUER): a multicentre, randomised, double-blind, placebo-controlled, phase 3b trial. Lancet Neurol. 2020;19(10):814-25.
56. Masoud AT, Hasan MT, Sayed A, et al. Efficacy of calcitonin gene-related peptide (CGRP) receptor blockers in reducing the number of monthly migraine headache days (MHDs): A network meta-analysis of randomized controlled trials. J Neurol Sci. 2021;427:117505.
57. Lu J, Zhang Q, Guo X, et al. Calcitonin Gene–Related Peptide Monoclonal Antibody Versus Botulinum Toxin for the Preventive Treatment of Chronic Migraine: Evidence From Indirect Treatment Comparison. Front Pharmacol. 2021;12:631204.
58. Di Fiore P, Bussone G, Galli A, et al. Transcutaneous supraorbital neurostimulation for the prevention of chronic migraine: a prospective, open-label preliminary trial. Neurol Sci. 2017;38(Suppl 1):201-6.
59. Ordás CM, Cuadrado ML, Pareja JA, et al. Transcutaneous Supraorbital Stimulation as a Preventive Treatment for Chronic Migraine: A Prospective, Open-Label Study. Pain Med Malden Mass. 2020;21(2):415-22.
60. Danno D, Iigaya M, Imai N, et al. The safety and preventive effects of a supraorbital transcutaneous stimulator in Japanese migraine patients. Sci Rep. 2019;9(1):9900.
61. Silberstein SD, Calhoun AH, Lipton RB, et al. Chronic migraine headache prevention with noninvasive vagus nerve stimulation: The EVENT study. Neurology. 2016;87(5):529-38.
62. Najib U, Smith T, Hindiyeh N, et al. Non-invasive vagus nerve stimulation for prevention of migraine: The multicenter, randomized, double-blind, sham-controlled PREMIUM II trial. Cephalalgia Int J Headache. 2022;42(7):560-9.
63. Brighina F, Piazza A, Vitello G, et al. rTMS of the prefrontal cortex in the treatment of chronic migraine: a pilot study. J Neurol Sci. 2004;227(1):67-71.
64. Rapinesi C, Del Casale A, Scatena P, et al. Add-on deep Transcranial Magnetic Stimulation (dTMS) for the treatment of chronic migraine: A preliminary study. Neurosci Lett. 2016;623:7-12.

CHAPTER 13

Management of Cluster Headache: An Update

Debashish Chowdhury, Sanjay Rao Kordcal, Samiran Chowdhury

ABSTRACT

Cluster headache (CH), an uncommon primary headache disorder, classified under a group of disorders known as trigeminal autonomic cephalalgias, is characterized by daily or near-daily one to eight bouts of extremely severe side-locked headaches with ipsilateral cranial autonomic symptoms and signs lasting for 30–180 minutes. These attacks typically occur episodically in clusters lasting weeks to months, followed by remission periods. In about 20% of patients, these remission periods may be absent or be <3 months when it is called chronic CH. During a CH attack, patients typically demonstrate motor restlessness and agitation. The pathophysiology of CH is uncertain but probably involves the hypothalamus (accounting for circadian and circannual rhythmicity) and activation of the trigeminovascular pain pathway along with the trigeminal autonomic reflex (accounting for headache and cranial autonomic symptoms). Treatment of CH consists of acute medications for aborting the attack and preventive treatment to decrease the headache frequency and intensity and to shorten the cluster period. Transitional preventives are also commonly prescribed as a bridge to buy time for the preventive medications to take effect. Though multiple evidence-based treatments are available for these three categories, efficacy, tolerability, and cost remain suboptimum, especially for patients with chronic CHs. More effective and safe treatment options need to be developed.

Keywords: Cluster headache, Acute treatment, Preventive treatment, Transitional treatment, Pathophysiology, Monoclonal antibodies against calcitonin gene-related peptide.

INTRODUCTION

Cluster headache (CH) is an uncommon headache disorder classified under the broad rubric of trigeminal autonomic cephalalgias (TACs), a term first coined by Goadsby and Lipton.[1] CH is characterized by unilateral extremely severe headache attacks, typical ipsilateral cranial autonomic symptoms/signs (CAS), and restlessness. Because of the extreme severity of headaches, TACs have been called the "worst headaches of humankind"[2] and the CH the "suicide headache."[3] The present chapter summarizes the recent updates regarding the management of CH.

DIAGNOSIS AND CLASSIFICATION

The International Classification of Headache Disorders, 3rd edition (ICHD-3) has laid down the diagnostic criteria and classification of CH (**Table 1**).[4] It is important to note that any one of five groups of cranial autonomic features and/or restlessness is required for diagnosis. Also, a CAS described in ICHD-3 beta, namely aural fullness, has been removed from the current classification. CH can occur in two forms, namely episodic and chronic. The definition of chronic CH (CCH) has been modified in ICHD-3. In episodic CH (ECH), attacks usually occur in bouts [cluster periods (CPs)] lasting from 2 weeks to 2 months but

TABLE 1: The International Classification of Headache Disorders, 3rd edition (ICHD-3) diagnostic criteria and the classification of cluster headache.	

Cluster headache	A. At least five attacks fulfilling criteria B–D
	B. Severe or very severe unilateral orbital, supraorbital and/or temporal pain lasting 15–180 minutes (when untreated)[1]
	C. Either or both of the following:
	  1. At least one of the following symptoms or signs, ipsilateral to the headache:
	    i. Conjunctival injection and/or lacrimation
	    ii. Nasal congestion and/or rhinorrhea
	    iii. Eyelid edema
	    iv. Forehead and facial sweating
	    v. Miosis and/or ptosis
	  2. A sense of restlessness or agitation
	D. Occurring with a frequency between one every other day and 8 per day[2]
	E. Not better accounted for by another ICHD-3 diagnosis

Episodic cluster headache	A. Attacks fulfilling criteria for cluster headache and occurring in bouts (cluster periods) B. At least two cluster periods lasting from 7 days to 1 year (when untreated) and separated by pain-free remission periods of ≥3 months.
Chronic cluster headache	A. Attacks fulfilling criteria for cluster headache, and criterion B below B. Occurring without a remission period, or with remissions lasting <3 months, for at least 1 year

may occasionally last long. When these pain-free periods are absent or last <3 months, the patient is diagnosed as suffering from CCH.

EPIDEMIOLOGY

A meta-analysis of population-based studies conducted by Fischera et al.[5] in 2008 estimated the pooled prevalence rate of CH as 0.1%. Although CH commonly affects patients during the third to fifth decade, the age range at presentation has varied from 6 to 74 years.[6] Initial reports suggested a high male predominance, but later studies have shown a male-to-female ratio of 3.4–2.4:1, respectively.[7] Many CH patients are smokers. ECH is the predominant subtype of CH. About 15–20% of patients have CCH. Twin and family studies have suggested a genetic basis for CH, but the degree of heritability is uncertain.

CLINICAL FEATURES

Clinical features of CH have been well characterized in many clinic-based studies.[6-10] Characteristically, CH patients have a severe headache attack (8–10 on the visual analog scale) that is abrupt in onset and can last up to 15–180 minutes (the average attack duration is 30–45 minutes). The headache peaks early, within 5–10 minutes in most attacks in >76% of cases. Usually, it also subsides rapidly. There can be 1–8 attacks per day. Headache is side locked in >80% of cases; however, it may be side-shifting in 15–20%. The orbit-temporal region is affected most often. The character of pain may be variable; many patients describe their pain as being neuralgic (stabbing, sharp, dull, and burning), while others may describe it as throbbing or pulsating. Less commonly, nausea, vomiting, photo, and phonophobia can occur. Photo and phonophobia are characteristically lateralized.

Cluster headache patients can have premonitory symptoms as well as aura. Premonitory symptoms such as blurred vision, watering from the eyes, localized pain, anxiety, and yawning have been reported in CH. Aura has been reported in 6–23% of patients. The most characteristic feature is the "clustering of attacks," for which it bears its name. The headache attacks occur in bouts or periods, usually lasting for weeks or months, followed by periods of complete remission. These are called CPs and remission periods, respectively. A strict circadian and circannual periodicity of attacks may be reported by 50% of patients. Nocturnal attacks may occur in 40–70% of patients. Alcohol (during CP), change in ambient temperature (hot), sleep, emotional stress, insomnia, relaxation, odors (especially of solvents and oil-based paints), smoking, fatigue, altitude, menstruation, flashing lights, histamine, and nitroglycerine have been noted as triggers in various studies.

The hallmark feature of CH is the presence of ipsilateral CAS, which are present only during the attacks (except ptosis which may persist for some time between the attacks). CAS were present in up to 98.8% of CH cases. Lacrimation (80–93%), followed by conjunctival injection (75%), was reported to be CH's most common autonomic feature. Motor restlessness was present in 38.3–94% of CH cases. 42–94% of patients felt a strong tendency to move about, and 50% punched their fists against the wall. Physical activity exacerbated pain in 7–45.8% of cases.

MANAGEMENT

Management of CH includes patient education, especially making them understand the periodic nature of the disease, the distinction between the episodic and the chronic forms, and the optimum use of abortive and preventive medications. They also need to be informed about the potential triggers, avoidance of which can be rewarding. Certain lifestyle habits have been associated with CH, such as excessive smoking, alcohol, and coffee consumption.

These should be addressed during the initial consultation. Many patients during a CP develop significant suicidal ideation, which needs to be addressed, and remedial measures need to be undertaken by the treating physicians. Acute (abortive), transitional, and preventive treatments are available for CH **(Table 2)**.

■ Acute Treatment of Cluster Attacks

Acute treatments abort a cluster attack episode once it has started. These treatments, however, do not affect the duration of the cluster bout. The acute treatment options for terminating a cluster attack are discussed here.

TABLE 2: Treatment options for cluster headache.					
	No. of open-label studies	No. of randomized controlled trial	Efficacy	Adverse effects/precautions and contraindications	Efficacy recommendations based on evidence
Acute treatments					
High-flow oxygen therapy	3	4	Headache relief rate at 15 minutes: 78% vs. 20% (placebo)[13]	Mask discomfort, nasal dryness, oral dryness, eye irritation	A
Sumatriptan injection 6 mg	4	2	Headache relief rate at 15 minutes: 74% vs. 26% (placebo)[21]	Local site reactions, nausea, chest tightness, fatigue, and drowsiness. Rarely vascular events such as TIA and MI can occur. Contraindicated in patients with history of TIA, MI, stroke, and PVD	A
Sumatriptan nasal spray 20 mg	1	1	Pain-free rates at 30 minutes: 47% vs. 18% (placebo)[25]	Chest pressure, bitter taste	B
Intranasal zolmitriptan 5 mg and 10 mg	1	2	Headache relief rates at 30 minutes: 48% for 5 mg; 63% for 10 mg vs. 30% (placebo)[27]	Altered taste sensation	A
Transitional preventive treatments					
Oral steroids	2	1	A treatment benefit of oral prednisolone compared to placebo (100 mg oral prednisone for 5 days followed by tapering of 20 mg every 3 days, or matching placebo) in reducing the CH attacks by 2.4 (95% CI −4.8 to −0.03; $p = 0.002$); complete cessation of cluster headache attacks occurred in 35% of patients compared to 7% receiving placebo at the end of 1 week[34]	Peptic ulcer disease, osteopenia, avascular necrosis, Cushing syndrome, predisposition to infections. Used with caution in patients with GI diseases, hepatic and renal impairment, older adults, and pediatric population	B
Injectable steroids	2	-	Statistically significant difference in attack frequency was noted in two open-label studies	Peptic ulcer disease, osteopenia, avascular necrosis, Cushing syndrome, predisposition to infections	U
GONB with steroids	16	2	85% patients in the first week after 3 days vs. 0 in the placebo group, and 61% remained attack-free at 4 weeks vs. none in the placebo group[35]	Local site reactions, local site bleeding, syncope, dizziness, alopecia	A

Continued

Continued

	No. of open-label studies	No. of randomized controlled trial	Efficacy	Adverse effects/precautions and contraindications	Efficacy recommendations based on evidence
Preventive treatments					
Verapamil	3	2	Significant decrease in attack frequency; 80% complete termination of pain in ECH by 2 weeks[40]	Heart block, hypotension, bradycardia, constipation, peripheral edema. cardiac monitoring with serial ECGs prior to dose escalation	C
Lithium	5	2	• One double-blind trial was negative[43] • 37% got relief compared with 50% receiving verapamil (measured by headache index).[39] 77% of patients achieved either a complete response or >50% reduction in attack frequency in a network meta-analysis of three open studies[45]	Prior to starting therapy, kidney function tests, thyroid function tests, and ECG are necessary. Serial monitoring of drug levels is indicated, and the dose has to be adjusted to maintain the level of lithium between 0.6 and 1.2 mEq/L. AEs are usually dose-related and include cardiovascular side effects such as bradycardia, heart block, and sick sinus syndrome; CNS effects like confusion, memory problems, tremors, hyperreflexia, ataxia, and delirium; renal side effects like nephrogenic diabetes insipidus and hypothyroidism	C
Topiramate	4	0	21–100% response rates in open-label studies	Paresthesias, renal stones, dizziness, cognitive effects, weight loss, mood disorder and anxiety. To be used in caution in older patients and those with hepatic/renal dysfunction	C
Melatonin	2	1	Significant decrease in attack frequency in a double blind trial	Nausea, dizziness. Not to be used in patients with autoimmune disorders and seizures	C
Gabapentin	4	0	Reduced attack frequency and duration of CP in CCH patients	Drowsiness, sexual dysfunction; dizziness, slowness, and constipation	U
Galcanezumab	2	2	Difference in mean change in weekly attack frequency between active and placebo was 3.4 attacks/week; 50% responder rate, 71% in the galcanezumab group and 53% in the placebo group in ECH; ineffective in CCH	Local site pain, nasopharyngitis, and injection site erythema, constipation	B

(A: established as effective; B: probably effective; C: possibly effective; U: insufficient evidence to make recommendation; CCH: chronic cluster headache; CI: confidence interval; CNS: central nervous system; CP: cluster period; ECH: episodic cluster headache; GI: gastrointestinal; GONB: greater occipital nerve block; MI: myocardial infarction; PVD: peripheral vascular disease; TIA: transient ischemic attack)

High-flow Oxygen Therapy

Several randomized controlled trials (RCTs) have shown the effectiveness of oxygen therapy (OT) as an acute treatment option for CH.[11-13] Cohen et al. found that a higher oxygen flow rate of 12 L/min was more effective compared to air at 15 minutes {78% has pain relief at 15 minutes [95% confidence interval (CI) 71-85% for 150 attacks]} versus [20% (95% CI 14-26%; for 148 attacks; $p < 0.001$)].[13] According to both the European Federation of Neurological Sciences (EFNS) and the American Headache Society (AHS) guidelines, high-flow OT has Level A evidence for the acute management of CH.[14-16] The high-flow OT should be delivered through a nonrebreather mask. The most effective mask type is still open to debate. A single-blinded, semi-randomized, placebo-controlled, crossover inpatient study compared 100% OT delivered by demand valve oxygen (DVO), O$_2$ptimask, or simple mask (15 L/min) or placebo delivered by DVO for 15 minutes. There was no difference between the three mask types for the primary endpoint of pain relief at 15 minutes. However, the post hoc analysis suggested that O$_2$ptimask and DVO decreased the need for rescue medication.[17] The mechanism of action of OT is presently unknown. It has been suggested that hyperoxia can inhibit dural plasma protein extravasation, and one study showed a significant reduction of calcitonin gene-related peptide (CGRP) concentration in the jugular vein after oxygen treatment.[18] It is noteworthy that hyperbaric oxygen treatment in CCH patients was not efficacious.[19] A recent international survey involving 3,251 CH patients found that OT is ineffective or minimally effective in 19% of patients.[20] OT is practically devoid of adverse effects (AEs). It should be avoided in patients with chronic obstructive airway disease.

Triptans

Triptans have a selective agonist effect on 5-HT$_{1B}$ and 5-HT$_{1D}$ serotonin receptors. These receptors are present ubiquitously in the brainstem and trigeminal complex. The probable pain relief mechanisms are inhibition of trigeminal nerve (TN) endings in large cerebral vessels, direct vasoconstriction of these associated vessels, and neuronal inhibition of more central hypothalamic lesions. They also influence the peripheral nociceptors inhibiting the release of neuropeptides, such as CGRP and substance P.

The triptans approved for use in CH include:
- Subcutaneous sumatriptan
- Intranasal sumatriptan
- Intranasal zolmitriptan

Subcutaneous Sumatriptan

A subcutaneous injection of 6 mg of sumatriptan is the most efficacious CH treatment. The Sumatriptan Cluster Headache Study Group conducted the first randomized placebo-controlled trial in 1991.[21] 39 CH patients were included in this study. Two cluster attacks were treated randomly with 6 mg of sumatriptan subcutaneously or placebo. The primary endpoint (freedom from pain or almost complete relief from headache within 10 or 15 minutes) was achieved in 74% of patients treated with sumatriptan versus 26% for placebo. In another dose comparison RCT, the authors found no benefit of a 12-mg subcutaneous (SC) sumatriptan injection over a 6-mg injection.[22] A Cochrane review reported pain-free results after 15 minutes for 48% with sumatriptan versus 17% with placebo, resulting in a number needed to treat (NNT) of 3.3.[23] A new formulation of 3 mg subcutaneous sumatriptan is now available in some countries and is helpful in migraine patients (a proof of concept RCT). However, its efficacy for acute cluster attacks remains to be established.

Intranasal Sumatriptan

Intranasal sumatriptan in a dose of 20 mg was first investigated as an abortive therapy for CH in an open-label pilot study in 2002. It was found to be less efficacious than subcutaneous sumatriptan.[24] A double-blind, randomized, placebo-controlled trial with 118 patients with 154 attacks was conducted. The responder rates at 30 minutes were 57% for sumatriptan and 26% for placebo ($p = 0.002$). Pain-free rates at 30 minutes were 47% for sumatriptan and 18% for placebo ($p = 0.003$). Sumatriptan was superior to placebo for most of the secondary outcomes.[25]

Intranasal Zolmitriptan

Two randomized placebo-controlled trials investigated the efficacy of intranasal zolmitriptan at two doses (5 mg and 10 mg) in the acute treatment of CH.[26,27] One study, which included 92 patients, achieved pain relief (from very severe-moderate to mild-none) in 62% of patients with 10 mg of zolmitriptan and 40% with 5 mg of zolmitriptan. The placebo response was 21% in the study.[26] In the second study, the primary endpoint (headache relief at 30 minutes) was met by 63% of patients treated with 10 mg, 50% with 5 mg, and 30% with placebo.[27] A meta-analysis of the above two studies included 121 patients.[28] An odds ratio for pain relief of 8.68 and 3.48 for 10 mg and 5 mg of zolmitriptan, respectively, was found.

Contraindications

Contraindications of triptan use include coronary artery disease, past myocardial infarction (MI), transient ischemic attacks (TIAs), poorly controlled hypertension, severe hepatic impairment, and concomitant use of ergotamine derivatives or monoamine oxidase (MAO) inhibitors.

Adverse Effects

Following SC injection, there are local injection site reactions. The most common adverse events associated with sumatriptan use are nausea, chest tightness, feeling of warmth, fatigue, and drowsiness. Rarely, it can lead to vascular events such as MI, TIA, ischemic colitis, and stroke. However, no MI or stroke has been reported following triptan use in CH. Nasal formulations can alter taste sensations in a few patients.

Other Agents for Acute Treatment

Somatostatin, an endogenously occurring 14-amino acid peptide, has been shown to inhibit the release of numerous vasoactive peptides, including CGRP and VIP. Two small, randomized, double-blind trials suggested the efficacy of somatostatin in CH.[29,30] Octreotide, a somatostatin analog with a half-life of approximately 1.5 hours, which can be given subcutaneously, has been studied for the acute treatment of CH. One Class II RCT examined the effect of SC octreotide in the acute treatment of CH.[31] Patients were instructed to treat two attacks of at least moderate pain severity, with at least a 24-hour break, using subcutaneous octreotide or a matching placebo. The headache response rate (RR) with subcutaneous octreotide was 52%, whereas that with placebo was 36%. Another somatostatin analog, pasireotide, was found to be nonefficacious in a phase 2 trial, which was terminated.

Dihydroergotamine aerosol spray in two to three aerosol doses (0.35 mg each) with deep inhalation at the onset of an attack has been found to decrease the intensity of the attack. However, the frequency and the duration of the attack were not reduced.[32]

Four sprays of intranasal lidocaine solution (4%) with the provision of using two more, if necessary, were used intranasally ipsilaterally as an abortive therapy for CH. 27% reported moderate relief, 27% mild relief, and 46% had no relief from the lidocaine; side effects were minimal. Thus, lidocaine spray was marginally helpful.[33]

■ Transitional Treatment

Transitional treatment is offered to ECH patients currently in their CP and CCH patients who require preventive therapy to reduce the frequency and severity of attacks. However, the preventives used in CH need slow up-titration of their doses to prevent AEs. This gives rise to the need for a treatment that will bridge the time until long-term preventive therapy becomes effective.

Corticosteroids

A few open-label trials have investigated the efficacy of corticosteroids as a transitional preventive therapy in CH. However, the AHS treatment guideline published in 2016 has a Level U guideline for corticosteroids as a prophylactic treatment because, at that time, no RCT was available.[15] According to the EFNS guidelines, 100 mg methylprednisolone (or equivalent corticosteroid) given orally or at up to 500 mg intravenous (IV)/day over 5 days (then tapering down) is recommended.[14] Obermann et al.[34] conducted a multicenter, double-blind, randomized, controlled trial between April 2013 and January 2018 in which they enrolled 118 episodic CH patients. Patients with ECH aged between 18 and 65 years and within a current pain episode for not >30 days received 100 mg oral prednisone for 5 days followed by tapering of 20 mg every 3 days or a matching placebo (17 days total exposure). All the patients received oral verapamil for long-term prevention. The primary endpoint was the mean number of attacks within the first week of treatment with prednisone compared with placebo. 109 patients were included in the modified intention-to-treat analysis. Participants in the prednisone group had a mean of 7.1 [standard deviation (SD) 6.5] attacks within the first week compared with 9.5 (6.0) attacks in the placebo group (difference −2.4 attacks, 95% CI −4.8 to −0.03; $p = 0.002$). These findings support the use of prednisone as a first-line treatment in parallel to the up-titration of verapamil.

Greater Occipital Nerve Block with Steroids

Greater occipital nerve block (GONB) has been used for various headache disorders, including CH. The rationale for using GONB as a headache treatment comes from the proximity of sensory neurons in the upper cervical spinal cord to trigeminal nucleus caudalis (TNC) neurons and the convergence of sensory input to TNC neurons from cervical and trigeminal fibers. GONB is believed to modulate the pain pathway. Two RCTs are available for the use of GONB in CH.[35,36] Ambrosini et al. reported that a mixture of long-acting and rapid-acting steroids (betamethasone) with 0.5 mL of 2% lignocaine, a single suboccipital injection, completely suppressed attacks in 85% (11/13) patients in the first week after 3 days versus 0/10 in the placebo group. Eight (61%) remained attack free at 4 weeks versus none in the placebo group.[35] Leroux et al., on the other hand, demonstrated the efficacy and safety of repeated suboccipital injections (2 or 3 times over 2–4 days) of only steroid (cortivazol) in a randomized, double-blind, placebo-controlled trial as add-on therapy in patients having frequent daily CH attacks (mean of >2 attacks per day for 3 days preceding the day of inclusion). The primary outcome was reducing the mean number of attacks per day to two or fewer during the second, third, and fourth days after the third injection (around 9–12 days after randomization). 95% of the patients, compared to 55% of the placebo group, achieved the primary outcome.[36]

■ Preventive Therapy

The established drugs used for long-term preventive treatment of CH are:
- Verapamil
- Lithium
- Melatonin
- Topiramate

Verapamil

Verapamil, a calcium-channel blocker, is the first-line maintenance preventive for CH. Due to its efficacy, relative safety, and ability to be coadministered with other acute/transitional treatments of CH with negligible drug interactions, it is considered a first-line therapy. Both the EFNS and the AHS recommend using verapamil in the long-term preventive treatment of CH. The putative mechanism of actions of verapamil includes the blockade of presynaptic calcium channels that prevents CGRP release, possibly inhibiting the CGRP-induced hyper-responsive state. Furthermore, calcium channels appear to play a role in the circadian rhythm, which is hypothesized to play a significant role in the pathophysiology of CH.

The use of verapamil as a preventive treatment was first investigated in 1983 by Meyer et al.[37] in a prospective open-label study. All the patients in the verapamil subgroup experienced reduced headache frequency. The dosage used in this study ranged between 160 and 720 mg/day. Following this, two open-label studies, one placebo-controlled study and one double-blind, double-dummy crossover trial, were conducted to investigate the efficacy of verapamil in CH.[38-41] Verapamil significantly reduced the cluster attack frequency and the need for abortive treatment.

The dose of verapamil used ranged from 200 to 960 mg. In clinical practice, it is usually started at a dose of 40–80 mg three times a day and gradually titrated upward till there is relief from headaches. Verapamil can lead to heart block. Hence monitoring of therapy with electrocardiogram (ECG) is required. Though an international Delphi study[42] on cardiac monitoring in verapamil therapy reached a consensus only on the requirement of an ECG prior to initiation of therapy, it is considered a good clinical practice to get an ECG done following dose increments every 2 weeks. Other AEs of verapamil include hypotension, constipation, bradycardia, peripheral edema, and gingival hyperplasia.

Lithium

Lithium is the second choice for the prophylactic treatment of CH. It has a more unfavorable side effect profile compared to verapamil. The effect of lithium on rapid eye movement (REM) sleep, its affinity to opiate receptors, and its effect on serotonin levels in the hypothalamus are some of the hypotheses that have been put forward to explain its efficacy in CH.

The efficacy of lithium in CH, except for one placebo-controlled trial,[43] has been mainly investigated in small open-label trials and case reports. A placebo-controlled trial showed no significant improvement with lithium therapy at the end of 1 week. However, lithium levels were low, and 1 week was considered too short to assess the preventive efficacy of lithium for CH. A retrospective case series showed that lithium treatment led to a significant reduction in attack frequency.[44] A network meta-analysis of three open-label studies on lithium in CH reported that 77% of patients on lithium achieved either a complete response or >50% reduction in attack frequency.[45]

The dose of lithium is 300–900 mg/day. Before starting treatment with lithium, it is essential to get kidney function tests and thyroid function tests. In patients above 50 years of age, an ECG is also necessary. Monitoring therapeutic levels includes trough plasma levels drawn 8–12 hours after the last dose. The therapeutic range is 0.6–1.2 mEq/L for chronic therapy. Monitoring should be done every 1–2 weeks until the desired therapeutic levels are reached. Then, lithium levels need to be checked every 2–3 months for 6 months. It is also essential to monitor patients for dehydration and lower the dose when there are signs of infection, excessive sweating, or diarrhea. Toxic levels are when the drug level is >2 mEq/L. Lithium can cause a wide variety of AEs. These are usually dose related and include cardiovascular side effects such as bradycardia, heart block, and sick sinus syndrome; CNS effects such as confusion, memory problems, tremors, hyperreflexia, ataxia, and delirium; renal side effects such as nephrogenic diabetes insipidus and hypothyroidism.

Topiramate

Topiramate is an antiseizure medication that blocks voltage-dependent sodium channels, enhances the activity of gamma-aminobutyric acid (GABA) at a non-benzodiazepines (BZDs) site, and antagonizes N-methyl-D-aspartate (NMDA)-glutamate receptor. There are predominantly open-label studies and case reports on the role of topiramate as a preventive therapy for CH. An initial open-label study with 10 patients showed a positive response at 3 weeks. Subsequent studies showed similar trends.[46-48] Topiramate is usually started at 25 mg. It gradually increases by 25–50 mg every 3–7 days to a maximum of 200 mg/day. The most common AEs due to topiramate therapy are paresthesias, cognitive effects, dizziness, and renal stones. Topiramate is associated with psychiatric disturbances such as aggressive behavior, mood disorder, and anxiety.

Melatonin

Cluster headache attacks often follow a circadian rhythm, and these effects are considered to be due to alterations in hypothalamic sleep regulation mechanisms. Hence, the use of melatonin to prevent CH was investigated. Two case series and one RCT[49] have investigated the effect of melatonin on CH. According to the AHS guidelines, melatonin has Level C evidence for its use as a preventive treatment option in CH.

■ Other Treatments

Sodium Valproate

A randomized, double-blind, placebo-controlled study on the effect of sodium valproate in CH included 96 patients

(17 CCH), 50 in the sodium valproate group and 46 in the placebo group.[50] Treatment was given for 2 weeks with a daily dose of 1,000–2,000 mg of sodium valproate. The primary study endpoint was at least a 50% reduction in the mean number of cluster attacks per week. There was no statistical difference between sodium valproate and placebo for this endpoint. Hence, valproate is not recommended in the treatment of CH.

Gabapentin

Four open-labeled studies have shown moderate efficacy of gabapentin in a dose of 1,000–1,800 mg/day in ECH and CCH.[51-54] Patients with CCH were refractory to established drugs. Gabapentin decreased the attack frequency as well as reduced the duration of CP. Thus, though no randomized trials are available, gabapentin may be considered in refractory CCH patients.

■ Newer Treatment Options in Cluster Headache

Monoclonal Antibodies Against Calcitonin Gene-related Peptide in Cluster Headache

Studies have been conducted on the efficacy of various monoclonal antibodies (mAbs) in CH. The mAbs investigated include galcanezumab, fremanezumab, and eptinezumab. CGRP levels were found to be raised in CH patients during their CPs. Increased CGRP levels were seen in the tears of CH patients compared to healthy controls. These returned to normal levels after abortive treatment for the attack. Galcanezumab, a humanized mAb against CGRP, has been investigated as a potential treatment for ECH and CCH.

Goadsby et al.[55] conducted a multicenter, randomized, double-blind, placebo-controlled trial in 2019 investigating the efficacy of 300 mg SC galcanezumab injection in preventing ECH. Patients who had at least one attack every other day, a minimum of four attacks, and a maximum of eight attacks during the baseline period, with CPs lasting for at least 6 weeks, were included in the study. They were assigned to receive 300 mg SC galcanezumab or placebo at baseline and 1 month. The primary endpoint was the mean change from baseline in the weekly frequency of CH attacks across weeks 1 through 3 after receipt of the first dose. The key secondary endpoint was the percentage of patients who had a reduction from baseline of at least 50% in the weekly frequency of CH attacks at week 3. Of 106 enrolled patients, 49 were randomly assigned to receive galcanezumab, and 57 received a placebo. The mean reduction in the weekly frequency of CH attacks across weeks 1 through 3 was 8.7 attacks in the galcanezumab group, as compared with 5.2 in the placebo group (difference, 3.5 attacks per week; 95% CI 0.2–6.7; $p = 0.04$). The percentage of patients with a reduction of at least 50% in headache frequency at week 3 was 71% in the galcanezumab group and 53% in the placebo group. They concluded that SC galcanezumab was effective as a preventive treatment for ECH.

Dodick et al.[56] conducted a prospective, double-blind, randomized, placebo-controlled trial of SC galcanezumab in CCH patients. 237 patients were enrolled in the study (172 males and 55 females). Up to six protocol-specified concomitant preventive medications were allowed if patients were on a stable dose for 2 months before the prospective baseline period. Patients were randomized 1:1 to monthly subcutaneous galcanezumab (300 mg) or placebo. 237 patients were randomized and treated (120 placebos; 117 galcanezumab). The primary endpoint was unmet; the mean change in weekly attack frequency was −4.6 placebo versus −5.4 galcanezumab ($p = 0.334$). Key secondary endpoints also were not met. They concluded that 300 mg SC galcanezumab is ineffective in preventing CCH.

Riesenberg et al.[57] conducted a Phase 3b open-label study to evaluate the long-term safety of galcanezumab in patients with CH who completed one of two Phase 3 double-blind studies in ECH or CCH. The study's primary endpoint was safety. 164 patients who had received at least one dose of 300 mg SC galcanezumab were enrolled. Treatment-emergent adverse events [$n = 119$ (72.6%)] were mainly mild to moderate, with nasopharyngitis the most reported (22.0%). One of 18 serious adverse events was judged as treatment related (constipation). Two patients (1.2%) reported suicidal ideation. Five patients (3.1%) discontinued due to an adverse event. The authors found galcanezumab was generally well tolerated and safe in CH patients.

In their retrospective open-label study, Mo et al.[58] investigated the preventive efficacy and tolerability of two 120 mg galcanezumab doses for ECH in clinical practices. 47 ECH patients were included in the study. The median time to the first occurrence of 100% reduction from baseline in CH attacks per week after galcanezumab therapy was 17 days (25 to 75% quartile range: 5.0 ~ 29.5) in all patients with ECH, 15.5 days (3.8 ~ 22.1) in 36 patients with galcanezumab therapy add-on conventional preventive therapy, 21.0 days (12.0 ~ 31.5) in 11 patients started galcanezumab as initial preventive therapy. They concluded that one 240 mg dose of galcanezumab with or without conventional therapy for the prevention of CH was considered effective and safe in clinical practice.

The most common AEs of galcanezumab included local site pain, nasopharyngitis, and injection site erythema. Constipation has also been noted in a small proportion of patients.

Other Monoclonal Antibodies

Erenumab was helpful in a patient with CH and a patient with CH with coexistent migraine in two single case reports. Fremanezumab had a negative trial for both ECH and CCH. IV eptinezumab is currently under investigation for its efficacy in CH.

Surgery, Neurostimulation, and Neuromodulation

Various surgeries were tried in patients of CCH who were refractory to the available drugs. Recent advances include various noninvasive and invasive neurostimulation/modulation devices **(Table 3)**. A brief summary follows.

Radiofrequency Lesioning, Radiosurgery, and Section

Destructive procedures have been used for refractory CH patients, especially patients with CCH. Although immediate improvement was provided by these procedures, such as surgical rhizotomy[59] or section[60] of the TN but sustained improvement was not maintained. Further, several complications were reported, such as severe hypoesthesia, anesthesia dolorosa, keratitis, and motor (mastication difficulties).

Microvascular Decompression

Microvascular decompression (MVD) of the TN or the nervous intermedius (NI) was done in a series of 28 CCH patients.[61] Initially, 73% of them reported an improvement of >50%. However, the favorable outcome did not maintain over time, despite repeated procedures. Targeting NI was more rewarding than targeting TN.

Stereotactic Radiosurgery of Intracisternal Portion of Trigeminal Nerve

Three case series are available involving 24 patients treated with stereotactic radiosurgery (SRS) with a mean follow-up of 3 years.[62-64] More than 50% improvement was seen in only 20% of patients, and up to 20% developed neuropathic pain.

Sphenopalatine Ganglion Neuromodulation

The CAS associated with CH attacks probably result from activating a trigeminal autonomic reflex. The

TABLE 3: Neuromodulation in cluster headache.

	Clinical trails	Efficacy	Adverse effects	Efficacy recommendations based on evidence
Sphenopalatine ganglion stimulation for treating acute attacks and prevention	One randomized, sham-controlled study in refractory CCH patients and one double-blind, randomized controlled trial in CCH patients	• 68% had a clinically significant improvement, but only 32% achieved pain relief in >50% of the treated attacks, and 43% experienced a reduction of >50% in attack frequency[67] • Pain relief, defined as reduction from a minimum of moderate pain to none or mild pain, at 15 minutes poststimulation was documented in 62% of CCH patients; the response in terms of median frequency reduction was at least 75%[68]	• Transient, mild/moderate loss of sensation within the maxillary (V-2) nerve • Four serious adverse events that were related to the procedure or implantation device: aspiration during intubation, nausea and vomiting, and venous injury or compromise and an infection	B
Noninvasive vagus nerve stimulation for treating acute attacks	One open-label randomized controlled study and two-double-blind sham-controlled RCTs	Odds of achieving pain-free attacks in 15 minutes (OR 9.8; 95% CI 2.2–44.1; $p = 0.01$) compared to sham stimulation in ECH[74]	Application-site discomfort and redness	A
Occipital nerve stimulation for prevention	All open-label studies*	An overall >50% responder rate of about 75%	Lead migration, local infection, and development of tolerance	C**
DBS of posterior hypothalamus for prevention	• Mainly open-label case series • One double-blind, randomized, placebo-controlled trial	• In a review of about 50 patients who underwent DBS for refractory CCH, 60% had at least 50% responder rate and 30% were almost pain free at the most extended follow-up[70] • No significant change in the weekly attack frequency during DB phase but long-term efficacy in >50% patients[71]	Intracerebral hemorrhage due to the implantation procedure subcutaneous infection, transient loss of consciousness, and micturition syncope	U

*Very difficult to perform a double-blind study as a mandatory clinical improvement requires feeling of paresthesia in the neck.
**Due to technical difficulty of performing a double-blind study, the recommendation relied on the available open-label studies.

(A: established as effective; B: probably effective; C: possibly effective; U: insufficient evidence to make recommendation; CCH: chronic cluster headache; DBS: deep brain stimulation; ECH: episodic cluster headache; OR: odds ratio; RCT: randomized controlled trial)

parasympathetic efferent component of this reflex is mediated, at least in part, through the sphenopalatine ganglion (SPG). SRS of the SPG and TN seems slightly more efficient than SRS of TN alone. In two series involving 25 patients,[65,66] thermolesion of the SPG, using a percutaneous infra-zygomatic approach, decreased the mean frequency of CCH attacks by half (mean follow-up 12 and 24 months, respectively). However, AEs were significantly high: epistaxis (80%), lesion of the maxillary division of the TN (40%), and transient hypoesthesia of the palatine area (90%). Encouraged by the results of the destructive procedures on the SPG, new nonlesional procedures targeting the SPG were developed and investigated.

The first case of chronic SPG stimulation with an implantable device was published in 2007. Subsequently, an implantable neuromodulation device specifically designed for acute SPG stimulation has been developed in order to abort the CH attacks on demand. The device is implanted in the pterygopalatine fossa along the posterior wall of the maxillary bone. It is fixed to the zygomatic process with a screwed plate, the lead being placed in contact with the SPG. A remote controller using radiofrequency energy activates it. A multicenter randomized, sham-controlled study using an SPG neurostimulator was undertaken in 28 patients suffering from refractory CCH.[67] Each CH attack was randomly treated with full, subperception, or sham stimulation. 67.1% of full stimulation-treated attacks had pain relief compared to 7.4 % of sham-treated and 7.3% of subperception-treated attacks ($p < 0.0001$). 19 of 28 (68%) patients experienced a clinically significant improvement, but only 32% achieved pain relief in >50% of the treated attacks, and 43% experienced a reduction of >50% in attack frequency. Most patients (81%) experienced transient, mild/moderate loss of sensation within the maxillary (V-2) nerve territory, resolving in most patients within 3 months. A recent RCT showed that the pain relief, defined as reduction from a minimum of moderate pain to none or mild pain, at 15 minutes poststimulation was documented in 62% of CCH patients; the response in terms of median frequency reduction was at least 75%.[68] Four serious adverse events that were related to the procedure or implantation device included aspiration during intubation, nausea, vomiting, and venous injury or compromise and an infection.

Deep Brain Stimulation

Functional imaging revealed that activation occurs in the posterior hypothalamus during the CH attacks. Leone et al.[69] used deep brain stimulation (DBS) to modulate this region in a patient with refractory CCH, which led to complete relief from attacks. Other case reports have highlighted DBS's role in managing refractory CCH. In a review of about 50 patients who underwent DBS for refractory CCH, 60% had at least 50% responder rate and 30% were almost pain free at the most extended follow-up.[70] Complications included gaze disturbances, autonomic disturbances, and intracranial hemorrhage. This prompted a double-blind, randomized, placebo-controlled trial of DBS in CCH. Fontaine et al.[71] conducted a randomized, placebo-controlled, double-blind, multicenter trial assessing the efficacy and safety of unilateral hypothalamic DBS in 11 patients with severe refractory CCH. Active and sham stimulation were compared during 1-month periods followed by a 1-year open-label extension. Change in the weekly attack frequency was the primary endpoint. The active and placebo groups observed no significant change in primary endpoint measurement. Three serious AEs were reported. The findings of this study thus did not support the efficacy of DBS in refractory CCH. Currently, DBS is not approved for use in refractory CCH.

Occipital Nerve Stimulation

Occipital nerve stimulation (ONS) delivers a continuous electrical stimulation to the greater occipital nerve (GON) and/or to the lesser occipital nerve (LON) via a subcutaneous chronically implanted electrode adjacent to the nerve and connected to a generator. It has been used for many refractory headache syndromes, including CCH. Open-labeled studies showed an overall >50% responder rate of about 75%.[70] ONS does not stop the CP once it has begun but decreases the frequency of the CH attacks and their intensity. ONS results in the feeling of paresthesia in the neck, a mandatory clinical improvement requirement. Hence, it is challenging to perform a placebo-controlled trial of ONS. Some patients described a headache recurrence following lead migration or electrode dysfunction (and a consequent lack of paresthesia), suggesting the actual effect rather than the placebo effect of the procedure. Three important problems with ONS are lead migration, local infection, and development of tolerance (requiring progressively increased stimulation intensity and rapid depletion of battery). ONS is a reasonable option in medically refractory CCH patients.

■ Noninvasive Vagal Nerve Stimulation

The vagus nerve consists of an intricate neuroendocrine-immune network that maintains homeostasis. It acts as a control center that integrates interoceptive information and responds with appropriate adaptive modulatory feedback. Invasive vagal nerve stimulation (VNS) for managing epilepsy and depression showed a serendipitous reduction in headache frequency and duration. The significant effects of VNS on headache possibly occur due to the following mechanisms: effects on autonomic nervous system functions; inhibition of cortical spreading depression (CSD); neurotransmitter regulation; and nociceptive modulation. Noninvasive VNS (nVNS), which stimulates the carotid vagus nerve with a handheld device (gammaCore), has demonstrated efficacy for acute migraine or CH attacks.

One open-label randomized controlled study[72] and two double-blind sham-controlled RCTs [The Acute Treatment of Cluster Headache Studies (ACT1 and ACT2)][73-75] have been conducted recently, both of which show that the efficacy of nVNS in pain relief is superior to placebo in ECH patients. In ACT1, gammaCore resulted in a higher RR (RR 3.2; 95% CI 1.6–8.2; $p = 0.014$), higher pain-free rate for >50% of attacks (RR 2.3; 95% CI 1.1–5.2; $p = 0.045$), and shorter duration of attacks [mean difference (MD) –30 minutes; $p < 0.01$] compared with the sham group. In ACT2, gammaCore resulted in higher odds of achieving pain-free attacks in 15 minutes [odds ratio (OR) 9.8; 95% CI 2.2–44.1; $p = 0.01$], lower pain intensity in 15 minutes (MD –1.1; $p < 0.01$), and higher rate of achieving responder status at 15 minutes for ≥50% of treated attacks (RR 2.8; 95% CI 1.0–8.1; $p = 0.058$) compared with the sham group.[71] Subsequently, an open-label study, The PREVention and Acute Treatment of Chronic Cluster Headache (PREVA), demonstrated the superiority of gammaCore plus standard of care over the standard of care alone in patients with CCH. No treatment-related severe adverse events were reported in trials involving nVNS (both in migraine and CH). The most common adverse drug events (ADEs) reported included application site discomfort and redness. nVNS is Food and Drug Administration (FDA) approved for the acute treatment of ECH.

Other Investigational Treatments

Two small open-labeled studies have found ketamine infusions moderately effective in CH patients.[76,77] A study using intranasal ketamine spray in CCH is underway. Onabotulinum toxin-A (OBT-A) in CH had mixed results. A small study involving 17 patients found that 59% had a >50% responder rate.[78] Another study, however, was negative.[79] OBT-A injection in SPG using a especially designed instrument is being investigated. A survey by Clusterbusters.org involving 496 CH patients reported good efficacy of indoleamine hallucinogens, namely psilocybin, lysergic acid diethylamide, and lysergic acid amide in shortening or aborting CP.[80] However, these agents are prohibited by regulatory agencies because of many serious AEs and high addiction potential. The Modified Atkins diet (MAD) role for 12 weeks was studied in 18 drug-resistant CCH patients in an open-label design. Eleven patients experienced a complete resolution of headache; four had a headache reduction of at least 50%.[81] Case reports of acupuncture in CH have been published; however, no major series or RCTs are available.[82] There are open-label studies of transcranial magnetic stimulation, direct current stimulation, spinal cord stimulation, and supraorbital nerve stimulation in CCH patients.[83] However, RCTs are required, which can be challenging because of the rarity of the disorder.

CONCLUSION

Although many options are available for treating acute attacks and preventing CH, these are suboptimum in efficacy, have many AEs, and do not have a rigorous evidence base. Because CH attacks cause significant distress and significantly impact the quality of life, better management options are required.

REFERENCES

1. Goadsby PJ, Lipton RB. A review of paroxysmal hemicranias, SUNCT syndrome and other short-lasting headaches with autonomic feature, including new cases. Brain. 1997;120(1):193-209.
2. Chowdhury D. Worst headaches of the humankind. Ann Indian Acad Neurol. 2018;Suppl 1:S1-2.
3. Horton B. Histaminic cephalgia. Lancet. 1952;72:92-8.
4. Headache Classification Committee of the International Headache Society (IHS). The International Classification of Headache Disorders, 3rd edition (beta version). Cephalalgia. 2013;33(9):629-808.
5. Fischera M, Marziniak M, Gralow I, et al. The incidence and prevalence of cluster headache: a meta-analysis of population-based studies. Cephalalgia. 2008;28(6):614-8.
6. Rozen TD, Fishman RS. Cluster headache in the United States of America: demographics, clinical characteristics, triggers, suicidality, and personal burden. Headache. 2012;52(1):99-113.
7. Gaul C, Christmann N, Schröder D, et al. Differences in clinical characteristics and frequency of accompanying migraine features in episodic and chronic cluster headache. Cephalalgia. 2012;32(7):571-77.
8. Bahra A, May A, Goadsby PJ. Cluster headache: a prospective clinical study in 230 patients with diagnostic implications. Neurology. 2002;58(3):354-61.
9. Schürks M, Kurth T, de Jesus J, et al. Cluster headache: clinical presentation, lifestyle features, and medical treatment. Headache. 2006;46(8):1246-54.
10. Blau JN. Behavior during a cluster headache. Lancet. 1993;342(8873):723-25.
11. Kudrow L. Response of cluster headache attacks to oxygen inhalation. Headache. 1981;21(1):1-4.
12. Fogan L. Treatment of cluster headache. A double-blind comparison of oxygen v air inhalation. Arch Neurol. 1985;42(4):362-3.
13. Cohen AS, Burns B, Goadsby PJ. High-flow oxygen for treatment of cluster headache: a randomized trial. JAMA. 2009;302(22):2451-7.
14. May A, Leone M, Afra J, et al. EFNS guidelines on the treatment of cluster headache and other trigeminal-autonomic cephalalgias. Eur J Neurol. 2006;13(10):1066-77.
15. Robbins MS, Starling AJ, Pringsheim TM, et al. Treatment of cluster headache: the American Headache Society evidence-based guidelines. Headache. 2016;56(7):1093-106.
16. Dirkx THT, Haane DYP, Koehler PJ. Oxygen treatment for cluster headache attacks at different flow rates: a double-blind, randomized, crossover study. J Headache Pain. 2018;19(1):94.
17. Petersen AS, Barloese MC, Lund NL, et al. Oxygen therapy for cluster headache. A mask comparison trial. A single-blinded,

placebo-controlled, crossover study. Cephalalgia. 2017;37(3):214-24.
18. Goadsby PJ, Edvinsson L. Human in vivo evidence for trigeminovascular activation in cluster headache. Neuropeptide changes and effects of acute attacks therapies. Brain. 1994;117(3):427-34.
19. Di Sabato F, Rocco M, Martelletti P, et al. Hyperbaric oxygen in chronic cluster headaches: influence on serotonergic pathways. Undersea Hyperb Med. 1997;24(2):117-22.
20. Pearson SM, Burish MJ, Shapiro RE, et al. Effectiveness of oxygen and other acute treatments for cluster headache: results from the Cluster Headache Questionnaire, an international survey. Headache. 2019;59(2):235-49.
21. Sumatriptan Cluster Headache Study Group. Treatment of acute cluster headache with sumatriptan. N Engl J Med. 1991;325(5):322-6.
22. Ekbom K, Monstad I, Prusinski A, et al. Subcutaneous sumatriptan in the acute treatment of cluster headache: a dose comparison study. The Sumatriptan Cluster Headache Study Group. Acta Neurol Scand. 1993;88(1):63-9.
23. Law S, Derry S, Moore RA. Triptans for acute cluster headache. Cochrane Database Syst Rev. 2013;2018(5):CD008042.
24. Schuh-Hofer S, Reuter U, Kinze S, et al. Treatment of acute cluster headache with 20 mg sumatriptan nasal spray--an open pilot study. J Neurol. 2002;249(1):94-9.
25. Van Vliet JA, Bahra A, Martin V, et al. Intranasal sumatriptan in cluster headache. Neurology. 2003;60(4):630-3.
26. Cittadini E, May A, Straube A, et al. Effectiveness of intranasal zolmitriptan in acute cluster headache: a randomized, placebo-controlled, double-blind crossover study. Arch Neurol. 2006;63(11):1537-42.
27. Rapoport AM, Mathew NT, Silberstein SD, et al. Zolmitriptan nasal spray in the acute treatment of cluster headache: a double-blind study. Neurology. 2007;69(9):821-6.
28. Hedlund C, Rapoport AM, Dodick DW, et al. Zolmitriptan nasal spray in the acute treatment of cluster headache: a meta-analysis of two studies. Headache. 2009;49(9):1315-23.
29. Sicuteri F, Geppetti P, Marabini S, et al. Pain relief by somatostatin in attacks of cluster headache. Pain. 1984;18(4):359-65.
30. Geppetti P, Brocchi A, Caleri D, et al. Somatostatin for cluster headache attack. In: Pfaffenrath V, Lundberg PO, Sjaastad O (Eds). Updating in Headache. Berlin, Heidelberg, New York, Tokyo: Springer-Verlag; 1985. pp. 302-5.
31. Matharu MS, Levy MJ, Meeran K, Goadsby PJ. Subcutaneous octreotide in cluster headache: randomized placebo-controlled double-blind crossover study. Ann Neurol. 2004;56(4):488-94.
32. Andersson PG, Jespersen LT. Dihydroergotamine nasal spray in the treatment of attacks of cluster headache: a double-blind trial versus placebo. Cephalalgia. 1986;6(1):51-4.
33. Robbins L. Intranasal lidocaine for cluster headache. Headache. 1995;35(2):83-4.
34. Obermann M, Nägel S, Ose C, et al. Safety and efficacy of prednisone versus placebo in short-term prevention of episodic cluster headache: a multicentre, double-blind, randomised controlled trial. Lancet Neurol. 2021;20(1):29-37.
35. Ambrosini A, Vandenheede M, Rossi P, et al. Suboccipital injection with a mixture of rapid- and long-acting steroids in cluster headache: a double-blind placebo-controlled study. Pain. 2005;118(1-2):92-6.
36. Leroux E, Valade D, Taifas I, et al. Suboccipital steroid injections for transitional treatment of patients with more than two cluster headache attacks per day: a randomised, double-blind, placebo-controlled trial. Lancet Neurol. 2011;10(10):891-7.
37. Meyer JS, Hardenberg J. Clinical effectiveness of calcium entry blockers in prophylactic treatment of migraine and cluster headaches. Headache. 1983;23(6):266-77.
38. Gabai IJ, Spierings EL. Prophylactic treatment of cluster headache with verapamil. Headache. 1989;29(3):167-8.
39. Bussone G, Leone M, Peccarisi C, et al. Double blind comparison of lithium and verapamil in cluster headache prophylaxis. Headache. 1990;30(7):411-7.
40. Leone M, D'Amico D, Frediani F, et al. Verapamil in the prophylaxis of episodic cluster headache: a double-blind study versus placebo. Neurology. 2000;54(6):1382-5.
41. Blau JN, Engel HO. Individualizing treatment with verapamil for cluster headache patients. Headache. 2004;44(10):1013-8.
42. Koppen H, Stolwijk J, Wilms EB, et al. Cardiac monitoring of high-dose verapamil in cluster headache: an international Delphi study. Cephalalgia. 2016;36(14):1385-8.
43. Steiner TJ, Hering R, Couturier EG, et al. Double-blind placebo-controlled trial of lithium in episodic cluster headache. Cephalalgia. 1997;17(6):673-5.
44. Stochino ME, Deidda A, Asuni C, et al. Evaluation of lithium response in episodic cluster headache: a retrospective case series. Headache. 2012;52(7):1171-5.
45. Pompilio G, Migliore A, Integlia D. Systematic literature review and Bayesian network meta-analysis of episodic cluster headache drugs. Eur Rev Med Pharmacol Sci. 2021;25(3):1631-40.
46. Mathew NT, Kailasam J, Meadors L. Prophylaxis of migraine, transformed migraine, and cluster headache with topiramate. Headache. 2002;42(8):796-803.
47. Láinez MJ, Pascual J, Pascual AM, et al. Topiramate in the prophylactic treatment of cluster headache. Headache. 2003;43(7):784-9.
48. Leone M, Dodick D, Rigamonti A, et al. Topiramate in cluster headache prophylaxis: an open trial. Cephalalgia. 2003;23(10):1001-2.
49. Leone M, D'Amico D, Moschiano F, et al. Melatonin versus placebo in the prophylaxis of cluster headache: a double-blind pilot study with parallel groups. Cephalalgia. 1996;16(7):494-6.
50. El Amrani M, Massiou H, Bousser MG. A negative trial of sodium valproate in cluster headache: methodological issues. Cephalalgia. 2002;22(3):205-8.
51. Ahmed F. Chronic cluster headache responding to gabapentin: a case report. Cephalalgia. 2000;20(4):252-3.
52. Leandri M, Luzzani M, Cruccu G, et al. Drug-resistant cluster headache responding to gabapentin: a pilot study. Cephalalgia. 2001;21(7):744-6.
53. Schuh-Hofer S, Israel H, Neeb L, et al. The use of gabapentin in chronic cluster headache patients refractory to first-line therapy. Eur J Neurol. 2007;14(6):694-6.
54. Vuković V, Lovrenčić-Huzjan A, Budišić M, et al. Gabapentin in the prophylaxis of cluster headache: an observational open label study. Acta Clin Croat. 2009;48(3):311-4.
55. Goadsby PJ, Dodick DW, Leone M, et al. Trial of galcanezumab in prevention of episodic cluster headache. N Engl J Med. 2019;381(2):132-41.
56. Dodick DW, Goadsby PJ, Lucas C, et al. Phase 3 randomized, placebo-controlled study of galcanezumab in patients with chronic cluster headache: results from 3-month double-blind treatment. Cephalalgia. 2020;40(9):935-48.
57. Riesenberg R, Gaul C, Stroud CE, et al. Long-term open-label safety study of galcanezumab in patients with episodic or chronic cluster headache. Cephalalgia. 2022;42(11-12):1225-35.

58. Mo H, Kim BK, Moon HS, et al. Real-world experience with 240 mg of galcanezumab for the preventive treatment of cluster headache. J Headache Pain. 2022;23(1):132.
59. Taha JM, Tew JM. Long-term results of radio frequency rhizotomy in the treatment of cluster headache. Headache. 1995;35(4):193-6.
60. Jarrar RG, Black DF, Dodick DW, et al. Outcome of trigeminal nerve section in the treatment of chronic cluster headache. Neurology. 2003;60(8):1360-2.
61. Lovely TJ, Kotsiakis X, Jannetta PJ. The surgical management of chronic cluster headache. Headache. 1998;38(8):590-4.
62. Donnet A, Tamura M, Valade D, et al. Trigeminal nerve radiosurgical treatment in intractable chronic cluster headache: unexpected high toxicity. Neurosurgery. 2006;59(6):1252-7; discussion 1257.
63. Kano H, Kondziolka D, Mathieu D, et al. Stereotactic radiosurgery for intractable cluster headache: an initial report from the North American Gamma Knife Consortium. J Neurosurg. 2011;114(6):1736-43.
64. McClelland S, Tendulkar RD, Barnett GH, et al. Long-term results of radiosurgery for refractory cluster headache. Neurosurgery. 2006;59(6):1258-62; discussion 1262.
65. Narouze S, Kapural L, Casanova J, et al. Sphenopalatine ganglion radio-frequency ablation for the management of chronic cluster headache. Headache. 2009;49(4):571-7.
66. Sanders M, Zuurmond WW. Efficacy of sphenopalatine ganglion blockade in 66 patients suffering from cluster headache: a 12- to 70-month follow-up evaluation. J Neurosurg. 1997;87(6):876-80.
67. Schoenen J, Jensen RH, Lantéri-Minet M, et al. Stimulation of the sphenopalatine ganglion (SPG) for cluster headache treatment. Pathway CH-1: a randomized, sham-controlled study. Cephalalgia. 2013;33(10):816-30.
68. Goadsby PJ, Sahai-Srivastava S, Kezirian EJ, et al. Safety and efficacy of sphenopalatine ganglion stimulation for chronic cluster headache: a double-blind, randomised controlled trial. Lancet Neurol. 2019;18(12):1081-90.
69. Leone M, Franzini A, Bussone G. Stereotactic stimulation of posterior hypothalamic grey matter for intractable cluster headache. N Engl J Med. 2001;345(19):1428-9.
70. Fontaine D, Vandersteen C, Magis D, et al. Neuromodulation in cluster headache. Adv Tech Stand Neurosurg. 2015;42:3-21.
71. Fontaine D, Lazorthes Y, Mertens P, et al. Safety and efficacy of deep brain stimulation in refractory cluster headache: a randomized placebo-controlled double-blind trial followed by a 1-year open extension. J Headache Pain. 2010;11(1):23-31.
72. Gaul C, Diener HC, Silver N, et al. Non-invasive vagus nerve stimulation for PREVention and Acute treatment of chronic cluster headache (PREVA): A randomised controlled study. Cephalalgia. 2016;36(6):534-46.
73. Silberstein SD, Mechtler LL, Kudrow DB, et al. Non-invasive vagus nerve stimulation for the ACute treatment of cluster headache: findings from the randomized, double-blind, sham-controlled ACT1 study. Headache. 2016;56(8):1317-32.
74. Goadsby PJ, de Coo IF, Silver N, et al. Non-invasive vagus nerve stimulation for the acute treatment of episodic and chronic cluster headache: A randomized, double-blind, sham-controlled ACT2 study. Cephalalgia. 2018;38(5):959-69.
75. Gaul C, Magis D, Liebler E, et al. Effects of non-invasive vagus nerve stimulation on attack frequency over time and expanded response rates in patients with chronic cluster headache: a post hoc analysis of the randomised, controlled PREVA study. J Headache Pain. 2017;18(1):22.
76. Granata L, Niebergall H, Langner R, et al. Ketamine i.v. for the treatment of cluster headaches: an observational study. Schmerz. 2016;30(3):286-8.
77. Moisset X, Giraud P, Meunier E, et al. Ketamine-magnesium for refractory chronic cluster headache: a case series. Headache. 2020;60(10):2537-43.
78. Lampl C, Rudolph M, Bräutigam E. Onabotulinumtoxin A in the treatment of refractory chronic cluster headache. J Headache Pain. 2018;19(1):45.
79. Crespi J, Bratbak D, Dodick DW, et al. Open-label, multi-dose, pilot safety study of injection of onabotulinumtoxinA toward the otic ganglion for the treatment of intractable chronic cluster headache. Headache. 2020;60(8):1632-43.
80. Schindler EA, Gottschalk CH, Weil MJ, et al. Indoleamine hallucinogens in cluster headache: results of the Clusterbusters Medication Use Survey. J Psychoact Drugs. 2015;47(5):372-81.
81. Di Lorenzo C, Coppola G, Di Lenola D, et al. Efficacy of modified Atkins ketogenic diet in chronic cluster headache: an open-label, single-arm, clinical trial. Front Neurol. 2018;9:64.
82. Fofi L, Allais G, Quirico PE, et al. Acupuncture in cluster headache: four cases and review of the literature. Neurol Sci. 2014;Suppl 1: 195-8.
83. Evers S, Summ O. Neurostimulation treatment in chronic cluster headache-a narrative review. Curr Pain Headache Rep. 2021;25(12):81.

CHAPTER 14

Uncommon Trigeminal Autonomic Cephalalgias: An Update

Sanjay Prakash, Ajai Kumar Singh

ABSTRACT

Trigeminal autonomic cephalalgias (TACs) are a group of four primary headaches that include cluster headache (CH), paroxysmal hemicrania (PH), short-lasting unilateral neuralgiform headache attacks (SUNHA), and hemicrania continua (HC). SUNHA includes two subtypes of headaches: Short-lasting unilateral neuralgiform headache with conjunctival injection and tearing (SUNCT) and short-lasting unilateral neuralgiform headache attacks with cranial autonomic symptoms (SUNA). Except for HC, all TACs are episodic headache syndromes. The TACs differ in the duration and frequency of headaches as well as the drugs used to treat these headaches. CH has the longest attack durations (15–180 minutes) and comparatively few attacks per day. PH has an intermediate attack frequency and an intermediate duration (2–30 minutes). SUNCT and SUNA have the shortest attack duration (1–600 seconds) and the highest attack frequency. HC is characterized by continuous, strictly unilateral pain in the trigeminal region, with variable exacerbations. PH and HC respond dramatically to indomethacin. Lamotrigine is the first-line drug for SUNCT/SUNA. Several alternative drugs and surgical interventions have been tried in patients who are refractory to first-line drugs.

Keywords: Trigeminal autonomic cephalalgias, Paroxysmal hemicrania, Hemicrania continua, SUNCT, SUNA, Indomethacin.

INTRODUCTION

Trigeminal autonomic cephalalgias (TACs) are primary headache diseases included in section-III of the International Classification of Headache Disorders, 3rd edition (ICHD-3).[1] **Box 1** provides an overview of TAC classification. TACs include four different primary headaches: cluster headache (CH), paroxysmal hemicrania (PH), short-lasting unilateral neuralgiform headache attacks (SUNHA), and hemicrania continua (HC). SUNHA includes two subtypes of headaches: SUNCT and SUNA.[1] All five TACs share three clinical features: (1) Severe or very severe unilateral pain in the trigeminal distribution, (2) ipsilateral cranial autonomic features (CAFs) in the trigeminal distribution, and (3) agitation or restlessness during attack. Each TAC is then identified based on: (1) The frequency and duration of attacks and (2) a response to a specific drug.[2] TACs are primarily treatable, although the medications used to treat them are exceedingly "selective." **Table 1** presents a comparison of the diagnostic criteria of all TACs. **Figures 1A to D** depict all four TACs diagrammatically. This chapter will focus on all five except CH.

PAROXYSMAL HEMICRANIA

■ Epidemiology

Sjaastad and Dale reported the first case of PH in 1974.[3] PH has been reported in all age groups worldwide. Despite this, epidemiological studies addressing the prevalence of PH are lacking. The response to indomethacin is an inherent component in the diagnostic criteria. Consequently, it is difficult to estimate the prevalence of (definite) PH in epidemiological studies. The estimated prevalence of PH is around 0.02%.[4] In various case series, the mean age at the onset of PH ranges from 31 to 42 years. However, no age

> **BOX 1: Classification of trigeminal autonomic cephalalgias (ICHD-3).**[1]
>
> 3.1 Cluster headache (CH):
>   3.1.1 Episodic CH
>   3.1.2 Chronic CH
> 3.2 Paroxysmal hemicrania (PH):
>   3.2.1 Episodic PH
>   3.2.2 Chronic PH
> 3.3 Short-lasting unilateral neuralgiform headache attacks (SUNHA):
>   3.3.1 Short-lasting unilateral neuralgiform headache attacks with conjunctival injection and tearing (SUNCT):
>   3.3.1.1 Episodic SUNCT
>   3.3.1.2 Chronic SUNCT
>   3.3.2 Short-lasting unilateral neuralgiform headache attacks with cranial autonomic symptoms (SUNA):
>   3.3.2.1 Episodic SUNA
>   3.3.2.2 Chronic SUNA
> 3.4 Hemicrania continua (HC):
>   3.4.1 Hemicrania continua, remitting subtype
>   3.4.2 Hemicrania continua, unremitting subtype
>
> (ICHD-3: International Classification of Headache Disorders, 3rd edition)

group is immune, and it can begin at any stage of life.[4,5] The age at onset ranged from 1 to 81 years. PH was once thought to be a female-predominant condition. In an earlier review, the female–male ratio was 2.3:1. Recent studies, however, do not support a female predominance, and it appears to affect both males and females equally.[4] In a recent systematic review of 22 pediatric PH cases, the ratio of boys to girls was 1.12:1.[6] Only one case of familial PH has been reported, and no genetic predisposition has yet been proposed.[7]

Clinical Features

Clinically, PH is characterized by recurrent, short-lasting, strictly unilateral headaches associated with CAFs and restlessness or agitation during attacks. Both the right and left sides of the head are affected with equal frequency. However, side-alternating attacks could occur in up to 15% of patients.[4,5] A few case reports of bilateral PH have also been reported.[5] Typically, pain originates behind and around the eye and may spread to the head, face, or neck. Nonetheless, some patients may experience predominant pain in locations other than the ocular or retro-ocular regions. There are a few case reports in the literature in which tooth pain or facial pain was the primary or

TABLE 1: A comparison of the ICHD-3 diagnostic criteria of all four TACs.[1]

Cluster headache	Paroxysmal hemicrania	SUNHA	Hemicrania continua
A. At least five attacks fulfilling criteria B–D	A. At least 20 attacks fulfilling criteria B–E	A. At least 20 attacks fulfilling criteria B–D	A. Unilateral headache fulfilling criteria B–D
B. Severe or very severe unilateral orbital, supraorbital, and/or temporal pain lasting 15–180 minutes (when untreated)	B. Severe unilateral orbital, supraorbital, and/or temporal pain lasting 2–30 minutes	B. Moderate or severe unilateral head pain, with orbital, supraorbital, temporal, and/or other trigeminal distribution, lasting for 1–600 seconds	B. Present for >3 months, with exacerbations of moderate or greater intensity

C. Either or both of the following:
1. At least one of the following symptoms or signs, ipsilateral to the headache:
  i. Conjunctival injection and/or lacrimation
  ii. Nasal congestion and/or rhinorrhea
  iii. Eyelid edema
  iv. Forehead and facial sweating
  v. Miosis and/or ptosis
2. A sense of restlessness or agitation
	C. Either or both of the following:
	1. At least one of the following symptoms or signs, ipsilateral to the headache:
	  i. Conjunctival injection and/or lacrimation
	  ii. Nasal congestion and/or rhinorrhea
	  iii. Eyelid edema
	  iv. Forehead and facial sweating
	  v. Miosis and/or ptosis
	2. A sense of restlessness or agitation
		C. At least one of the following five cranial autonomic symptoms or signs ipsilateral to the pain:
		1. Conjunctival injection and/or lacrimation
		2. Nasal congestion and/or rhinorrhea
		3. Eyelid edema
		4. Forehead and facial sweating
		5. Miosis and/or ptosis
			C. Either or both of the following:
			1. At least one of the following symptoms or signs ipsilateral to the headache:
			  i. Conjunctival injection and/or lacrimation
			  ii. Nasal congestion and/or rhinorrhea
			  iii. Eyelid edema
			  iv. Forehead and facial sweating
			  v. Miosis and/or ptosis
			2. A sense of restlessness or agitation, or aggravation of the pain by movement

Continued

Continued

Cluster headache	Paroxysmal hemicrania	SUNHA	Hemicrania continua
D. Occurring with a frequency between one every other day and eight per day	D. Occurring with a frequency of >5 per day	D. Occurring with a frequency of at least one a day	
	E. Prevented absolutely by therapeutic doses of indomethacin		D. Responds absolutely to therapeutic doses of indomethacin
E. Not better accounted for by another ICHD-3 diagnosis	F. Not better accounted for by another ICHD-3 diagnosis	E. Not better accounted for by another ICHD-3 diagnosis	E. Not better accounted for by another ICHD-3 diagnosis

(ICHD-3: International Classification of Headache Disorders, 3rd edition; SUNHA: short-lasting unilateral neuralgiform headache attacks; TACs: trigeminal autonomic cephalalgias)

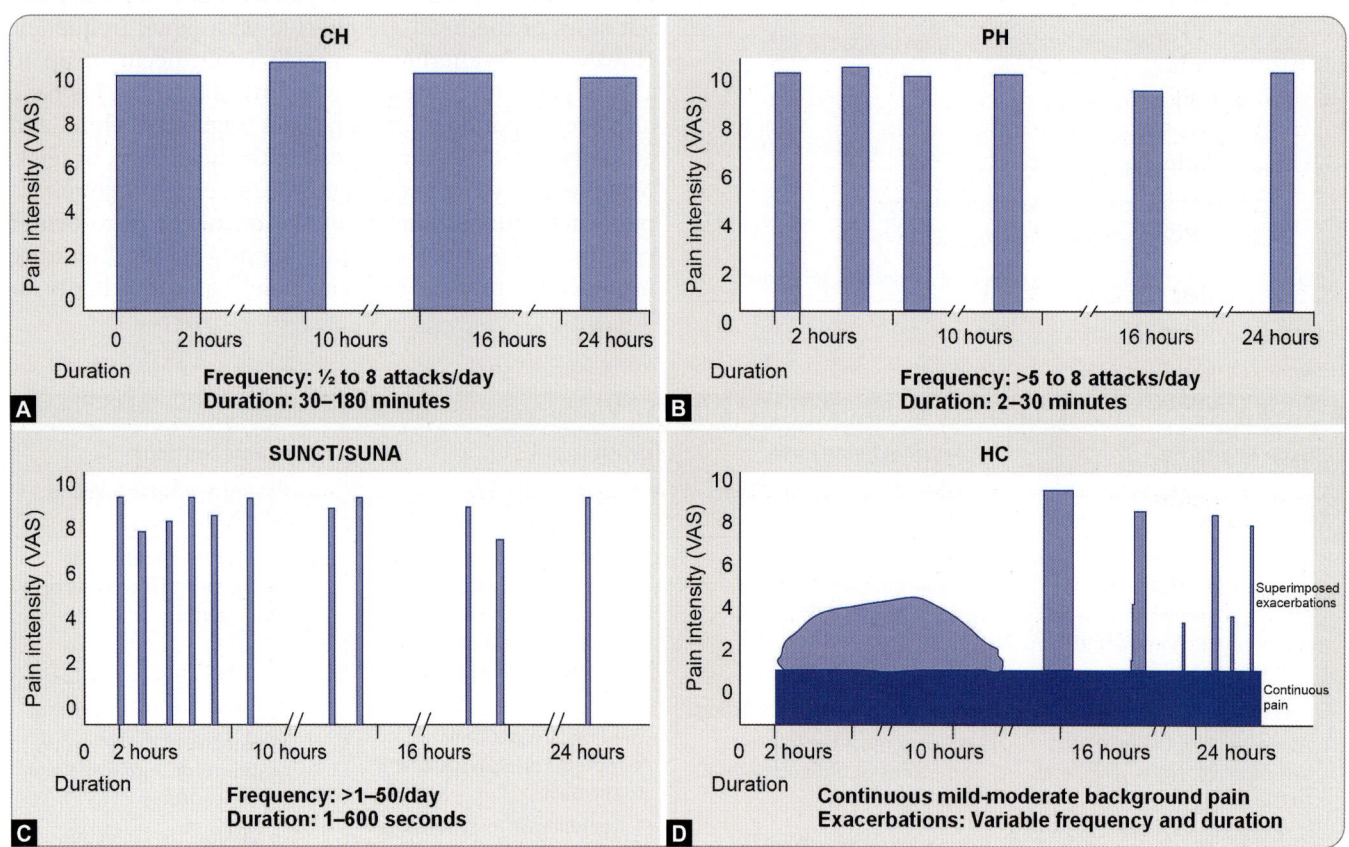

FIGS. 1A AND B: Diagrammatic representation of trigeminal autonomic cephalalgias: (A) Cluster headache—frequency: ½ to 8 attacks/day; duration: 30–180 minutes; pain intensity (VAS): 8–10; (B) Paroxysmal hemicrania—frequency >5 to 8 attacks/day; duration: 2–30 minutes; pain intensity (VAS): 8–10; (C) SUNCT/SUNA—frequency: >1–50/day; duration: 1 second to 10 minutes; pain intensity (VAS): 7–10; (D) Hemicrania continua—superimposed severe exacerbations (variable duration and intensity), continuous, mild–moderate background pain.
(SUNA: short-lasting unilateral neuralgiform headache attacks with cranial autonomic symptoms; SUNCT: short-lasting unilateral neuralgiform headache with conjunctival injection and tearing; VAS: visual analog scale)

presenting symptom of PH.[4] Most often, headache episodes start abruptly and without any warning, and they get worse quickly. The severity of headache is comparable to that of CH. Approximately 90% of patients classify their headache as severe or very severe.[8,9] In one study, 65% of patients rated the severity of their most painful attacks as a 10 (out of 10) on a visual analog scale (VAS).[9] These patients described their pain as the most painful they had ever felt, comparing it to childbirth and duodenal ulcer perforation.[9]

Like CH, >90% of patients with PH report CAFs during attacks. However, only 35% of patients exhibit CAFs during each episode.[4] Lacrimation, conjunctival injection, rhinorrhea, and nasal congestion are the common CAFs. During headache attacks, 50–80% of patients may experience agitation or restlessness.[4] According to ICHD-3, the duration of PH attacks should last from 2 to 30 minutes. However, most attacks last 10–30 minutes. Attacks lasting longer than 30 minutes, though, are not unusual. About 24–75% of patients may feel attacks of >30 minutes' duration. Similarly, up to 41% of individuals may experience attacks that last under 2 minutes.[4] According to the ICHD-3, there must be more than five attacks per day on more than half of the occasions. Attacks typically occur 7–13 times per day, on average. However, a significant proportion of patients (9–37%) may not get more than five attacks in a day.

Classification of Paroxysmal Hemicrania

There are two types of PH: Episodic PH (EPH) and chronic PH (CPH). CPH is either continuous for more than a year or occurs with a brief period of remission (remissions lasting <3 months). EPH must have at least two attacks that last between 7 days to a year (when left untreated), separated by at least 3 months of pain-free remission.[1] The CPH accounts for 80% of cases of PH. Typically, the EPH develops into CPH, but the opposite can also happen.[10]

Secondary Paroxysmal Hemicrania

Secondary PH is frequently linked to tumors or vascular disease. One of the most significant causes of PH and other TACs is pituitary gland abnormalities, especially pituitary tumor. The vascular pathologies include carotid artery dissection, aneurysm of the carotid artery, and cerebral venous thrombosis. Other reported secondary PH are demyelinating lesions in brain, orbital metastasis, and phosphodiesterase inhibitor administration.[4,11]

Management

The duration of PH attacks is too short to start abortive therapies. However, some attacks may last longer, necessitating therapy to stop a persistent attack. Subcutaneous sumatriptan and oxygen inhalation have been tried during attacks. However, the results are conflicting.[4] The primary goal of treatment is to prevent attacks (prophylactic therapy) **(Table 2)**. A response to indomethacin is a must in the diagnostic criteria of PH. The intramuscular indomethacin 50–100 mg (INDOTEST) has been proposed as a diagnostic test for both PH and HC.[16] A trial of oral indomethacin is the more popular regimen. The ICHD-3 recommends starting with at least 150 mg of indomethacin per day.[1] The dose can be increased up to 225 mg daily. Patients may require a lower maintenance dose over time. Moreover, about 20% of cases may have episodic variety of PH. Therefore, every 3–6 months, it is suggested to gradually reduce the dose in order to find the lowest effective dose and EPH.[4]

Patients who experience side effects from indomethacin may be offered a trial of various other drugs and interventions. Other drugs that have been effective in a subset of patients with PH are other nonsteroidal anti-inflammatory drugs (NSAIDs) (naproxen, diclofenac, aspirin, ketoprofen, and piroxicam derivatives), cyclooxygenase-2 (COX-2) inhibitors (celecoxib and rofecoxib), calcium channel blockers (verapamil, flunarizine, and nicardipine),

TABLE 2: Overview of preventive treatment of PH, SUNCT/SUNA, and HC.[4,5,12-15]			
	Paroxysmal hemicrania	**SUNHA**	**Hemicrania continua**
First-line drug	Indomethacin (150–225 mg/day)	Lamotrigine (200–700 mg/day)	Indomethacin (150–225 mg/day)
Second-line drug	• NSAIDs (aspirin, naproxen, diclofenac, and piroxicam) • Cyclooxygenase-2 inhibitors (Celecoxib)	• Oxcarbazepine • Topiramate • Duloxetine	• Topiramate • Cyclooxygenase-2 inhibitors (Celecoxib)
Other medications	• Calcium channel blockers (verapamil, flunarizine, and nicardipine) • Antiepileptic drugs (topiramate, carbamazepine lamotrigine, and gabapentin)	• Carbamazepine • Gabapentin • Pregabalin • Mexiletine • Lidocaine patches	• Steroids • Ibuprofen • Acetyl salicylic acid • Gabapentin • Melatonin • Piroxicam
Surgical interventions	• Peripheral nerve block • Sphenopalatine ganglion blockade • Deep brain stimulation • Occipital nerve stimulation • Vagus nerve stimulation	• Microvascular decompression of the trigeminal nerve • Deep brain stimulation • Occipital nerve stimulation • Ablation of trigeminal neuralgia • Peripheral nerve block	• Peripheral nerve block • Sphenopalatine ganglion block • Occipital nerve stimulation • Vagus nerve stimulation • Botulinum toxin

(HC: hemicrania continua; NSAIDs: nonsteroidal anti-inflammatory drugs; PH: paroxysmal hemicrania; SUNA: short-lasting unilateral neuralgiform headache attacks with cranial autonomic symptoms; SUNCT: short-lasting unilateral neuralgiform headache with conjunctival injection and tearing; SUNHA: short-lasting unilateral neuralgiform headache attacks) antiepileptic drugs (topiramate, carbamazepine, lamotrigine, and gabapentin), and miscellaneous (dihydroergotamine, methysergide, acetazolamide, and lithium).[2,4,9] Several surgical approaches have been tried in patients with PH who were unable to tolerate indomethacin and were refractory to other oral medications. Surgical procedures include peripheral nerve block [greater occipital nerve (GON)], sphenopalatine ganglion blockade, hypothalamic deep brain stimulation, occipital nerve stimulation, and noninvasive vagus nerve stimulation.[2]

SUNHA (SUNCT AND SUNA)

In 1978, Sjaastad and colleagues reported the first case of SUNCT.[1,17] The ICHD-2 added SUNCT as a form of TAC. The ICHD-2 appendix section made reference to SUNA and speculated that SUNCT might be a subtype of SUNA.[18] However, SUNCT and SUNA were classified as independent disease entities in ICHD-3 and were grouped together under the umbrella term SUNHA.[1] However, a number of recent studies suggest that both headache disorders share the same phenotype and lack significant clinical differences.[10,19] Now, it has been recommended that both disorders be put into a single diagnostic category.

■ Epidemiology

The incidence and prevalence of SUNHA are largely unknown. According to a study done in Australia, the estimated prevalence was 6.6 per 100,000 people.[20] SUNHA often manifests in the fourth or fifth decade of life; however, onset can occur at any age between 2 and 88 years.[21,22] SUNCT occurs mostly in males, whereas SUNA is more common in females. However, when SUNCT and SUNA are combined, SUNHA is a male-predominant disease.[12,21]

■ Clinical Features

Both SUNCT and SUNA are characterized by abrupt, brief attacks of severe unilateral orbital, periorbital, or temporal pain accompanied by ipsilateral CAFs. The pain may spread to the V2/V3 division of the trigeminal nerves and, in rare cases, to extratrigeminal nerves. Around 6% of SUNHA patients may experience side-shifting pain. Moreover, there have been reports of SUNA affecting both sides at the same time.[4] Like the pain of trigeminal neuralgia (TN), the pain of SUNHA is described as stabbing, sharp, burning, or like electric shocks. Pain can come in the form of a single stab, a cluster of stabs, or prolonged saw tooth-like attacks.[23] According to ICHD-3, the duration of SUNCT or SUNA attacks should last from 1 to 600 seconds. Single stabs typically last 58 seconds on average. The mean duration of group of stabs is 396 seconds (range 10 seconds to 20 minutes). Sawtooth pattern-like pain typically lasts for 1,100 seconds (range 10 seconds to 120 minutes).[12,23] Longer attacks of pain with a sawtooth pattern lasting for 1–2 hours may create diagnostic confusion with CH. The majority of patients (85–95%) rate their headaches as severe or extremely severe (VAS: 8–10).[23]

In SUNCT, both conjunctival injection and lacrimation must be present. Conjunctival injection or lacrimation may be among the autonomic symptoms in SUNA, but not both.[4] Both SUNA and SUNCT may have other types of CAFs, including rhinorrhea, nasal congestion, ptosis, mitosis, eyelid edema, facial sweating, and/or flushing. Conjunctival injection or lacrimation may also occur in people with TN. It is milder and less frequent though. Moreover, rhinorrhea is very rare in TN.[24]

The majority of patients with SUNHA had both spontaneous and triggered attacks. The triggers for SUNHA include touching the face, cold wind exposure, bathing or taking a shower, washing or combing hair, chewing or eating, brushing teeth, shaving, talking, and coughing. There are several triggers that are similar between SUNHA and TN. Triggers are nearly universal in TN, with 91–99% of patients reporting attack triggers.[25] However, a sizable fraction of SUNHA patients, 30–50% of all SUNHA cases, exhibit totally spontaneous attacks.[10,12,19] Even a mild form of a trigger can cause an attack in TN patients. Attacks in SUNHA, though, may require a little "rougher" triggers.[24] After triggering an attack, no more attacks can be provoked for a few seconds or minutes in TN. This period is called postictal refractory period. SUNHA does not show a refractory period after exposure to a trigger.[10,12] The most common misdiagnosed condition for SUNHA is TN. **Table 3** shows a comparison between SUNHA and TN.

■ Classification of SUNCT and SUNA

Both SUNCT and SUNA have episodic and chronic variants, i.e., episodic SUNCT and episodic SUNA, and chronic SUNCT and chronic SUNA. Chronic SUNCT or SUNA is either continuous for more than a year or occurs with a remission lasting <3 months. Episodic SUNCT or SUNA must have at least two attacks that last between 7 days to a year (when left untreated), separated by at least 3 months of pain-free remission.[1] The chronic variant accounts for 80–90% of all cases of SUNHA.[10,12]

■ Secondary SUNCT and SUNA

Several cases of secondary SUNCT have been reported in the literature. It is likely that symptomatic SUNCT is more common than primary SUNCT.[11,12,21] The most common secondary SUNHA is vascular compression of the trigeminal nerve. In a review of 201 cases, 16.9% of SUNHA patients had vascular compression of the trigeminal nerve.[21] A neurovascular conflict with the trigeminal nerve was detected in 88% of patients with SUNHA who had a magnetic resonance imaging (MRI) with dedicated views of the trigeminal nerve.[21] Other causes of secondary SUNHA are pituitary gland tumors, posterior fossa lesions, and orbital pathologies.

TABLE 3: Differentiating features of TN and SUNHA.[12,24,25]		
	Trigeminal neuralgia	SUNHA (SUNCT/SUNA)
Site of pain	Mainly V2—distribution. Over time spread to involve V1 and V3	Typically, V1—distribution sites are stationary over time
Severity	Very severe	Moderate to severe
Cranial autonomic features	• Conjunctival injection, lacrimation—occasional and mild • Rhinorrhea—extremely rare	• Conjunctival injection, lacrimation—frequent and marked • Rhinorrhea—common
Duration	Shorter than a SUNCT (1–120 seconds)	Longer than a TN (1–600 seconds)
Triggers	91–99% of patients report triggered attacks. Just a minimal touch or a puff of wind triggers an attack	30–50% of patients may not have triggers. Slightly "rougher" stimulus may be necessary, e.g., rubbing of the skin
Refractory period	Postictal refractory period—present	No refractory period
Nocturnal attacks	Frequent	Rare (1–2% of attacks)
Agitation	Less agitation	More agitation
Treatment response	Carbamazepine has dramatic effect	Lamotrigine is effective

(SUNA: short-lasting unilateral neuralgiform headache attacks with cranial autonomic symptoms; SUNCT: short-lasting unilateral neuralgiform headache with conjunctival injection and tearing; SUNHA: short-lasting unilateral neuralgiform headache attacks; TN: trigeminal neuralgia)

▪ Management

Abortive therapies are useless in SUNHA because the attacks are brief. Lamotrigine is the first-line drug for the prevention of SUNHA. Second-line preventive therapies include topiramate, oxcarbazepine, carbamazepine, and duloxetine. Other drugs that may be effective are gabapentin, pregabalin, mexiletine, and zonisamide.[12,13] It may take a few days or weeks for patients to see effects from the preventive therapy. Transitional therapies may be useful in such circumstances. Transitional therapies include intravenous lidocaine, GON blocks, and corticosteroids. Surgical intervention is advised for patients whose medical treatment has failed. Microvascular decompression of the trigeminal nerve should be done if MRI suggests neurovascular conflict with the trigeminal nerve. Patients who are medically intractable and do not have neurovascular compression can benefit from peripheral and central neurostimulation, such as occipital nerve stimulation and deep brain stimulation of the ventral tegmental region. Destructive procedures of the trigeminal nerve, such as percutaneous trigeminal ganglion compression, trigeminal ganglion thermocoagulation, retrogasserian glycerol rhizolysis, and gamma-knife surgery, are other options in refractory chronic SUNHA. Nerve block, mainly GON block, can also be tried in intractable chronic SUNHA.[12]

HEMICRANIA CONTINUA

▪ Epidemiology

Probably the first authors to describe the clinical phenotype of HC were Medina and Diamond in 1981. Sjaastad and Spierings later used the term "Hemicrania Continua." The prevalence and incidence of HC are mostly unknown. In 1838 parishioners in the Vågå study, Sjaastad and Bakketeig noted 18 patients (1.0%) with clinical characteristics resembling HC. The prevalence of HC ranges from 1.3 to 2.3% (mean = 1.7%) of all headache patients presenting to a neurology or headache clinic.[14] HC was the fourth most common cause of side-locked headaches in a pooled analysis of side-locked headaches. HC is most likely the second-most frequent TAC in a clinical setting.[5] HC usually manifests during the fourth or fifth decade of life. However, it can start at any stage of life. Age at onset ranged from 5 to 76 years. HC, like migraine and tension-type headache, is more prevalent among women. There are two documented case reports of HC in the same family. But no genetic susceptibility has yet been proposed.[26]

▪ Clinical Features

Clinically, HC is defined as a strictly unilateral, mild-to-moderate, continuous headache with superimposed severe exacerbations in the trigeminal distribution. Around 2% of HC patients may experience side-shifting pain. There have also been a few reports of bilateral HC.[27,28] Pain in HC, like other TACs, is primarily located in the first division of the trigeminal nerve (orbital, supraorbital, or temporal). However, pain may spread to other divisions of the trigeminal nerves and, in rare cases, to extra trigeminal nerves. In a few patients, the pain was predominantly localized in the V2/V3 distribution of the trigeminal nerve (teeth, oral cavity, mandible, ear, temporomandibular joint, and ear).

In HC, the headache has two components: (1) Continuous background pain, and (2) severe superimposed exacerbations. The most consistent and essential component of HC is "continuous background pain." Typically, the background pain is mild to moderate (VAS: 3.3–5.2) and has no significant impact on daily activities. Patients may not disclose the history of background pain and may instead emphasize only severe superimposed exacerbations. The most common reason for a delayed or incorrect diagnosis of HC is a failure to obtain a history of background pain.[29] Superimposed exacerbations vary greatly in terms of character, intensity, duration, frequency, and associated features. The frequency and duration of attacks in CH, PH, and SUNCT/SUNA—all follow a predictable pattern. However, the frequency and duration of exacerbations in HC are highly variable and do not follow any pattern. Exacerbations might last anything from a few seconds to 2 weeks. The frequency of exacerbations ranges from >20 attacks per day to one attack per 4 months. Exacerbations are typically severe to very severe (VAS: 5–10). Approximately 50% of patients may experience nocturnal exacerbations. However, it is unclear whether exacerbations have a circadian pattern.[14]

Exacerbations of headaches may be accompanied by CAFs, restlessness or agitation, and migrainous features. CAFs are noted in eye/eye lid (conjunctival injection, lacrimation, ptosis, eyelid edema, and meiosis), nose (nasal congestion and rhinorrhea), and face/forehead (sweating). In a pooled analysis and a systematic review, about 70% of the cases had at least one CAFs.[14,29] This prevalence is marginally lower than the prevalence of CAFs seen in patients with CH and PH, where it is observed in over 90% of cases. Furthermore, CAFs may be subtle in some patients, and patients may be unaware of its presence. Consequently, an objective evaluation of autonomic features is necessary during exacerbations phase. The two most common CAFs are lacrimation (73%) and conjunctival injection (70%).[14,29] A characteristic trait shared by all TACs is a feeling of agitation or restlessness. During exacerbations, patients have difficulty staying motionless and rarely lie down comfortably. The prevalence of restlessness or agitation in HC ranged from 10 to 69% in different studies, and it is lower than found in PH and CH.[14] The most common form of restlessness is to rub, press, or hold the aching part. Other common forms of restlessness include rolling on the bed or the floor, walking back and forth, pacing or rocking, and putting something on the aching part. Suicidal ideation is also experienced by a few patients during exacerbations.

During exacerbations of HC, migraine symptoms such as nausea, vomiting, photophobia, and phonophobia are fairly common. The prevalence of at least one migrainous symptom ranges from 17 to 90% (with an average pooled prevalence of 60%). Approximately half of the patients may meet the migraine criteria during HC exacerbations.[14] Because of this, HC is commonly confused with migraine. The most common misdiagnosed condition for HC is side-locked migraine. **Table 4** shows a comparison between HC and side-locked migraine.

Classification of Hemicrania Continua

There are two types of HC based on whether the patient gets any symptom-free days or not: (1) Remitting subtype and (2) unremitting subtype. Unremitting HC is characterized by continuous pain for at least a year with no symptom-free intervals.[1] In remitting HC, the patient is symptom free for at least 1 day. The remitting type accounts for 10–22% of all cases of HC. About 50–60% of cases of unremitting HC are chronic from the beginning, and 25–35% progress from the remitting form to the continuous phase.[14,15]

TABLE 4: Differentiating features of side-locked migraine and hemicrania continua.[15]

Features	Side-locked migraine	Hemicrania continua
Age at onset	Second to third decade	Fourth to fifth decade
Sites of pain	Variables	First division of trigeminal nerve
Continuous pain	No. Pain-free period present	Present. No pain-free period
Duration of exacerbations/attacks	Attacks of <4 hours—uncommon	Extremely variable. Attack of <4 hours—very common
Intensity of pain	Moderate to severe	Very severe—intolerable
Cranial autonomic features	Rare, not prominent, bilateral, and no itchy eye	Common, prominent, ipsilateral, and itchy eye
Restlessness or agitation	Absent. Patient prefers to lie down	Present. Patient cannot lie down. Cannot be motionless
Suicidal thoughts	Not reported yet	May occur during exacerbations
Response to indomethacin	Response—variables	Immediate and dramatic
Effects on skipping the effective drug	Reappearance is not immediate on skipping the drug	Reappearance of headache even after missing one dosage

Secondary Hemicrania Continua

About 80 cases of secondary HC have been reported in the literature, and they involve >25 different pathologies. Both intracranial and extracranial structures, including the skull, neck, nose, sinuses, eyes, ears, teeth, mouth, and vessels, can cause HC-like headaches. The most common secondary HC is post-traumatic HC, followed by postsurgery, dissection, prolactinoma, carcinoma lung, and nasopharyngeal carcinoma.[15]

Management

A "complete" response to a therapeutic dose of indomethacin is considered "sine qua non" for HC. INDOTEST (by intramuscular indomethacin) can be done to observe the immediate response. The initial oral dose of indomethacin must be 150 mg/day, similar to PH. However, some patients may require a higher dose, up to 300 mg daily. Over time, up to 77% of patients might need a lower maintenance dose. Therefore, it is recommended to gradually reduce the dose every 3–6 months in order to identify the lowest effective dose and remitting subtype of HC.[14,15]

About 20–75% of people could experience side effects from indomethacin and need to take different medications. Case reports and open-label trials have proven the efficacy of several medicines. It includes topiramate, COX-2 inhibitors (celecoxib and rofecoxib), ibuprofen, piroxicam, naproxen, aspirin, acemetacin, melatonin, gabapentin, verapamil, and steroids.[14,15] However, the responses to any of these medications are unpredictable. The most effective medicine can only be discovered through trial and error. However, headaches reappear within a few hours to a few days of missing the effective drugs (indomethacin or others), and some authors consider it a "strong testimony" for HC.[29]

Surgical interventions should be tried in patients who could not take indomethacin and did not respond to other oral medicines, and have tried a number of medical treatments. Surgical procedures include peripheral nerve block, sphenopalatine ganglion blockade, occipital nerve stimulation, radiofrequency ablation of dorsal root ganglion or sphenopalatine ganglion, vagus nerve stimulation, and botulinum toxin.[15]

PATHOPHYSIOLOGY OF PAROXYSMAL HEMICRANIA, SUNHA, AND HEMICRANIA CONTINUA

All TACs share a common pathophysiology. Both peripheral and central processes are implicated in the generation of attacks. A variety of hypothalamic nuclei and circuits, including orexinergic, somatostatinergic, serotoninergic, and opioidergic pathways, are involved in the generation of TAC. Trigeminovascular nociceptive pathways, which include the trigeminal autonomic reflex, are the final pathways for the symptoms of these disorders. Dysfunctions in the hypothalamus and related circuits modify the inputs to the trigeminovascular system and the trigeminal autonomic reflex.[30]

Positron emission tomography (PET) and functional MRI studies have demonstrated the involvement of various parts of the hypothalamus and other brain structures in various TACs. There was activation of the ipsilateral posterior hypothalamic gray matter area in patients with CH. PET study in patients with PH has demonstrated activation of the contralateral posterior hypothalamus, ventral midbrain, red nucleus, and substantia nigra. Patients with HC have been shown to have activation in the contralateral posterior hypothalamus, ipsilateral ventrolateral midbrain, ipsilateral dorsal rostral pons, and bilateral pontomedullary junction. The activation of the hypothalamus is variables in patients with SUNHA. Studies have demonstrated bilateral, contralateral, and even ipsilateral hypothalamic activation in patients with SUNHA.

REFERENCES

1. Headache Classification Committee of the International Headache Society (IHS). The International Classification of Headache Disorders, 3rd edition. Cephalalgia. 2018;38:1-211.
2. Wei DY, Ong JJY, Goadsby PJ. Overview of trigeminal autonomic cephalalgias: Nosologic evolution, diagnosis, and management. Ann Indian Acad Neurol. 2018;21(Suppl 1):S39-44.
3. Sjaastad O, Dale I. Evidence for a new (?), treatable headache entity. Headache. 1974;14:105-8.
4. Prakash S, Patell R. Paroxysmal hemicrania: An update. Curr Pain Headache Rep. 2014;18(4):407.
5. Osman C, Bahra A. Paroxysmal hemicrania. Ann Indian Acad Neurol. 2018;21(Suppl 1):S16.
6. Bemanalizadeh M, Oskouei HB, Hadizadeh A, et al. Paroxysmal hemicrania in children and adolescents: A systematic review. Headache. 2022;62(8):952-66.
7. Cohen AS, Matharu MS, Goadsby PJ. Paroxysmal hemicrania in a family. Cephalalgia. 2006;26(4):486-8.
8. Prakash S, Belani P, Susvirkar A, et al. Paroxysmal hemicrania: A retrospective study of a consecutive series of 22 patients and a critical analysis of the diagnostic criteria. J Headache Pain. 2013;14(1):26.
9. Cittadini E, Matharu MS, Goadsby PJ. Paroxysmal hemicrania: A prospective clinical study of 31 cases. Brain. 2008;131(Pt 4): 1142-55.
10. Lambru G, Rantell K, Levy A, et al. A prospective comparative study and analysis of predictors of SUNA and SUNCT. Neurology. 2019;93(12):e1127-37.
11. Chowdhury D. Secondary (symptomatic) trigeminal autonomic cephalalgia. Ann Indian Acad Neurol. 2018;21(Suppl 1):S57.
12. Levy A, Matharu MS. Short-lasting unilateral neuralgiform headache attacks. Ann Indian Acad Neurol. 2018;21(Suppl 1): S31.
13. Lambru G, Stubberud A, Rantell K, et al. Medical treatment of SUNCT and SUNA: A prospective open-label study including single-arm meta-analysis. J Neurol Neurosurg Psychiatry. 2021;92(3): 233-41.
14. Prakash S, Patel P. Hemicrania continua: Clinical review, diagnosis and management. J Pain Res. 2017;10:1493-509.
15. Prakash S, Rawat KS. Hemicrania continua: An update. Neurol India. 2021;69(7):160.
16. Antonaci F, Pareja JA, Caminero AB, et al. Chronic paroxysmal hemicrania and hemicrania continua. Parenteral indomethacin: The 'indotest'. Headache. 1998;38(2):122-8.
17. Sjaastad O, Russell D, Hørven I, et al. Multiple Neuralgiform, Unilateral Headache Attacks Associated with Conjunctival Injection and Appearing in Clusters. A Nosological Problem. Proceedings of the Scandinavian Migraine Society; 1978. p. 31.
18. Headache Classification Subcommittee of the International Headache Society. The International Classification of Headache Disorders: 2nd edition. Cephalalgia. 2004;24 Suppl 1:9-160.
19. Zhang S, Cao Y, Yan F, et al. Similarities and differences between SUNCT and SUNA: A cross-sectional, multicentre study of 76 patients in China. J Headache Pain. 2022;23(1):137.
20. Williams MH, Broadley SA. SUNCT and SUNA: Clinical features and medical treatment. J Clin Neurosci. 2008;15:526-34.
21. Favoni V, Grimaldi D, Pierangeli G, et al. SUNCT/SUNA and neurovascular compression: New cases and critical literature review. Cephalalgia. 2013;33(16):1337-48.

22. Cesaroni CA, Pruccoli J, Bergonzini L, et al. SUNCT/SUNA in pediatric age: A review of pathophysiology and therapeutic options. Brain Sci. 2021;11(9):1252.
23. Cohen AS, Matharu MS, Goadsby PJ. Short-lasting unilateral neuralgiform headache attacks with conjunctival injection and tearing (SUNCT) or cranial autonomic features (SUNA)—A prospective clinical study of SUNCT and SUNA. Brain. 2006;129: 2746-60.
24. Antonaci F, Fredriksen T, Pareja JA, et al. Shortlasting, unilateral, neuralgiform, headache attacks with conjunctival injection, tearing, sweating, and rhinorrhea: The term and new viewpoints. Front Neurol. 2018;9:262.
25. Lambru G, Zakrzewska J, Matharu M. Trigeminal neuralgia: A practical guide. Pract Neurol. 2021;21(5):392-402.
26. Huang H, Newman LC. Hemicrania continua in a family: A report of two cases. Headache. 2021;61(7):1132-5.
27. Prakash S, Rathore C. Side-locked headaches: An algorithm-based approach. J Headache Pain. 2016;17:95.
28. Al-Khazali HM, Al-Khazali S, Iljazi A, et al. Prevalence and clinical features of hemicrania continua in clinic-based studies: A systematic review and meta-analysis. Cephalalgia. 2023;43(1):03331024221131343.
29. Prakash S, Rathore C, Rana K, et al. A long-term prospective observational study in 31 patients with hemicrania continua. Cephalalgia Reports. 2019;2:251581631882469.
30. Prakash S, Hansen JM. Mechanisms of cluster headache and other trigeminal autonomic cephalalgias. In: Martelletti P, Timothy J, Steiner TJ (Eds). Handbook of Headache: Practical Management, 1st edition. Berlin: Springer Verlag; 2011. pp. 330-40.

CHAPTER 15

Tension-type Headache: Still an Enigma

Menka Jha, Sanjeev Kumar Bhoi, Debashish Chowdhury

ABSTRACT

Tension-type headache (TTH) is the most common form of primary headache. The pathophysiology and management of which is still less studied as compared to migraine. The two subtypes of TTH are episodic TTH (ETTH) and chronic TTH (CTTH), which differ in their pathogenesis. Peripheral mechanism (myofascial nociception) and environmental factors play more important role in ETTH, whereas genetic and central factors (sensitization and inadequate endogenous pain control) are more significant for the CTTH. TTH is a more difficult headache to treat, which requires both pharmacologic and nonpharmacologic measures. ETTH can be managed by simple analgesics and nonsteroidal anti-inflammatory drugs (NSAIDs), whereas CTTH requires multimodal approach. Combination of preventive medications such as amitriptyline and nonpharmacologic measures such as stress management, relaxation, and physical therapies are required for the management of CTTH. Despite these measures, the outcome is less than satisfactory in the majority. There is a huge socioeconomic burden of TTH in the society, but it still remains an enigma for the treating physicians. More research in the understanding of its pathophysiology is required, which can lead to improvement in the management of TTH, especially the chronic form.

Keywords: Chronic TTH, Episodic tension-type headache, Pathophysiology, Central sensitization, Amitriptyline, Trigger point, Disability, Economic burden.

INTRODUCTION

Tension-type headache (TTH) is the most common form of the primary headaches,[1] though less well understood and less medical attention is sought than the other headache subtypes. Patients usually self-diagnose and self-treat unless they have a concurrent migraine or transition from episodic to frequent or the chronic form of TTH.

The characteristic feature of TTH is mild-to-moderate head pain lasting minutes to weeks. The typical pain is pressing or tightening in quality, bilateral in location, and does not worsen with routine physical activity. The hallmark of TTH is the absence of systemic features such as nausea, vomiting, and photo- and phonophobia found in other headache types, such as migraine. Hence, TTH is also called a "featureless" headache. The diagnosis requires the exclusion of other organic disorders. The treatment options for TTH especially the CTTH are not too many and the outcome is not rewarding, resulting from the lag in scientific understanding of TTH pathophysiology as compared to migraine. In recent decades, researches relating to the structural and functional brain alterations in TTH patients, however, have helped to understand the pathophysiological aspects better. Unfortunately, there is no recent breakthrough in the major therapeutics of TTH, though it is much waited for this neglected subgroup of headache patients. Few reviews in the recent past have given some insight on the pathophysiology and management of TTH,[2-5] but it still remains to be an enigma.

EPIDEMIOLOGY

Despite being the most prevalent headache subtype, there is still a lack of widespread epidemiologic studies of TTH compared to migraine. Majority of the published literature is from high-income countries.

The Global Burden of Disease (GBD) 2016 rated TTH as the third most prevalent disorder with 1.89 billion individuals estimated to have TTH.[6] The global prevalence of patients with active TTH was reported to be 26% (22.7–29.5) with 23.4% in men and 27.1% in women.[7,8] In a population-based study from the United States, the prevalence of episodic TTH (ETTH) peaked in the third decade (30–39 years) and decreased slightly with age.

Data for disease burden of TTH from East and Southeast Asia, Middle East, and North African region were extracted from the GBD 2019, which reported high burden of TTH. There was variation between the study findings and also between the World Bank region and country income level.[7] The methodological and socioeconomic factors might have been contributory.

The epidemiological data on TTH from India is sparse. A population-based survey in southern India (Karnataka state) has shown the crude 1-year prevalence of TTH to be 34.8% (age-standardized 1-year prevalence was 35%). The prevalence was similar between gender but higher among rural areas. The prevalence declined from 40% in those aged 18–25 years to 28.7% in those over 56.[9]

Associated Comorbidities

Psychiatric comorbidities are common in chronic daily headaches, the prevalence ranging from 64–90% (mostly in the form of anxiety and mood disorders). In general, persons with CTTH have increased levels of affective distress, such as depression, anxiety, and anger. These patients also report more headache-related disability. Greater depressive symptomatology in TTH patients is particularly common in women, older persons, and those with more extensive headache histories. Among the Indian population, psychiatric comorbidity was present in 36.4% of patients with CTTH.[10]

Relationship with Migraine

Migraine and TTH may be considered related conditions with shared environmental and lifestyle factors. In the general population, 94% of migraineurs have TTH, and 56% of these have frequent ETTH. In contrast, TTH occurs with similar prevalence in patients with and without migraine, which leads to the assumption that migraine can trigger TTH, whereas TTH may not trigger a migraine. In a population study that compared the clinical characteristics of TTH, the 1-year prevalence and male-to-female ratios of TTH were similar in individuals with and without migraine. However, the frequency and duration of TTH attacks were greater in persons with migraine compared with persons without migraine.

Circadian and Sleep Disturbances

A significant diurnal variation in headache intensity was shown in TTH through the utilization of computerized ecological momentary assessment (EMA), with headache being weakest in the morning, worsening toward the evening, and peaking afterward. Sleep disturbances are common in both migraine and TTH and may contribute to the overall disability and reduced quality of life. A Korean study reported CTTH being associated with higher excessive daytime somnolence (EDS) prevalence compared to ETTH and without headache.[11] Furthermore, the subjects with TTH with EDS had more severe TTH symptoms compared to TTH without EDS.

Emergency Department Visits due to Tension-type Headache

In the TEDDi study,[12] TTH was overdiagnosed in emergency visits due to headache; the majority had another primary headache, and some had secondary headaches including life-threatening conditions. Only a minority of patients fulfilled the International Classification of Headache Disorders (ICHD) criteria of TTH. Inconsistencies in prior medical history or anamnesis were frequent.

Disability and Economic Burden of Tension-type Headache

The prevalence of TTH is greater than migraine and the overall economic cost of TTH is higher. The effects of TTH on the individual include physical suffering, loss of quality of life, and economic effects, but these are difficult to quantify. The absenteeism resulting from TTH is considerable and can be as high as three times more than that seen in migraine. The disability is higher in patients with psychiatric comorbidities. Globally, TTH accounts for 6.5% of all the years lived with disability (YLD) (7.7% in females and 5.1% in males) (GBD 2016).[6]

CLASSIFICATION

As per ICHD-3, there are three main subtypes of TTH based on the frequency of headache episodes **(Tables 1 and 2)**.[13]
1. Infrequent ETTH—with headache episode less than once a month
2. Frequent ETTH—with headache episodes 1–14 days a month
3. Chronic TTH (CTTH)—with headache occurring for 15 days or more a month

This division is relevant for several reasons. The underlying pathophysiology, impact on daily living, and therapeutic options differ among the subtypes.[14] Each of the subtypes is additionally classified as occurring with or without

TABLE 1: ICHD-3 diagnostic criteria for TTH.*[15]	
Infrequent (a) or frequent (b) TTH	**Chronic TTH**
A. At least 10 episodes of headache (a) fulfilling criteria B–D	A. Headache occurring on ≥15 days/month on average for >3 months (≥180 days/year), fulfilling criteria B–D
B. Lasting from 30 minutes to 7 days	B. Lasting hours to days, or unremitting
C. At least two of the following characteristics: 1. Bilateral location 2. Pressing or tightening (nonpulsatile) quality 3. Mild or moderate pain intensity 4. Not aggravated by routine physical activities such as walking or climbing stairs	C. At least two of the following characteristics: 1. Bilateral location 2. Pressing or tightening (nonpulsatile) quality 3. Mild or moderate pain intensity 4. Not aggravated by routine physical activities such as walking or climbing stairs
D. Both of the following: 1. No nausea and/or vomiting 2. No more than one of photophobia or phonophobia	D. Both of the following: 1. No more than one of photophobia, phonophobia, or mild nausea 2. Neither moderate or severe nausea nor vomiting
E. Not better accounted for by another ICHD-3 diagnosis	E. Not better accounted for by another ICHD-3 diagnosis

(ICHD-3: International Classification of Headache Disorders, 3rd edition; TTH: tension-type headache)
(a) Infrequent TTH is defined as pain on <1 day/month on average.
(b) Frequent TTH is defined as pain on 1–14 days/month on average for >3 months.

*NB: Each type is additionally classified as occurring with or without pericranial muscle tenderness. Pericranial tenderness is detected and recorded by manual palpation by small rotating movements with the index and middle fingers, and by firm pressure. Palpometer may be used and summated local tenderness scores of various muscles such as frontal, temporal, masseter, pterygoid, sternocleidomastoid, splenius, and trapezius can be generated. ICHD recommends a scale of 0–3 for scoring. There is also a category of probable TTH involving all the above three categories (infrequent, frequent, and chronic) where all the criteria for diagnosis are fulfilled except one.

TABLE 2: Differentiation of chronic headache of the two subtypes.		
Chronic headache subtype	**Number of headache days/month**	**Number of episodes of migraine**
Chronic migraine	≥15 days/month	≥8 days/month of migraine
Pure chronic tension-type headache (TTH)	≥15 days/month	Nil
Chronic TTH	≥15 days/month	≤8 days/month of migraine

pericranial muscle tenderness.[15] There is also a category of probable TTH involving all the above three categories where all the criteria for diagnosis are fulfilled except one.

PATHOPHYSIOLOGY

The pathogenesis is probably multifactorial and varies between the subtypes of TTH **(Table 2)**. It has been suggested that the peripheral and environmental factors more important in ETTH, whereas genetic and central factors possibly play a significant role in the chronic variety **(Flowchart 1)**.[14]

■ Genetic Factors

In contrast to migraine, hereditary factors seem to play a minor role in the pathogenesis of ETTH. However, genetic factors may be more important in the development of CTTH than ETTH.

■ Peripheral Factors

Peripheral sensitization of myofascial nociceptors plays an important role in the development of ETTH. Myofascial factors can be further described in two groups, namely pericranial tenderness and myofascial trigger points (TrPs).

Pericranial Tenderness

Pericranial tenderness most probably arises from the activation of peripheral nociceptors. Nociceptors around the blood vessels in striated muscle, tendon insertions, and fascia have been suggested as the source of pain.[14] The frequency and intensity of TTH correlate positively with pericranial muscle tenderness.[16] The possible peripheral mechanisms include inflammatory reaction, decreased blood flow, increased muscle activity, and muscle atrophy.

Myofascial Trigger Points

Myofascial trigger point is a hyperirritable spot associated with a taut band of a skeletal muscle, painful on compression and stretch. Active TrPs cause clinical symptoms, whereas latent TrPs might produce other muscle dysfunctions like fatigue, and restricted range of motion rather than pain. A nonblinded study found that TTH subjects had a greater number of either active or latent TrPs than healthy subjects. In a further blinded study, CTTH was associated with active TrPs in various head and neck muscles. CTTH subjects with active TrPs had greater headache intensity, duration, and frequency than those with latent TrPs. A therapeutic approach based on TrP management needs to be evaluated in CTTH patients.

■ Central Factors

Continuous myofascial nociception may induce central changes (central sensitization) probably at both the

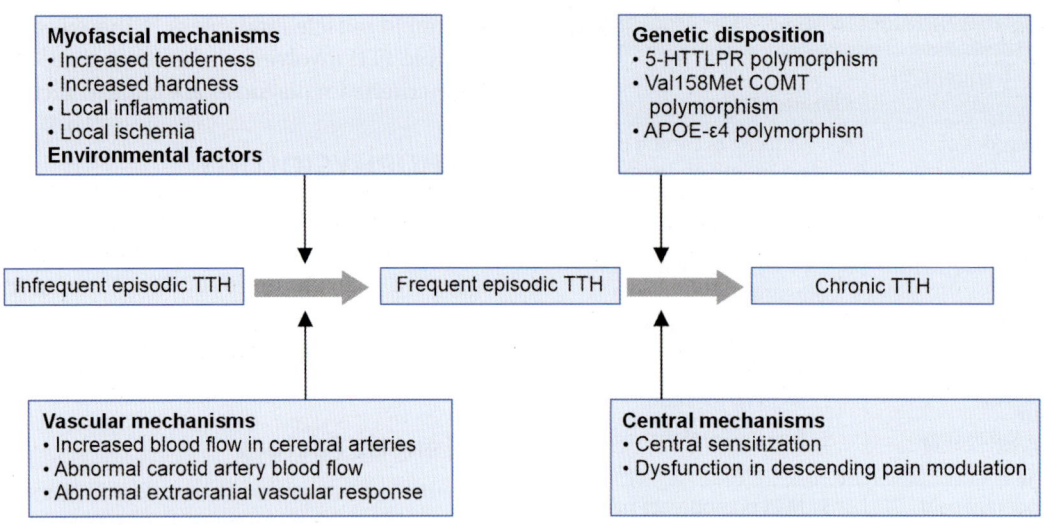

FLOWCHART 1: Proposed pathophysiological model of chronic tension-type headache (TTH).

supraspinal level and spinal dorsal horn/trigeminal nucleus in patients with CTTH.[11] The likely changes include both increased central excitability and attenuated central pain inhibition. This in turn may lead to a further increase in pericranial tenderness. Thus, in the chronic pain state, increased tenderness is caused by both peripheral nociception and central sensitization.

Pain Perception Studies in Tension-type Headache

Pain thresholds can be studied using pressure and electrical and thermal (heat and/or cold) stimuli. For each stimulus modality, pain detection threshold and pain tolerance threshold can be measured. The *pain detection threshold* is the lowest possible stimulus causing the sensation of pain. The *pressure tolerance threshold* is the maximal painful stimulus that a person can tolerate. Pain report is another measure that includes fixed stimulus (threshold and suprathreshold), temporal summation, and DNIC studies (descending inhibitory control studies). Studies of pain threshold in patients with ETTH revealed mixed responses. While the majority of these studies reported normal pain detection threshold, only two studies reported decreased pressure–pain detection threshold in ETTH of frequent type.[17,18] In contrast, the majority of studies reported lower pressure and thermal and electrical pain threshold in CTTH patients as compared with the controls.[16,19] Studies on pressure pain tolerance threshold and suprathreshold testing have also demonstrated similar results in CTTH patients and might be even more sensitive than threshold measurement in the evaluation of central sensitization [increased excitability of neurons in the central nervous system (CNS)] in TTH patients.[14]

Few studies on temporal summation have been reported in TTH; two of these did not find any significant difference,[19,20] whereas a recent study by Cathcart et al.[21] has demonstrated increased temporal summation in the CTTH patients. DNIC studies found decreased nociceptive flexion reflex (NFR) thresholds in patients with CTTH compared to controls, pointing to dysfunction of DNIC in CTTH.[21]

Imaging Studies

Abnormal brain functions have been demonstrated in TTH patients using resting-state functional magnetic resonance imaging (fMRI) study and functional connectivity study.[22] Using voxel-based morphometry (VBM), Schmidt-Wilcke et al. have demonstrated a decrease in the volume of gray matter brain structures involved in pain processing in patients with CTTH. This decrease correlated positively with the duration of the headache. The most likely explanation put forward was that the central sensitization generated by prolonged input from pericranial myofascial structures might have caused these changes. Other studies have also suggested alteration in brain structure and gray matter volume in TTH patients.[23] Further white matter tracking have shown abnormalities in patients with TTH. Overall, these studies need to be interpreted in the context of central mechanisms of pain generation in CTTH and to be integrated with the existing models for current understanding of TTH pathophysiology.

DIAGNOSIS

The diagnosis of TTH relies only upon clinical profile and no diagnostic tests are specific for TTH. Thus, a detailed history taking along with a thorough clinical examination is mandatory to rule out secondary causes.

Head pain in TTH is usually described as dull, pressure-like, and wearing a tight band around their head or heaviness of head. The headache does not worsen during routine physical activities, which is in sharp contrast to migraine. The head pain location is usually bilateral in 90% of the patients, mild to moderate in intensity. The headache starts at some point in the day with possible aggravation toward the end of the day.

While photophobia and phonophobia can often be present, only one of them is allowed by the diagnostic criteria for ETTH. Nausea and vomiting, if present, rule out the diagnosis of TTH, though mild-to-moderate anorexia may be present in 20% of TTH patients.[23] Mild nausea may be allowed for CTTH patients as long as there is no photophobia or phonophobia. Cranial autonomic features are uncommon. Precipitating and aggravating factors are similar to migraine, such as stress, lack of sleep, and fasting, and are not very helpful to distinguish the two subtypes.

Physical examination should include manual palpation of the pericranial muscles to identify tender points and trigger points, as described earlier in the pathophysiological subsection, which is increased in TTH patients. Manual palpation is performed by applying firm pressure with second and third digits with small rotatory movements on the pericranial muscles, frontal, temporal, masseter, pterygoid, sternocleidomastoid, splenius, and trapezius muscles.[15] Electromyography (EMG) studies have shown decreased relaxation of pericranial muscles at rest. Pericranial tenderness is associated with both the intensity and frequency of TTH attacks. The rest of the physical examination should be normal and should be thoroughly looked into to rule out the secondary causes. Neuroimaging is not indicated in most patients who have a stable headache pattern for over 6 months and a normal neurological examination.

DIAGNOSTIC CHALLENGES

■ Episodic Tension-type Headache

Differentiating TTH from mild migraine without aura is sometimes challenging when patients underreport symptoms by poorly describing them or when TTH-like headaches are more severe than the typical TTH and associated with photophobia or phonophobia. In the spectrum study, 32% of the patients initially diagnosed as ETTH were rediagnosed with migraine or probable migraine when their headache diaries were reviewed.[24]

■ Chronic Tension-type Headache

Chronic TTH must be differentiated from other primary chronic daily headaches of long duration and infrequently from secondary headache disorders. One of the three clinical situations can occur in patients presenting with long duration headaches equal to or more than 15 days a month with migrainous and/or TTH phenotype. They can have any of these three diagnoses and the clinicians must be careful to diagnose them correctly as depicted in **Table 2**.

New daily persistent headache, an uncommon primary headache disorder that is characterized by headache that, unambiguously, is daily, and is remembered as an unremitting headache from <24 hours after its first onset is clearly distinguishable from CTTH if proper history is taken.

■ Secondary Headache

These may pose a diagnostic challenge for both episodic and chronic TTH. The features of a slowly growing brain tumor may be nonspecific and vary widely with tumor location and size. One should carefully look for subtle neurological deficits on physical examination.

■ Medication Overuse Headache

It should be suspected in patients who have frequent or daily headaches despite or because of the regular use of headache medications. It is typically preceded by an episodic headache disorder, usually migraine or TTH, which requires frequent and excessive amounts of acute symptomatic medications for management.

TREATMENT

The treatment of TTH can be divided into two broad groups, namely pharmacologic and nonpharmacologic. The usefulness of a headache diary cannot be overemphasized and often helpful for the physician. It helps to document the progression of the frequency and severity and sometimes specific headache triggers can be identified. While suspecting medication overuse, it can be very useful in the true estimation of drug intake and reality check.

■ Pharmacological

Acute pharmacotherapy—most of the patients of infrequent ETTH do not report to the physician and self-medicate with over-the-counter analgesics.

For patients with frequent ETTH, simple analgesics and nonsteroidal anti-inflammatory drugs (NSAIDs) are the mainstays of acute management. Aspirin (500 mg or 1,000 mg) and acetaminophen (1,000 mg) both are effective for acute pain management and superior to placebo. NSAIDs such as ibuprofen (200–400 mg) and naproxen sodium (375–550 mg) can be used and have been demonstrated to be more effective and better tolerated than other NSAIDs.[25]

The addition of caffeine, codeine, sedatives, and tranquilizers in the combination therapy should be avoided to prevent the risk of dependency, abuse, and chronification of headache.[25] Opiate and muscle relaxants also need to be avoided.

Frequent intake of NSAIDs and simple analgesics (≥10 days/month) and combination analgesics should be avoided to prevent the development of medication overuse headache. Some patients with ETTH may also have associated migraine, which may respond to triptans.

Chronic pharmacotherapy should be considered in all patients with CTTH, in those with ETTH and frequent attack (>8 headache days/month), and in those with headache-related disability.

Amitriptyline is the most extensively used and efficacious drug for the preventive treatment of TTH. Since 1964, it has been the mainstay in the treatment of CTTH patients and several studies support its use. It is generally well tolerated, though some side effects like dry mouth, drowsiness, and weight gain can be seen. Mechanism of action in TTH prevention includes serotonin reuptake inhibition, potentiation of endogenous opioids, N-methyl-D-aspartate receptor (NMDAR) antagonism, and blockade of ion channels. It should be started at a low dose (10–25 mg/day) and titrated by 10–25 mg weekly till a therapeutic effect is seen or side effects appear.

The usual goal of preventive treatment includes a reduction in headache frequency and intensity and improved response to abortive treatment. It is a reasonable practice to continue a successful preventive regimen for 6 months and then slowly reducing the dose, observing the headache frequency. A decrease in the daily dose by 20–25% every 2–3 days might avoid rebound headaches.

Mirtazapine, a noradrenergic and serotonergic antidepressant, is efficacious in situations where amitriptyline is either ineffective or contraindicated. The usual dose is 15–30 mg/day and has been shown to reduce the headache index by 34% more than placebo in difficult to treat patients.

Muscle relaxants, centrally acting muscle relaxants such as tizanidine (6–18 mg/day), may have some benefit, though not recommended routinely. A recent open randomized study has shown that a combination of tizanidine (4 mg/day) and amitriptyline (20 mg/day) during the first 3 weeks of treatment gave faster relief from head pain than amitriptyline alone.

Anticonvulsant (topiramate), in an open study, has shown to be effective at a dose of 100 mg/day, although this result needs to be confirmed in a randomized controlled trial.

Botulinum toxin type A: The results of a few controlled trials have been conflicting and mostly negative. The use of botulinum toxin at present is not recommended for CTTH prevention.[26]

Trigger-point injection (lidocaine): Limited data from small randomized controlled trials suggest a promising role in decreasing headache frequency and total acute medication use infrequent ETTH and CTTH patients. It requires more research in establishing its role.

Nonpharmacological

As pharmacological interventions are not optimally effective, there is an increased interest in nonpharmacologic interventions in recent years.

Behavioral treatments[27] include the following methods:
- Regulation of sleep, exercise, and meals
- Cognitive behavioral therapy
- Relaxation
- Biofeedback
- Combination of the above

Relaxation training and EMG biofeedback therapies have been shown to reduce headache activity by nearly 50%, both alone and in combination. Cognitive behavioral interventions such as stress management programs can effectively reduce TTH activity. They have been shown to be more useful when combined with biofeedback or relaxation therapies.

In a randomized control trial from North India to assess the effectiveness of progressive muscle relaxation and deep breathing exercises on pain, disability, and sleep quality among patients with CTTH showed out of the 169 randomly selected patients, 84 performed the intervention and reported less pain severity and disability and better sleep quality after 12 weeks.[28] The combination of stress management therapy and amitriptyline (≤100 mg/day) was more effective than either therapy used alone.

The headache index score was reduced by 50% in 65% of the patients on the combination arm compared with 38% on tricyclics, 35% on stress management, and 29% of the placebo arm.[29]

The improvement seen after behavioral treatment might appear slowly compared with tricyclics; however, it is maintained for more extended periods.[14]

Physical therapy: Its components include positioning, exercise program, hot and cold packs, massage, ultrasound, and transcutaneous electrical nerve stimulation (TENS). Adding craniocervical training to classical physiotherapy might be better than physiotherapy alone.

Acupuncture: Most trials are limited by a small sample size and reported conflicting results. Acupuncture methods include needle acupuncture, laser acupuncture, and both, and have shown effectiveness as compared to placebo.[30]

FUTURE TARGETS

Calcitonin gene-related peptide (CGRP)-receptor antagonists has emerged as a key neuropeptide in migraine pathophysiology and have been approved as therapies for migraine. Whether they have a role in the treatment of TTH, requires future clinical trials.

Neuropeptide substance P: It colocalizes with CGRP in trigeminal ganglia neurons.[31] The nociceptive effect is mediated by binding to G protein-coupled neurokinin-1 (NK-1) receptor. The exact role of substance P in TTH, however, remains unclear.

Nitric oxide synthase (NOS) inhibitors: NG-monomethyl-L-arginine hydrochloride was found to reduce headache and pericranial tenderness and hardness in CTTH patients. Also, the nitric oxide (NO) donor glyceryl trinitrate-induced TTH in these patients. Hence, the inhibition of NOS may become a novel target in the treatment of CTTH.

CONCLUSION

Considering the prevalence of TTH and its socioeconomic burden, elucidation of pathophysiological mechanisms and therapeutics has received lesser attention than in migraine. In addition to the existing models of peripheral generation of pain in TTH due to excessive muscle contraction, ischemia, and inflammation of head and neck muscles, central mechanisms are being proposed based on neurophysiological and advanced neuroimaging studies. Once there is a better understanding of how to modulate these peripheral and central sensitization processes, effective control for head pain in TTH may be achieved. Though ETTH is well controlled with analgesics, CTTH requires a combination of pharmacologic and nonpharmacologic intervention for optimal results. However, the outcome still remains less than satisfactory.

KEY MESSAGE

Tension-type headache is the most common primary headache. There is no biomarker, so diagnosis is based on clinical history and examination and evaluation to rule out secondary headache causes. CTTH is more disabling and less responsive to current pharmacological therapy, so needs more attention from health authorities, clinical researchers, or industrial pharmacologists.

ACKNOWLEDGMENT

We thank Mrs Monalisa Dash for secretarial help.

REFERENCES

1. Stovner LJ, Hagen K, Jensen R, et al. The global burden of headache: A documentation of headache prevalence and disability worldwide. Cephalgia. 2007;27:193-210.
2. Jensen RH. Tension-Type Headache—the Normal and Most Prevalent Headache. Headache. 2018;58:339-45.
3. Chowdhury D. Tension-type headache. Ann Indian Acad Neurol. 2012;15:83-8.
4. Bhoi SK, Jha M, Chowdhury D. Advances in the understanding of Pathophysiology of TTH and its management. Neurol India. 2021;69(7):116-23.
5. Ashina S, Mistikostas DD, Lee MJ, et al. Tension-type headache. Nat Rev Dis Primers. 2021;7:24.
6. GBD 2016 Headache Collaborators. Global, regional, and national burden of migraine and tension-type headache, 1990–2016: A systematic analysis for the Global Burden of Disease Study 2016. Lancet Neurol. 2018;17:954-76.
7. Stovner LJ, Hagen K, Linde M, et al. The global prevalence of headache: An update with analysis of the influences of methodological factors on prevalence estimates. J Headache Pain. 2022;23(1):34.
8. GBD 2019 Diseases and Injuries Collaborators. Global burden of 369 diseases and injuries in 204 countries and territories, 1990–2019: A systematic analysis for the Global Burden of Disease Study 2019. Lancet. 2020;396(10258):1204-22.
9. Kulkarni GB, Rao GN, Gururaj G, et al. Headache disorders and public ill-health in India: Prevalence estimates in Karnataka State. J Headache Pain. 2015;16:67.
10. Singh AK, Shukla R, Trivedi JK, et al. Association of psychiatric comorbidity and efficacy of treatment in chronic daily headache in Indian population. J Neurosci Rural Pract. 2013;4:132-9.
11. Kim KM, Kim J, Cho SJ, et al. Excessive Daytime Sleepiness in Tension-Type Headache: A Population Study. Front Neurol. 2019;10:1282.
12. García-Azorín D, Farid-Zahran M, Gutiérrez-Sánchez M, et al. Tension-type headache in the Emergency Department Diagnosis and misdiagnosis: The TEDDi study. Sci Rep. 2020;10:2446.
13. Headache Classification Committee of the International Headache Society (IHS). The International Classification of Headache Disorders, 3rd edition (beta version). Cephalalgia. 2013;33:629-808.
14. Bendtsen L. Central sensitization in tension-type headache-possible pathophysiological mechanisms. Cephalalgia. 2000;20:486-508.
15. Headache Classification Committee of the International Headache Society (IHS). The International Classification of Headache Disorders, 3rd edition. Cephalalgia. 2018;38:1-211.
16. Ashina S, Babenko L, Jensen R, et al. Increased muscular and cutaneous pain sensitivity in cephalic region in patients with chronic tension-type headache. Eur J Neurol. 2005;12:543-49.
17. Schmidt-Hansen PT, Svensson P, Bendtsen L, et al. Increased muscle pain sensitivity in patients with tension-type headache. Pain. 2007;129:113-21.
18. Mørk H, Ashina M, Bendtsen L, et al. Induction of prolonged tenderness in patients with tension-type headache by means of a new experimental model of myofascial pain. Eur J Neurol. 2003;10:249-56.
19. Fernández-de-Las-Peñas C, Cuadrado ML, Arendt-Nielsen L, et al. Increased pericranial tenderness, decreased pressure pain threshold, and headache clinical parameters in chronic tension-type headache patients. Clin J Pain. 2007;23:346-52.
20. Buchgreitz L, Egsgaard LL, Jensen R, et al. Abnormal pain processing in chronic tension-type headache: A high-density EEG brain mapping study. Brain. 2008;131:3232-38.
21. Cathcart S, Winefield AH, Lushington K, et al. Noxious inhibition of temporal summation is impaired in chronic tension-type headache. Headache. 2010;50:403-12.

22. Wang P, Du H, Chen N, et al. Regional homogeneity abnormalities in patients with tension-type headache: A resting-state fMRI study. Neurosci Bull. 2014;30:949-55.
23. Husøy AK, Håberg AK, Rimol LM, et al. Cerebral cortical dimensions in headache sufferers aged 50–66 years: A population-based imaging study in the Nord-Trøndelag Health Study (HUNT-MRI). Pain. 2019;160:1634-43.
24. Lipton RB, Cady RK, Stewart WF, et al. Diagnostic lessons from the spectrum study. Neurology. 2002;58:S27-31.
25. Ashina S, Ashina M. Current and potential future drug therapies for tension-type headache. Curr Pain Headache Rep. 2003;7:466-74.
26. Jackson JL, Kuriyama A, Hayashino Y. Botulinum toxin A for prophylactic treatment of migraine and tension headaches in adults: A meta-analysis. JAMA. 2012;307:1736-45.
27. Penzien DB, Rains JC, Lipchik GL, et al. Behavioral interventions for tension-type headache: Overview of current therapies and recommendation for a self-management model for chronic headache. Curr Pain Headache Rep. 2004;8:489-99.
28. Gopichandran L, Srivastsava AK, Vanamail P, et al. Effectiveness of Progressive Muscle Relaxation and Deep Breathing Exercise on Pain, Disability, and Sleep Among Patients with Chronic Tension-Type Headache: A Randomized Control Trial. Holist Nurs Pract. 2021:1-12.
29. Holroyd KA, O'Donnell FJ, Stensland M, et al. Management of chronic tension-type headache with tricyclic antidepressant medication, stress management, and their combination: A randomized controlled trial. JAMA. 2001;285:2208-15.
30. Melchart D, Streng A, Hoppe A, et al. Acupuncture in patients with tension-type headache: Randomised controlled trial. BMJ. 2005;331:376-82.
31. Edvinsson L, Uddman R. Neurobiology in primary headaches. Brain Res Brain Res Rev. 2005;48:438-56.

Role of Greater Occipital Nerve Blocks in Headache Disorders

Ashish Kumar Duggal, Ruby Chopra

ABSTRACT

Headache is a common and disabling condition with significant impact on quality of life. Despite significant advances, there is an urgent requirement for more effective and affordable treatments for this debilitating condition. Peripheral nerve blocks have been used for many years to treat headache disorders in acute and outpatient settings. According to recent studies, greater occipital nerve (GON) blocks have been found to be effective in treating chronic migraines (CMs) and cluster headaches (CHs). GON block's effectiveness may be attributed to its ability to modulate the trigeminocervical complex and the ascending pain pathways. GON block with lidocaine is an effective, safe, and affordable treatment option for CM with a 50% responder rate in the range of 40–50% and decrease in monthly headache days in the 7–15 days range. It is equally effective in patients with medication overuse headaches. GON block, combined with steroids and local anesthetic, has been found to effectively abort a CH attack in up to 61% of patients. GON block is also effective in cervicogenic headaches and occipital neuralgia. In patients who do not respond well to GON block, peripheral nerve blocks that target other branches of the fifth cranial nerve (such as the supratrochlear, supraorbital, and auriculotemporal nerves) may be utilized.

Keywords: Headache, Chronic migraine, Cluster headache, Greater occipital nerve, Peripheral nerve blocks, Cervicogenic headache, Occipital neuralgia.

INTRODUCTION

Headache is one of the most prevalent, disabling, and undertreated conditions in neurological clinical practice, significantly impacting quality of life and a considerable burden on health resources.[1] Although several advancements have been made in managing headache disorders, such as gepants and monoclonal antibodies against calcitonin gene-related peptide (CGRP), there is a substantial unmet need for safe, effective, and economically viable treatment options in resource-limited settings like India. Patients with primary headaches complain of pain in the frontal and temporal (trigeminal innervation) and posterior (occipital nerves innervation) regions. This is due to the anatomical link between cervical and trigeminal afferents within the trigeminocervical complex (TCC).[2] Because of this, peripheral nerve blocks targeting the branches of the trigeminal and occipital nerves have been used to treat headaches for decades.[3,4] The most widely used procedure for pain relief in primary and secondary headache disorders has been the greater occipital nerve (GON) block.[5] GON block has additional advantages of safety, low cost, easy technique, and little potential for drug-to-drug interactions.[6] This review will discuss the rationale behind using GON block in various headache disorders, the evidence base for common indications, and the method for GON block, including the technique, drug constituents, frequency of administration, and potential pitfalls.

■ Rationale for the Use of GON Block in Headache Disorders

The trigeminovascular system regulates the cranial vasculature and is a critical element in the pathophysiology of various primary headache disorders, including migraine and cluster headaches (CHs). The forehead and upper periocular areas are innervated by peripheral branches of the first division of the trigeminal nerve (V1), mainly the supraorbital and the supratrochlear nerves. The temples are primarily supplied with nerves by the auriculotemporal nerve branch, which is part of the mandibular division of the trigeminal nerve (V3). The upper cervical and occipital region is supplied by posterior cervical branches of C2/C3 roots, namely the greater, lesser, and third occipital nerves.[7] The peripheral axons of the trigeminal nerve also project to the dura mater and cranial vessels, while the central branches project to the TCC in the brainstem **(Fig. 1)**. The TCC consists of the trigeminal nucleus caudalis and the spinal cord's dorsal horns at levels C1 and C2.[8] Activation of the hypothalamus and cortical spreading depression cause neurogenic inflammation in the meningeal vessels, which causes the release of CGRP and other neurotransmitters. As a result, nociceptive fibers of the trigeminal nerve (CN V) stimulate the TCC. The TCC further acts as a relay station for the pain impulses to the thalamus and cortical centers, including somatosensory, insular, motor, parietal association, retrosplenial, auditory, visual, and olfactory cortices.[9] These cortical areas are involved in processing the nociceptive signals' cognitive, emotional, and sensory aspects. This is responsible for the characteristic-associated symptoms of migraine, such as photophobia, phonophobia, cognitive dysfunction, osmophobia, and allodynia.[10] The

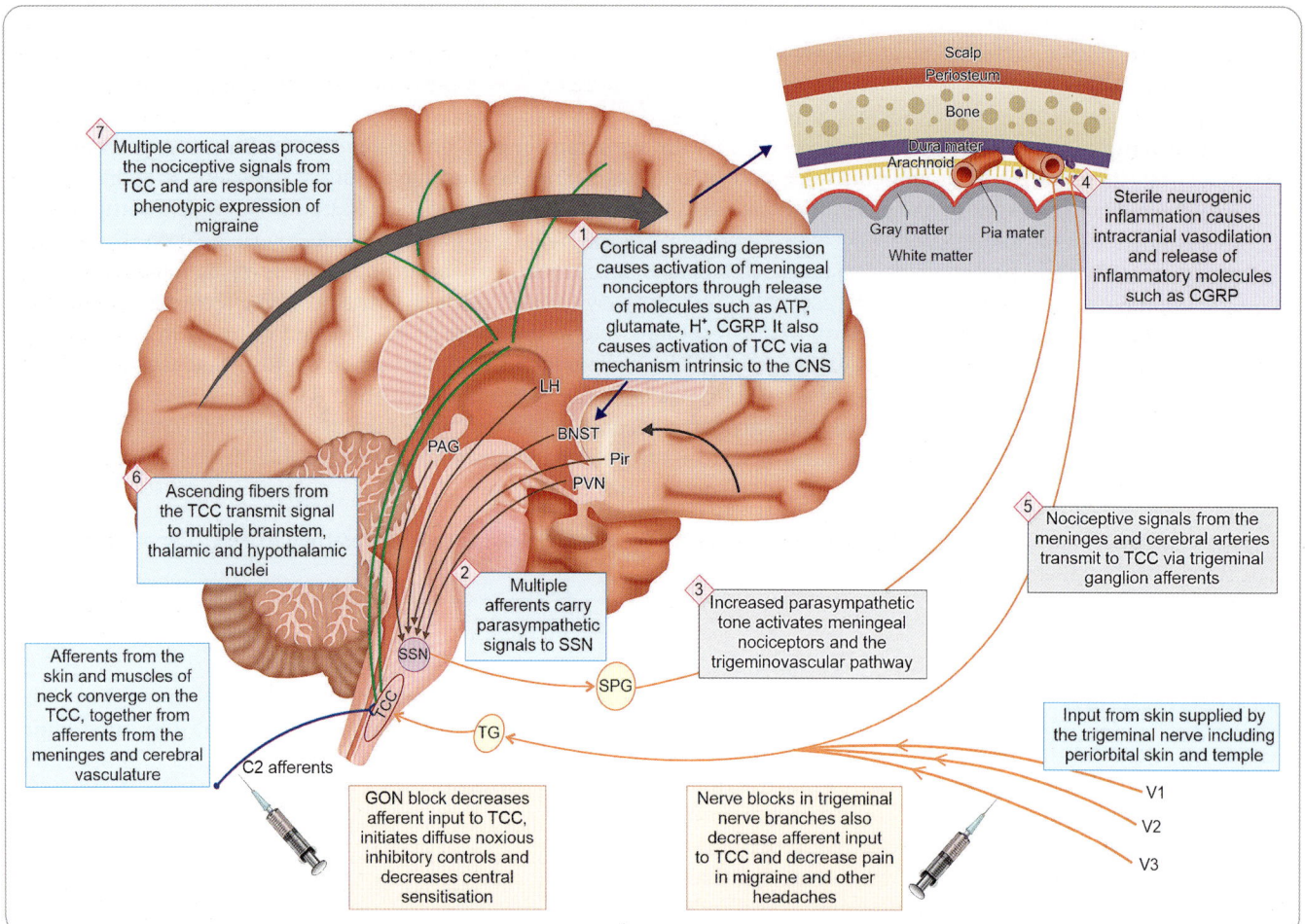

FIG. 1: Mechanism of action of GON block and other peripheral nerve blocks in migraine. Cortical spreading depression and multiples afferents from the hypothalamus, thalamus, and PAG activate the SSN to cause parasympathetic activation. This causes release of inflammatory mediators such as CGRP, which activate the A–delta and C fibers of trigeminal nerve. These nociceptive impulses converge on the trigeminocervical complex. Other afferents from the trigeminal nerve and cervical nerves (GON and LON) also converge on the TCC. Blocking these impulses from cervical and trigeminal afferents decreases the nociceptive input to TCC and decreases central sensitization, responsible for pain relief with peripheral nerve blocks.

(ATP: adenosine triphosphate; BNST: bed nucleus of stria terminals; CGRP: calcitonin gene-related peptide; CNS: central nervous system; GON: greater occipital nerve; LH: lateral hypothalamus; LON: lesser occipital nerve; PAG: periaqueductal gray; Pir: piriform cortex; PVN: paraventricular nucleus of hypothalamus; SPG: sphenopalatine ganglion; SSN: superior salivatory nucleus; TCC: trigeminocervical complex; TG: trigeminal ganglion) afferents of the skin and muscles of the neck converge on the TCC together with the afferents from the meninges and cerebral vasculature. GON block decreases the afferent input to the TCC, initiates diffuse noxious inhibitory controls, and decreases central sensitization. The decrease in the afferent input to TCC is responsible for the acute effect, and the central modulation is responsible for the prolonged effect of the GON block.[11]

An occipital nerve block can consist of a local anesthetic (LA) with or without corticosteroid injected into the occipital nerve.[12] Lidocaine and bupivacaine block the Na+ channels in a frequency- and voltage-dependent manner, causing decreased cellular excitability.[13] In chronic painful conditions, there may be an accumulation of voltage-gated Na+ channels resulting in axonal hyperexcitability and consequent central sensitization.[14] Lidocaine stops the nociceptive firing in the first-order neurons and reduces axonal hyperexcitability.[15] This effect is not dependent on the anesthetic action and may persist for many days and may be one of the reasons for the dissociation between pharmacokinetics and analgesia.[16] Corticosteroids can be beneficial for CHs and cervicogenic headaches (CeHs). However, their effectiveness in treating migraines is unclear, as conflicting results have been reported. Corticosteroids probably act by inhibiting the synthesis or release of several proinflammatory substances, a direct membrane-stabilizing effect, reversible inhibition of nociceptive C-fiber transmission, and modulation of nociceptive input within the dorsal horn substantia gelatinosa neurons.[17] Studies have shown that methylprednisolone can inhibit neurotransmission in healthy C fibers and reduce heat and mechanical pain sensitivity in nerve injury models.[18]

EVIDENCE FOR THE USE OF GREATER OCCIPITAL NERVE BLOCK IN VARIOUS HEADACHE DISORDERS

■ Acute Migraine and Status Migrainosus

Triptans and nonsteroidal anti-inflammatory drugs (NSAIDs) form the mainstay of acute migraine management. Patients with severe, long-lasting attacks may require emergency department (ED) visits and injectable therapy in the form of triptans, NSAIDs, or antiemetics. However, the management of acute migraine with currently available mediations is far from satisfactory with <25% of patients achieving freedom from headache and remaining headache free for 48 hours.[19] There is a substantial unmet need for an acute migraine intervention that can deliver rapid, complete, and sustained headache relief without causing side effects. The rapid onset of pain relief provided by anesthetic nerve blocks makes them ideal for acute headache presentations, where timely management is essential, reducing the need for opiate-based therapies. However, GON block has been used for patients with acute migraine with somewhat conflicting results **(Table 1)**.[20-25] The studies of GON

TABLE 1: Studies evaluating GON block for management of acute migraine.				
Author	Design	Number of patients	Site/Protocol/Outcome	Efficacy
Allen et al. (2017)	Retrospective	562	• All patients were in acute pain at the time of GON block • Technique not mentioned • Used lidocaine (2.4 mL); bupivacaine (6.3 mL) or combination; 99% patients also received steroid • Outcome assessed—pre- and post NPRS; (significant improvement defined as >50% NPRS point reduction)	• >30% improvement in NPRS = 82%, >50% improvement in NPRS = 58% • 59% patients received >1 GON block • NNT = 2.6
Korucu et al. (2018)	• RCT • GON block vs. Placebo (NS injected into GON area) vs. IV dexketoprofen and metoclopramide	60 (20 each group)	• 1 mL of 0.5% bupivacaine around GON—medial one-third of distance between OP and MP—U/L or B/L • PSS (1–10): Pre-treatment and at 5, 15, 30, and 45 minutes	PSS: 9 → 1 at 45 minutes for GON and NSAID group vs. 9 → 3 in the placebo group ($p = 0.03$)
Cuadrado et al. (2017)	Prospective observational	18 (MA)	• Patients with prolonged aura (>2 hours) • B/L GON block with 0.5% bupivacaine • Outcome—aura resolution (complete or partial)	• Complete resolution of aura in 59.1% • Partial response in 27.3%

Continued

Continued

Author	Design	Number of patients	Site/Protocol/Outcome	Efficacy
Friedman et al. (2018)	Sham-controlled RCT	• 15 (sham) • 13 (bupivacaine)	• Patients with acute migraine refractory to metoclopramide • B/L GON block with 6 mL bupivacaine (0.5%) vs. sham—0.5 mL bupivacaine 0.5% injected intradermally in GON area. Primary outcome—headache freedom @ 30 minutes	• Headache freedom @ 30 minutes 31% vs. 0% ($p = 0.03$) • Sustained headache relief for 48 hours—23% vs. 0%
Ebied et al.	Retrospective observational study	190	• Outcome—NPRS before and after the injection • Method of administration—at the discretion of neurologist	• Significant immediate relief = 27% • Postintervention NPRS of 0–2 = 42%
Friedman et al. (2020)	• Double-dummy, double-blind, parallel-arm, noninferiority RCT • GON block vs. IV metoclopramide	99 (51 to GON block, 48 to metoclopramide)	• B/L GON block with 6 mL bupivacaine (0.5%) vs. IV metoclopramide 10 mg • Outcome—mean improvement in NPRS at 1 hour	• Mean improvement—5.0 (GON block) vs. 6.1 (metoclopramide) • Sustained headache relief (22% vs. 38%) • Sustained headache freedom (6% vs. 15%)

(B/L: bilateral; GON: greater occipital nerve; IV: intravenous; MP: mastoid process; NPRS: Numerical Pain Rating Scale; NS: normal saline; NSAID: nonsteroidal anti-inflammatory drug; OP: occipital protuberance; PSS: pain scale score; RCT: randomized controlled trial; U/L: unilateral)

block in the acute management of migraine had several methodological flaws—small sample size, variable study populations, and outcomes. Moreover, only one study by Friedman used the endpoints described by International Headache Society, i.e., pain freedom at 2 hours, and none of the studies evaluated freedom from most bothersome symptom at 2 hours as an outcome.[23] Overall, GON block was as effective as standard treatment (NSAID + antiemetic), with almost 30–50% of patients achieving pain freedom or significant pain relief with GON block. A major limitation of the use of GON block in acute migraine has been the experience of the physician injecting the drug. Friedman et al. found that when patients were given GON block by an experienced physician (>7 prior GON block injections), there was a consistent benefit in headaches.[23,25] Therefore, training ED physicians in the procedure is essential for better outcomes. On the basis of limited available data, GON block can be used as a rescue therapy in patients with severe migraine who do not respond to first-line medications.

■ Preventive Treatment of Migraine

Until recently, preventive treatment for episodic migraine and chronic migraine (CM) was based on repurposed drugs such as antihypertensive, antiepileptics, calcium channel blockers, and antidepressants. The main problem with preventive migraine therapy is the significant adverse effects (AEs) of the drugs and poor compliance of the patients. The advent of CGRP antagonists and monoclonal antibodies against CGRP has been a game changer because we have migraine-specific therapy available for the first time.[26] However, these are expensive therapies, and may not be suitable for resource-limited countries like India. GON block has emerged as an attractive option for the preventive treatment of migraine. Recent trials and systemic meta-analysis have established the efficacy of GON block as a preventive strategy for migraine **(Table 2)**.[27-36] Overall GON block has been effective in decreasing the frequency and severity of headaches with a 50% responder rate in the range of 40–50%, and decrease in monthly headache days in the range of 7–15 days, and a decrease in monthly migraine days in the range of 6–10 days. There has been a significant improvement in disability and quality of life, as suggested by a substantial improvement in Headache Impact Test-6 (HIT-6) and Migraine Disability Assessment Scale (MIDAS) scores. One common problem in the trials has been the issue of blinding. This has been achieved by intradermal injection of LA or by application of lidocaine jelly. There has been heterogeneity in the dose and choice of anesthetic agent used across different studies. Two of the more recent trials by Chowdhury et al. have found that 40 mg lidocaine (2 mL of 2% lidocaine) has been very effective.[35,36] In the limited data available, the addition of steroids to the injecting solution has not had a significant effect. Patients with medication overuse headache (MOH) have a similar response to those who do not have MOH.[36]

Most of the studies have used bilateral GON block in migraine patients. GON block + topiramate was more efficacious combination than topiramate alone, the only oral agent approved for use in CM.[35] Based on the data available, it can be recommended that GON block is effective

TABLE 2: Studies evaluating the efficacy of GON block as a preventive treatment for migraine (episodic and chronic).

Author	N (Active/Placebo)	Study group	Agent used	Site	Protocol	Outcome	Efficacy
Ashkenazi 2008	37	Transformed migraine (MOH—not excluded)	4.5 mL of lidocaine 2%, 4.5 mL of bupivacaine 0.5%, and 1 mL saline vs. 4.5 mL of lidocaine 2%, 4.5 mL of bupivacaine 0.5%, and 40 mg triamcinolone	B/L GON (medial third to the distance b/w Po and mastoid process) + TPI	Single injection Assessment—20 minutes, 4 weeks	Headache severity, neck pain, photophobia, and phonophobia at 20 minutes duration of effect	43% vs. 50% decrease in headache score at 20 minutes Duration of response: 14.3 vs. 5.5 days Analgesic use ↓ by 19 vs. 10 doses per month
Kashipazha 2014	48	EM + CM + MOH	1 mL of lidocaine (2%) + saline vs. 1 mL of lidocaine + steroid (triamcinolone)	B/L GON (medial third to the distance b/w Po and mastoid process)	Once/month × 2 months Assessment—2 weeks, 1 and 2 months	Headache severity, frequency and duration at 2, 4, and 8 weeks	No difference b/w groups Severity : ↓50% Frequency: ↓50% and analgesic ↓45% at 2 weeks
Dilli 2015	63	EM + CM	2.5 mL BPV + 20 mg MP vs. saline + 0.25 mL lidocaine (1%)	U/L or B/L GON block (medial third to the distance b/w Po and mastoid process)	Single injection Assessment—4 weeks	Number with >50% reduction in frequency of moderate/severe headache	30% in both groups GON block not effective
Inan 2015	72	CM MOH excluded	1.5 mL BPV vs. Saline	2 cm lateral, 2 cm inferior to Po	1/week × 4 1/month × 2 Followed by open label Follow-up—3 months	Headache days (N), duration, pain scores	Frequency: 51% vs. 21% at 1 month Duration: 25% vs. 12% @ 1 month Severity: 36% vs. 17% @ 1 month At 3 months: frequency ↓ by 61% in both groups
Palamar et al. (2015)	23 (11/12)	Refractory CM MOH excluded	1.5 mL of 0.5% BPV vs. saline	USG-guided—GON block medial to the occipital artery U/L—as determined by patient to be more affected side	Once Follow-up—1 month	Pre- and postinjection VAS	Significant drop in VAS in the treatment group (3.93 ± 1.80 → 1.55 ± 1.42). However, postinjection VAS of treatment group not statistically significant from placebo group
Cuadrado et al. (2017)	36 (18/18)	CM MOH excluded	2 mL BPV (0.5%) vs. saline	3 cm below and 1.5 cm lateral to the inion B/L	Once Follow-up—1 week	Headache days Response rate: Patients showing a reduction in moderate or severe headache days >50% Mean headache days Mean medication use days Increase in mean PPT	Headache days (−2 vs. −0.4 days, $p = 0.02$) 50% responder rate (55.6% vs. 27.8%: $p = 0.008$) Medication use days (−1.4 vs. − 0.9: NS) PPT ↑ in GON block group and ↓ in Placebo group

Continued

Continued

Author	N (Active/Placebo)	Study group	Agent used	Site	Protocol	Outcome	Efficacy
Gul et al.	44 (22/22)	CM MOH excluded	1.5 mL of BPV (0.5%) + 1 mL saline vs. 2.5 mL saline	2 cm lateral and inferior to EOP B/L	1/week for 4 weeks Follow-up—3 months	Frequency of headache days/month VAS	Headache days First month (10.9 vs. 15.5) Second month (6.1 vs. 18.2) Third month (6.3 vs. 19.1) VAS First month (5.6 vs. 6.8) Second and third month—difference NS
Flamer et al.	40 (20/20)	CM MOH not excluded	1 mL of 0.5% bupivacaine with epinephrine and methylprednisolone acetate (40 mg)	USG-guided proximal (C2 vertebral level) or distal (superior nuchal line) GON block given either unilaterally or bilaterally	Once Assessment at 3 months	NRS @ 1 month	NRS pain score was significantly reduced after 24 hours and 1 week in both the groups and at 1 and 3 months in the proximal group only
Chowdhury et al. (2022)	125 (41/44/40)	CM MOH not excluded	Topiramate (100 mg/day) vs. Topiramate (100 mg/day) + GON block (40 mg lidocaine (2%) and 80 mg MP × 1 dose followed by lidocaine for 2 months vs. topiramate plus GON block with 40 mg lidocaine (2%) injections monthly for 3 months	Medial third to the distance b/w Po and mastoid process B/L	Once a month for 3 months Assessment @ 3 months	Change in monthly migraine days 50% responder rate Mean change in MHD Monthly AMT days Mean change in HIT-6 and MIDAS	MMD: −7.3 vs. −9.6 vs. −10.1 ($p < 0.001$) Responder rate: 39% vs. 71.4% vs. 63.2% MHD: −11.5 vs. −15.2 vs. −14.7 AMT: −7.4 vs. −8.9 vs. −8.4 HIT-6: −12.1 vs. −17.6 vs. −15.8 MIDAS: −27 vs. −31.8 vs. −32.1
Chowdhury et al. (2023)	44 (22/22)	CM MOH not excluded	2 mL of 2% (40 mg) lidocaine vs. 2 mL of 0.9% NS	Medial third to the distance b/w Po and mastoid process B/L	Once a month for 3 months Assessment @ 3 months	Change in mean MHD Change in mean MMD 50% responder rate Mean change in MHD Monthly AMT days Mean change in HIT-6 and MIDAS	MHD: −7.2 days vs. −3 days MMD: −6.4 days vs. −1.8 days Responder rate: 40.9% vs. 9.1% AMT: −5.9 vs. −2.9 HIT-6: −7.3 vs. −1.9 MIDAS: −20.2 vs. −7.3

(AMT: acute migraine treatment; B/L: bilateral; BPV: bupivacaine; b/w: between; CM: chronic migraine; EM: episodic migraine; GON: greater occipital nerve; HIT-6: Headache Impact Test-6; MIDAS: Migraine Disability Assessment test; MHD: monthly headache days; MMD: monthly migraine days; MOH: medication overuse headache; NRS: Numerical Rating Scale; NS: not significant; Po: external occipital protuberance; PPT: pressure pain threshold; TPI: trigger point injections; USG: Ultrasonography; VAS: Visual Analog Scale) in the management of CM. Moreover, just like botulinum toxin, the effects of GON block tend to accrue over time. The putative mechanism for such an effect may involve the modulation of the trigeminocervical pain pathway rather than the direct action of GON block in causing local anesthesia. GOB has also demonstrated efficacy in the older population with headache disorders, whose comorbidities might preclude the use of first-line preventative medications.[37] It can be used for short-term prevention of CM, till the oral medications take effect, and it can be used as a long-term preventive when alternative medications are ineffective, intolerable, or contraindicated. GON block is also an attractive option for patients who do not want to take regular oral pills or have poor compliance. It can be a cheaper alternative to botulinum toxin in preventing CM and can be particularly useful in middle- and low-income countries.

Transitional Treatment of Cluster Headache

Treatment strategies for CHs are classified as therapies for acute relief to abort individual attacks, short-term preventive treatment (transitional treatment), and long-term preventive therapies.[38] GON block in CH has been primarily used as a short-term preventive treatment, though there are case reports that GON block may provide pain relief for 2–3 hours during an acute attack of CH.[39,40] The evidence for using GON block comes from two well-conducted randomized controlled trials (RCTs). Ambrosini et al. conducted a placebo-controlled study by enrolling 23 patients in an active phase of CH [within 1 week of onset of CH in episodic CH (ECH)], devoid of contraindications for steroid treatment. 13 patients [9 ECH; 4 chronic CH (CCH)] were injected with 2.5 mL of a mixture containing a long-acting salt of betamethasone (dipropionate 12.46 mg) and a rapid-acting salt of betamethasone (disodium phosphate 5.26 mg) mixed with 0.5 mL xylocaine 2% (verum group). The control group (10 patients—7 ECH, 3 CCH) received a placebo injection containing 2 mL of physiological saline and 0.5 mL xylocaine 2% (placebo group). Patients taking prophylactic therapy (4 verapamil, 1 lithium) were allowed to continue. 11 out of 13 patients (84.6%) had a complete response (freedom from attacks for 1 week after 72 hours postinjection). Additionally, 8/13 (61%) patients were pain-free for the entire period of follow-up (4 weeks), with some patients being pain-free for as long as 26 months.[41] In another randomized, double-blind, placebo-controlled trial, suboccipital injections with cortivazol 3.75 mg ipsilateral to the CH attack side were performed three times, each 48–72 hours apart for the short-term prophylaxis of ECH and CCH in comparison to the same injection series with the same volume using normal saline in 43 patients with ECH and CCH. The prophylactic therapy (verapamil in ECH and unspecified in CCH) was continued, but further addition of prophylactic therapy was permitted only 15 days after the initial injection. The primary endpoint was a decrease in attack frequency to <2 attacks/day on the second, third, and fourth day after the third injection. 95% of patients in the cortivazol group achieved the primary endpoint compared to 55% in the placebo group. However, remission rates at day 30 were much the same between groups, though cortivazol induced a 7-day remission at a median of 7 days earlier than the placebo.[42] So, these two studies and several other retrospective and prospective open labelled studies have demonstrated that GON blockade reduces the frequency, severity and duration of individual CH attacks, particularly when a combination of steroids and LA is used. A response is more likely with concurrent long-term prophylactic medications like verapamil or lithium and where higher injectate volumes are used.[43,44] However, the dose necessary for efficacy must be determined, for which well-designed RCTs are required. The number of injections required to terminate an attack of a cluster is also not established. There may be individual variation since studies have shown that some patients may respond with one injection while others may require multiple GON blocks before a response can be seen. It has been speculated that the systemic effect of injected steroids may be responsible for the beneficial effect of GON block. However, attacks often resume when oral steroids are tapered down, whereas such a rebound was not reported with GON block. GON block-containing steroids and LA are safe and well tolerated, with only transient adverse events in these trials. American Headache Society also recommends the use of GON block containing a combination of LA and steroids as a short-term preventive therapy which can be used in patients who do not respond to a short course of steroids or have a contraindication to systemic steroids.[45] Care should be taken about the systemic absorption of steroids, especially with repeated injections. Rozen et al. reported that one patient with CH developed unilateral avascular necrosis after receiving 30 injections, although the link between the treatment and the pathology was unclear.[43]

Trigeminal Autonomic Cephalalgias Other than Cluster Headache

There is a single case report evaluating the role of GON block in short-lasting unilateral neuralgiform headache with conjunctival injection and tearing (SUNCT). Porta-Ertesam et al. observed complete remission of headache for 48 hours after the GON block in a patient of SUNCT and improvement of headache attacks persisted for nearly 3 weeks.[46] However, Miller et al. used multiple cranial nerve blocks (MCNB) [GON, lesser occipital nerve (LON), supraorbital, supratrochlear, and auriculotemporal nerves] in patients with SUNCT who had not responded to GON block and other traditional treatments. They found that 9/16 (56.3%) patients responded to MCNB with a decrease in attack frequency by 95.7% with response lasting up to 4 weeks.[47] MCNB can be utilized in refractory SUNCT/SUNA patients who do not respond to GON block alone. Miller et al. reported similar results in five patients with hemicrania continua who had not responded to GON block.[47]

■ Tension-type Headache

Peripheral nerve blocks have not been found to be useful in treatment of tension-type headache.[48] Rather trigger point injections in the pericranial and neck muscles may be an attractive option in refractory patients.[49]

OTHER UNCOMMON PRIMARY HEADACHES AND NEURALGIAS

Occipital neuralgia (ON) is characterized by paroxysmal electric, shock-like, sharp, or shooting pain in the distribution of the occipital nerves (GON and/or LON). The pain often worsens with local palpation and is temporarily relieved by anesthetic infiltration of the nerves. It may be accompanied by changes in sensation in the area of GON or LON.[50] ON may be caused by chronic entrapment of occipital nerves by muscles in the posterior neck and scalp, or by secondary causes such as previous surgery, vascular compression, or infectious diseases.[51,52] Block of GON and LON, preferably with a steroid, is both diagnostic and therapeutic. The duration of effect is variable, usually lasting for days to years and most patients do not require a repeat block. In patients who do not respond, a repeat block (with LA alone) once a week for 3 weeks may be used.[53] GON block has been reported to be beneficial in orgasmic headache and hypnic headache in single case reports.[54,55]

■ Cervicogenic Headache

The International Classification of Headache Disorders, 3rd edition (ICHD-3) defines CeH as headache caused by a cervical spine disorder that usually, but not invariably, is accompanied by neck pain. It is characterized by chronic hemicranial pain usually beginning in the suboccipital region and spreading anteriorly to the ipsilateral orbital, frontal, and temporal areas. Pain is usually unilateral headache without side shift and is often triggered by neck movement or sustained awkward posture. Treatment modalities include physical therapy and anesthetic injections of the lateral atlantoaxial joint, the C2-3 zygapophyseal joint (and the overlying third occipital nerve), and/or the C3-4 zygapophyseal joint, which have a diagnostic value as well.[56] Occipital nerve blocks have been tried and may provide temporary benefit in pain. Inan et al. found that GON block with lidocaine and bupivacaine was as effective as C2/C3 spinal rami blocks in 28 patients with CeH.[57] Naja et al. did an RCT comparing GON and LON block with a mixture of lidocaine, bupivacaine, epinephrine, fentanyl, and clonidine compared with saline injections in the suboccipital area. There was a statistically significant improvement in pain intensity, frequency, and duration, as well as a decrease in analgesic use was observed at 2 weeks in the block group compared to the placebo group.[58] Lauretti et al. compared the classical GON block technique with the proximal suboccipital compartment technique, with different amounts of injectate (5, 10, and 15 mL). A significant decrease in the pain score and rescue analgesic consumption and an improved quality of life were seen in all subcompartmental groups for 24 weeks compared to only 2 weeks with the classic technique.[59] A systematic review by Goyal et al. concluded that occipital nerve blocks (GON and LON) showed only limited evidence, as most of the studies were noncontrolled and yielded only transient benefits.[60] They may be used when anesthetic blocks of the upper cervical spinal nerves are not feasible.

■ Other Secondary Headaches

The use of GON block has been studied in open-label studies for postdural puncture headache (PDPH). It has been found to provide almost immediate relief, though the effects may not last and patients may need to receive repeat blocks. If conservative treatments fail to alleviate headaches, GON block can be used for PDPH. It has also been found to be beneficial for post-traumatic headaches in pediatric patients.

■ Injection Technique for Greater Occipital Nerve Block and Other Peripheral Nerve Blocks

The GON is responsible for providing sensation to the back of the scalp. Its origin is from the medial branch of the second cervical nerve's posterior division, and it travels obliquely between the obliquus capitis inferior and semispinalis capitis muscles. This nerve penetrates both muscles near their attachments to the occipital bone before finally reaching the trapezius muscle and ending at the scalp's medial area **(Fig. 2)**.[61] It is recommended that patients eat and drink before their procedure to decrease the likelihood of experiencing a syncopal episode. To reduce discomfort during injections, a topical anesthetic cream can be applied a few minutes prior to the procedure. This is particularly effective for injections targeting the supraorbital, supratrochlear, and auriculotemporal nerves. To administer the injection, the patient should sit comfortably on a chair with their head slightly flexed. The clinician should stand behind the patient. If the patient has experienced vasovagal episodes from pain or past injections, it is best to have them lie on their side to prevent sudden drops in blood pressure and syncope. The GON injection can be done through

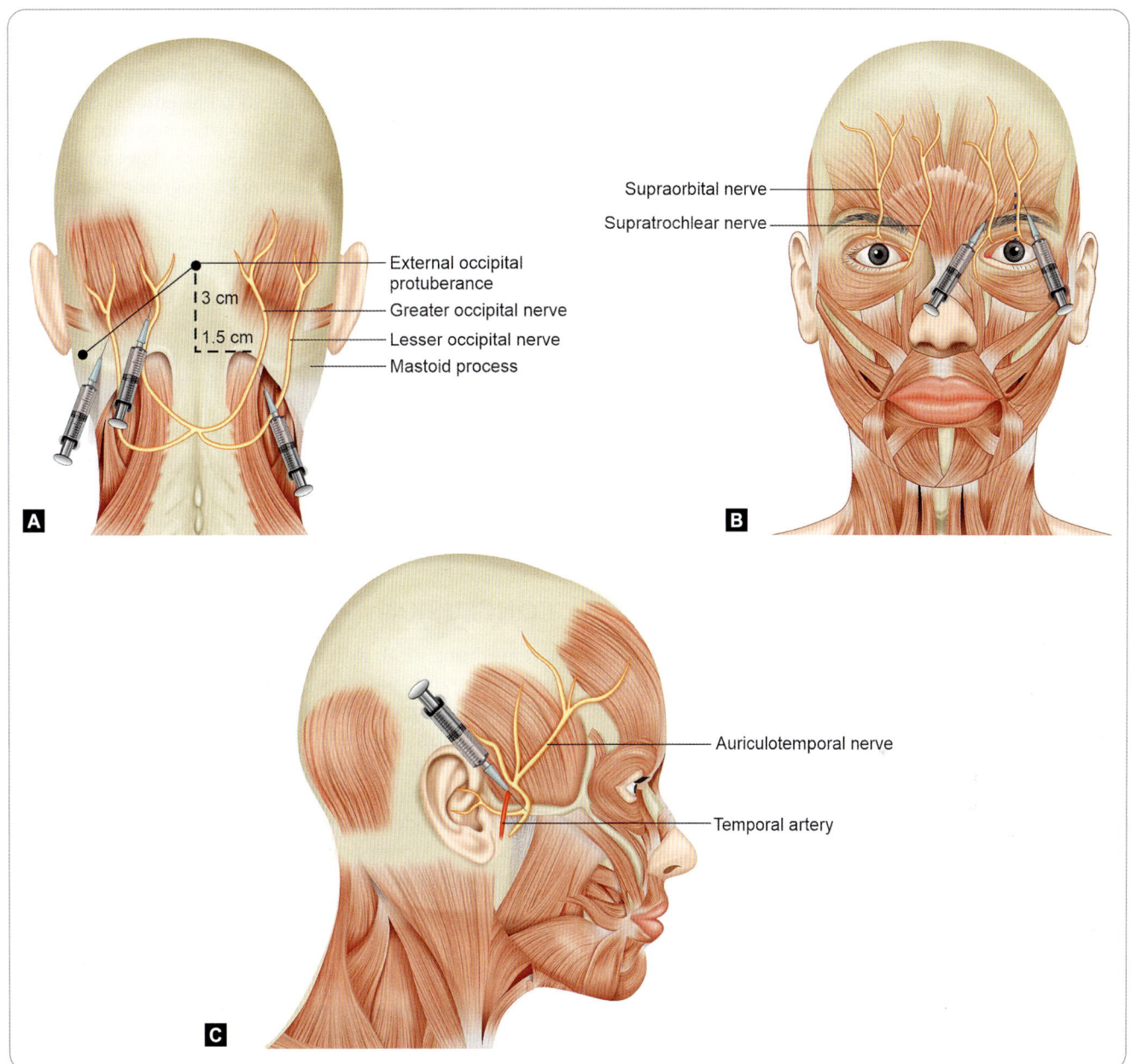

FIGS. 2A TO C: Anatomical landmarks and injection sites for peripheral nerve blocks in headache disorders. (A) Greater occipital nerve (GON) is injected at a point one-third from the external occipital protuberance (EOP) along the occipital ridge (distal injection). GON can also be injected at the proximal site, i.e., 3 cm below and 1.5 cm lateral to the EOP. Lesser occipital nerve is injected on the line between mastoid and EOP at a point two-thirds from the EOP. (B) Supratrochlear nerve is injected at the superior orbital ridge finger breadth lateral to the procures muscles. For the supraorbital nerve, the needle is injected in the mid-pupillary line in the corrugator muscle, at the superior margin of the orbit. (C) For the auriculotemporal nerve, the needle is injected 2 mm anterior to the temporal artery just anterior to the tragus.

two approaches—distal and proximal. To find the GON using the distal approach, locate a point that is one-third medially between the occipital protuberance (inion) and the mastoid process. This point should be approximately 2 cm lateral and 1.5–2.0 cm below the inion along the occipital ridge **(Fig. 2)**. When administering a nerve injection, it is important to consider the position of the occipital artery, which typically runs lateral to the GON to prevent accidental puncture. For the proximal approach, locate where the occipital nerve emerges from muscle approximately 3 cm below and 1.5 cm lateral to the inion **(Fig. 2)**.[62] This method has an added advantage as it can infiltrate the paraspinal muscles and allow for a greater amount of anesthetic solution to be administered.[63] However, most studies have used the distal approach, and studies which compared the two techniques did not find any significant difference in the efficacy. Palpating for the point of maximal tenderness may improve accuracy. A 2-5 mL syringe is typically used with a 25-30-G needle. To administer the injection properly, insert the needle gently and perpendicular to the skin until firm resistance is felt. This indicates that the needle tip has reached the periosteum. Then withdraw the needle slightly and aspirate to ensure that there is no arterial drawback. Finally, redirect the needle slightly upward and gently distribute the solution in a fan-like pattern. Alternatively, the solution can be injected with the needle in the same position, which is sufficient if injecting a reasonable volume of anesthetic. The patient may experience a burning sensation during the anesthetic administration, but it should go away in a few minutes when the anesthetic effect starts working. Withdraw the needle and apply pressure to the site with gauze to minimize bleeding. **Table 3** provides a detailed list of the dosage of LAs and steroids that are utilized for GON block. After the injection, check for numbness in the GON dermatome area. This should happen within 5 minutes of lidocaine injection and 10-15 minutes after bupivacaine injection. This can be done by using a pin on the sensory area served by the GON, away from the injection site, and checking for sharpness or bluntness comparing it with an area not served by the GON. It is important to note that pain relief may take time, and the full effect of the pain reliever may not be felt until at least 20 minutes after injection. Additionally, the benefits of GON block typically increase over time.

Patients who need multiple injections can be injected once every 2-4 weeks, depending on their response. For instance, patients with MOH may require additional treatment within a period of 2-4 weeks. Alternatively, when using GON block as a preventative measure for CM, longer intervals of 1 month or more may be adequate. The time interval between injections should be personalized to the patient's individual response pattern. When using steroids to treat migraines, limiting injections to no more than once every 3 months is recommended. Patients with CH may require a shorter interval of 2-3 injections on alternate days until a cluster is aborted. Before determining that GON block has not been effective for migraine patients, it is recommended to administer at least three injections spaced 2-4 weeks apart as a trial. If the patient fails to respond to GON block, then other nerves can be infiltrated or steroids may be added **(Table 4 and Flowchart 1)**.

ADVERSE EFFECTS AND PITFALLS

Greater occipital nerve block is generally considered safe if the precautions mentioned above are followed. AEs are minimal and generally transient **(Table 5)**. Corticosteroid injections can cause local and systemic AEs such as hair loss, skin thinning, darkening, bone tissue death, and Cushing's syndrome, especially with frequent and high doses.[64,65]

CONCLUSION

Greater occipital nerve block is a safe and effective procedure for patients with frequent, disabling, and refractory headaches. While the evidence is robust for some headache disorders (CM, CH, and CeH), it has been used in several other headaches with variable results. It is often difficult to identify which patients will respond to GON block, but an adequate trial should be given before labeling a patient as a nonresponder. Patients with poor response to GON block can be given blocks in other peripheral nerves—LON, supratrochlear nerve, supraorbital nerve, and the auriculotemporal nerve.

TABLE 3: Dosing of local anesthetic and steroids in greater occipital nerve (GON) block.			
Headache disorder	**Local anesthetic**	**Volume**	**Comments**
Migraine	• Lidocaine (2%); 20 mg/mL • Bupivacaine (0.5%); 5 mg/mL • Combination of lidocaine and bupivacaine in a ratio of 1:1–1:3	• 1.5–3 mL (usually 2 mL); 40 mg on each side • 1.5–3 mL (usually 2 mL), 10 mg on each side • Total volume of 2 mL (1 mL lidocaine + 1 mL bupivacaine) or (0.5 mL lidocaine + 1.5 mL bupivacaine)	• Lidocaine maximum dose: 4.5 mg/kg. Do not use >300 mg (15 mL) of 2% lidocaine per session • Maximum dose of bupivacaine: 2 mg/kg (maximum 175 mg per session) • If methylprednisolone is given—40 mg/mL (1–2 mL) + 2 mL of LA on each side (total volume 3–4 mL) • Maximum dose of methylprednisolone 160 mg per session
Cluster headache	Lidocaine 2 mL or bupivacaine 2 mL on the symptomatic side	Methylprednisolone 40 mg/mL: 2 mL on the symptomatic side	Other steroids can be used: • Triamcinolone—40 mg • Betamethasone—18 mg • Dexamethasone—4 mg

Role of Greater Occipital Nerve Blocks in Headache Disorders

TABLE 4: Other peripheral nerve blocks used in headache disorders.

Nerve injected	Location and technique	Syringe/Needle/Dose of anesthetic	Comments
Supraorbital	The needle is inserted at the corrugator muscle, at the superior margin of the orbit in the mid pupillary line to a depth of 3–4 mm	1 mL/25–30 G/0.2–1 mL of LA	Patient should be lying supine with neck in neutral position
Supratrochlear nerve	The needle is inserted at the medial aspect of the corrugator muscle, a finger breadth lateral to the procerus, to a depth of 3–4 mm	1 mL/25–30 G/0.2–1 mL of LA	Pressure should be applied to avoid periorbital hematoma
Auriculotemporal nerve	Palpate for the temporal artery along its course anterior to the tragus and inject 2 mm anterior to it at a depth of 4–6 mm	1–2 mL/25–30 G/0.5–1 mL	Patient supine and facing away from injection sit
Lesser occipital nerve	The needle is inserted two-thirds of the distance between EOP and mastoid. The needle is inserted perpendicular to the skin, stopping once the periosteum is reached	• Lidocaine 2% (1 mL), bupivacaine 0.5% (1 mL) • Total injection volume = 2 mL/25–30 G/2–5 mL	Commonly injected along with GON

(EOP: external occipital protuberance; GON: greater occipital nerve; LA: local anesthetic)

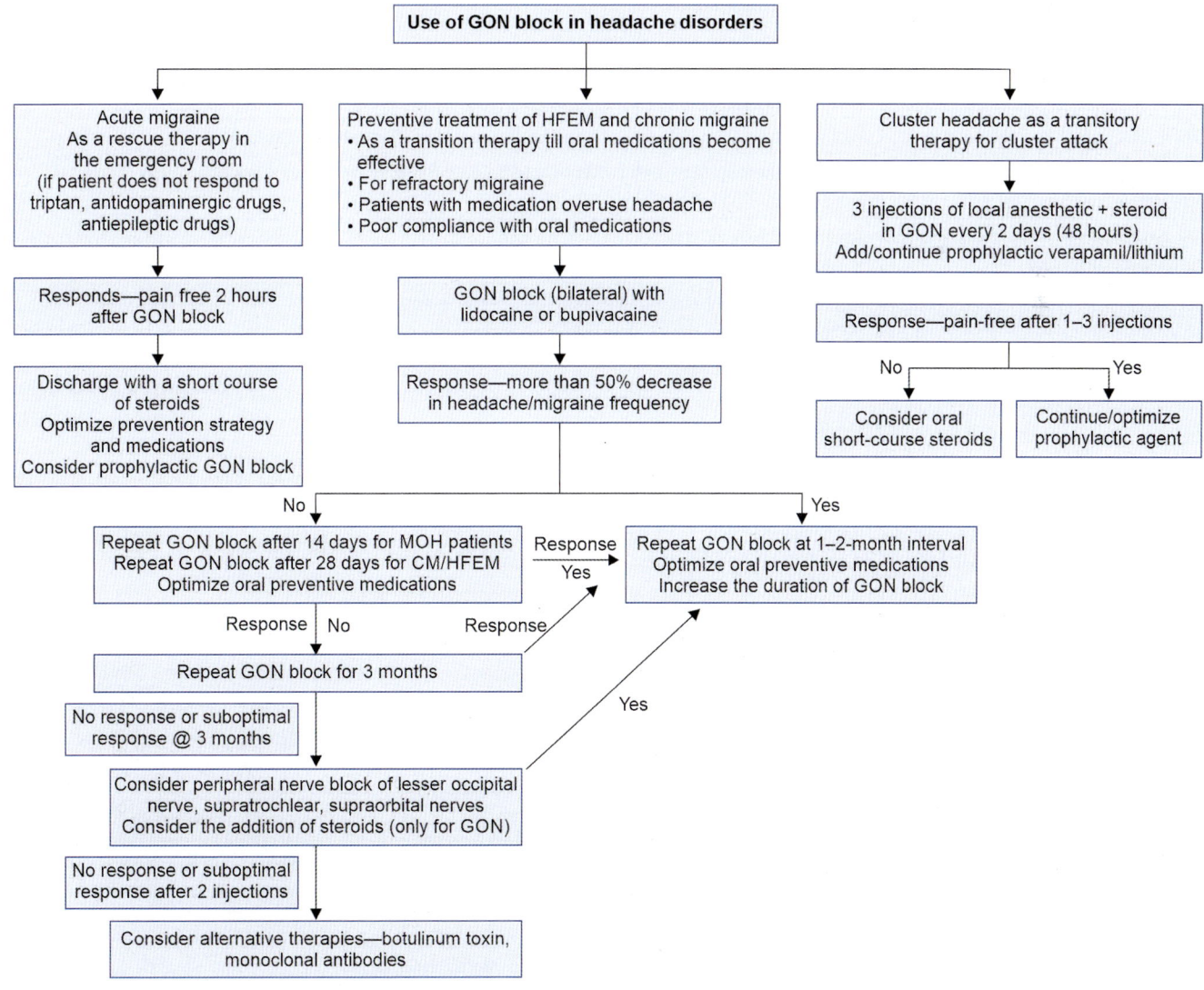

FLOWCHART 1: Use of GON block in migraine and CH.
(CH: cluster headache; GON: greater occipital nerve; HFEM: high-frequency episodic migraine; MOH: medication overuse headache)

TABLE 5: Adverse effects and pitfalls of GON block injections.

Potential adverse effects	Concern and action
Local anesthesia allergy	• Can cause allergic reactions, including anaphylaxis • PNB with LA is contraindicated • Use corticosteroids only • For anaphylactic shock, 0.3–0.5 mg adrenaline, life support, and transfer
Elderly population	• Can develop hypotension—reduce the concentration of anesthetic, give the injection in the supine position • Can develop hypertension—limit the number of nerves to be blocked in a single session, restrict PNB to unilateral GON injection if possible
Pregnancy	• Use lidocaine (FDA category B) over bupivacaine (FDA category C) • Avoid betamethasone and dexamethasone (accelerate fetal lung development) • Caution is warranted in the use of any corticosteroids in the pregnant population
Prior vasovagal attacks	• Perform PNB in supine position, where feasible • Where possible, no blockades on fasting patients • Limit the number of nerves to be blocked in a single session • In a vasovagal episode, place the patient in the Trendelenburg position; if no response, start atropine and fluid replacement
Prior syncopal attacks	• Use bupivacaine instead of lidocaine • Reduce the concentration of the anesthetic agent • Allow for extra time in the supine position after the procedure as a precaution
Open skull defect or craniotomy	Can cause intracranial diffusion of anesthetic agent, so PNB contraindicated
Anticoagulation therapy Antiplatelet therapy	Can develop hematoma—extra attention to palpate for (and avoid) neighboring arteries (occipital, temporal). Compress at each PNB site for 5–10 minutes
Cosmetic concerns—alopecia and cutaneous atrophy	• Avoid corticosteroids • If methylprednisolone must be used, a dose <80 mg in GON region
Local pain	• Apply an anesthetic cream to the site before the injection • Perform infiltration slowly, with a fine-gauge needle • Avoid lateral motions • Limit steroid use • Local cold application
Lesion to peripheral nerve	If the patient experiences sharp radiating pain, remove the needle and insert it again
Local infection	• Avoid infiltration if infection is present • Aseptic measures (sterile technique, local antiseptic)
Local anesthetic systemic toxicity	Use small doses and volumes. Avoid intravascular infiltration

(FDA: Food and Drug Administration; GON: greater occipital nerve; LA: local anesthetic; PNB: peripheral nerve block)

REFERENCES

1. Stovner LJ, Nichols E, Steiner TJ, et al. Global, regional, and national burden of migraine and tension-type headache, 1990–2016: a systematic analysis for the global burden of disease study 2016. Lancet Neurol. 2018;17:954-76.
2. Bartsch T, Goadsby PJ. The trigeminocervical complex and migraine: Current concepts and synthesis. Curr Pain Headache Rep. 2003;7:371-6.
3. Wolff HG (Ed). Wolff's Headache and Other Head Pain, 1st edition. New York: Oxford University Press; 1948.
4. Saadah HA, Taylor FB. Sustained headache syndrome associated with tender occipital nerve zones. Headache. 1987;27:201-5.
5. Ashkenazi A, Levin M. Greater occipital nerve block for migraine and other headaches: is it useful? Curr Pain Headache Rep. 2007;11(3):231-5.
6. Chowdhury D, Mundra A. Role of greater occipital nerve block for preventive treatment of chronic migraine: A critical review. Cephalalgia Reports. 2020;3:1-20.
7. Kwon HJ, Kim HS, Jehoon O, et al. Anatomical analysis of the distribution patterns of occipital cutaneous nerves and the clinical implications for pain management. J Pain Res. 2018;11:2023-31.
8. May A, Goadsby PJ. The trigeminovascular system in humans: pathophysiologic implications for primary headache syndromes of the neural influences on the cerebral circulation. J Cereb Blood Flow Metab. 1999;19:115-27.
9. Dodick DW. A Phase-by-Phase Review of Migraine Pathophysiology. Headache. 2018;58 Suppl 1:4-16.
10. Burstein R, Noseda R, Borsook D. Migraine: Multiple processes, complex pathophysiology. J Neurosci. 2015;35:6619-29.

11. Selekler MH. Greater occipital nerve blockade: Trigeminocervical system and clinical applications in primary headaches. Agri. 2008;20:6-13.
12. Tang Y, Kang J, Zhang Y. Influence of greater occipital nerve block on pain severity in migraine patients: a systematic review and meta-analysis. Am J Emerg Med. 2017;35:1750-4.
13. Hille B. Local anesthetics: Hydrophilic and hydrophobic pathways for the drug-receptor reaction. J Gen Physiol. 1977;69:497-515.
14. Strassman AM, Raymond SA, Burstein R. Sensitization of meningeal sensory neurons and the origin of headaches. Nature. 1996;384:560-4.
15. Wood JN, Boorman JP, Okuse K, et al. Voltage-gated sodium channels and pain pathways. J Neurobiol. 2004;61:55-71.
16. Attal N, Rouaud J, Brasseur L, et al. Systemic lidocaine in pain due to peripheral nerve injury and predictors of response. Neurology. 2004;62:218-25.
17. Li JY, Xie W, Strong JA, et al. Mechanical hypersensitivity, sympathetic sprouting, and glial activation are attenuated by local injection of corticosteroid near the lumbar ganglion in a rat model of neuropathic pain. Reg Anesth Pain Med. 2011;36:56-62.
18. He L, Üçeyler N, Krämer HH, et al. Methylprednisolone prevents nerve injury-induced hyperalgesia in neprilysin knockout mice. Pain. 2014;155(3):574-80.
19. Friedman BW, Bijur PE, Lipton RB. Standardizing emergency department-based migraine research: An analysis of commonly used clinical trial outcome measures. Acad Emerg Med. 2010;17: 72-9.
20. Allen S, Mb Bch BAO, Mookadam F, et al. Greater occipital nerve block for acute treatment of migraine headache: a large retrospective cohort study. J Am Board Fam Med. 2018;31:211-8.
21. Korucu O, Dagar S, Çorbacioglu ŞK, et al. The effectiveness of greater occipital nerve blockade in treating acute migraine-related headaches in emergency departments. Acta Neurol Scand. 2018;138(3):212-8.
22. Cuadrado ML, Aledo-Serrano Á, López-Ruiz P, et al. Greater occipital nerve block for the acute treatment of prolonged or persistent migraine aura. Cephalalgia. 2017;37(8):812-8.
23. Friedman BW, Mohamed S, Robbins MS, et al. A randomized, sham-controlled trial of bilateral greater occipital nerve blocks with bupivacaine for acute migraine patients refractory to standard emergency department treatment with metoclopramide. Headache. 2018;58:1427-34.
24. Ebied AM, Nguyen DT, Dang T. Evaluation of Occipital Nerve Blocks for Acute Pain Relief of Migraines. J Clin Pharmacol. 2020;60(3):378-83.
25. Friedman BW, Irizarry E, Williams A, et al. A randomized, double-dummy, emergency-department-based study of greater occipital nerve block with bupivacaine vs intravenous metoclopramide for treatment of migraine. Headache. 2020;60:2380-8.
26. Vandervorst F, Deun LV, Dycke AV, et al. CGRP monoclonal antibodies in migraine: An efficacy and tolerability comparison with standard prophylactic drugs. J Headache Pain. 2021;22(1):128.
27. Ashkenazi A, Matro R, Shaw JW, et al. Greater occipital nerve block using local anaesthetics alone or with triamcinolone for transformed migraine: a randomised comparative study. J Neurol Neurosurg Psych. 2008;79:415-7.
28. Kashipazha D, Nakhostin-Mortazavi A, Mohammadianinejad SE, et al. Preventive effect of greater occipital nerve block on severity and frequency of migraine headache. Global J Health Sci. 2014;6(6):209-13.
29. Dilli E, Halker R, Vargas B, et al. Occipital nerve block for the short-term preventive treatment of migraine: a randomized, double-blinded, placebo-controlled study. Cephalalgia. 2015;35:959-68.
30. Inan LE, Inan N, Ö Karadaş, et al. Greater Occipital Nerve blockade for the treatment of chronic migraine: a randomized, multicenter, double-blind, and placebo-controlled study. Acta Neurol Scand. 2015;132:270-7.
31. Palamar D, Uluduz D, Saip S, et al. Ultrasound-guided greater occipital nerve block: an efficient technique in chronic refractory migraine without aura? Pain Physician. 2015;18:153-62.
32. Cuadrado ML, Aledo-Serrano Á, Navarro P, et al. Short-term effects of greater occipital nerve blocks in chronic migraine: a double-blind, randomised, placebo-controlled clinical trial. Cephalalgia. 2017;37:864-72.
33. Gul HL, Ozon AO, Karadas Ö, et al. The efficacy of greater occipital nerve blockade in chronic migraine: a placebo-controlled study. Acta Neurol Scand. 2017;136:138-44.
34. Flamer D, Alakkad H, Soneji N, et al. Comparison of two ultrasound-guided techniques for greater occipital nerve injections in chronic migraine: a double-blind, randomized, controlled trial. Reg Anesth Pain Med. 2019;44:595-603.
35. Chowdhury D, Mundra A, Datta D, et al. Efficacy and tolerability of combination treatment of topiramate and greater occipital nerve block versus topiramate monotherapy for the preventive treatment of chronic migraine: A randomized controlled trial. Cephalalgia. 2022;42(9):859-71.
36. Chowdhury D, Tomar A, Deorari V, et al. Greater occipital nerve blockade for the preventive treatment of chronic migraine: A randomized double-blind placebo-controlled study. Cephalalgia. 2023;43(2):3331024221143541.
37. Hascalovici JR, Robbins MS. Peripheral nerve blocks for the treatment of headache in older adults: a retrospective study. Headache J Head Face Pain. 2017;57:80-6.
38. Gordon A, Roe T, Villar-Martínez MD, et al. Effectiveness and safety profile of greater occipital nerve blockade in cluster headache: a systematic review. J Neurol Neurosurg Psychiatry. 2023:jnnp-2023-331066.
39. Anthony M. The role of the occipital nerve in unilateral headache. In: Rose F (Ed). Advances in Headache Research. London: John Libbey; 1987. pp. 257-62.
40. Gelener P. Acute treatment of cluster headache with great occipital nerve blockade. Noro Psikiyatr Ars. 2019;56:224-5.
41. Ambrosini A, Vandenheede M, Rossi P, et al. Suboccipital injection with a mixture of rapid- and long-acting steroids in cluster headache: a double-blind placebo-controlled study. Pain. 2005;118:92-6.
42. Leroux E, Valade D, Taifas I, et al. Suboccipital steroid injections for transitional treatment of patients with more than two cluster headache attacks per day: a randomised, double-blind, placebo-controlled trial. Lancet Neurol. 2011;10:891-7.
43. Rozen TD. High-volume anesthetic suboccipital nerve blocks for treatment refractory chronic cluster headache with long-term efficacy data: An observational case series study. Headache. 2019;59:56-62.
44. Anthony M. Arrest of attacks of cluster headache by local steroid injection of the occipital nerve. In: Rose FC (Ed). Migraine: Clinical and Research Advances. London: Karger; 1985. pp. 169-73.
45. Blumenfeld A, Ashkenazi A, Napchan U, et al. Expert consensus recommendations for the performance of peripheral nerve blocks for headaches - a narrative review. Headache J Head Face Pain. 2013;53:437-46.
46. Porta-Etessam J, Cuadrado M, Galan L, et al. Temporal response to bupivacaine bilateral great occipital block in a patient with SUNCT syndrome. J Headache Pain. 2010;11:179.
47. Miller S, Lagrata S, Matharu M. Multiple cranial nerve blocks for the transitional treatment of chronic headaches. Cephalalgia. 2019;39(12):1488-99.

48. Leinisch-Dahlke E, Jürgens T, Bogdahn U, et al. Greater occipital nerve block is ineffective in chronic tension type headache. Cephalalgia. 2005;25:704-8.
49. Robbins MS, Kuruvilla D, Blumenfeld A, et al.; Peripheral Nerve Blocks and Other Interventional Procedures Special Interest Section of the American Headache Society. Trigger point injections for headache disorders: expert consensus methodology and narrative review. Headache. 2014;54(9):1441-59.
50. Headache Classification Committee of the International Headache Society (IHS). The International Classification of Headache Disorders, 3rd edition (beta version). Cephalalgia. 2013;33:629-808.
51. Bogduk N. The neck and headaches. Neurol Clin. 2004;22(1): 151-71, vii.
52. Narouze S. Occipital Neuralgia Diagnosis and Treatment: The Role of Ultrasound. Headache. 2016;56(4):801-7.
53. Ward JB. Greater occipital nerve block. Semin Neurol. 2003;23(1): 59-62.
54. Rehmann R, Tegenthoff M, Zimmer C, et al. Case report of an alleviation of pain symptoms in hypnic headache via greater occipital nerve block. Cephalalgia. 2017;37:998-1000.
55. Vanderhoek MD, Hoang HT, Goff B. Ultrasound-guided greater occipital nerve blocks and pulsed radiofrequency ablation for diagnosis and treatment of occipital neuralgia. Anesth Pain Med. 2013;3:256-9.
56. Verma S, Tripathi M, Chandra PS. Cervicogenic Headache: Current Perspectives. Neurol India. 2021;69(Supplement):S194-S198.
57. Inan N, Ceyhan A, Inan L, et al. C2/C3 nerve blocks and greater occipital nerve block in cervicogenic headache treatment. Funct Neurol. 2001;16:239-43.
58. Naja ZM, El-Rajab M, Al-Tannir MA, et al. Occipital nerve blockade for cervicogenic headache: a double-blind randomized controlled clinical trial. Pain Pract. 2006;6:89-95.
59. Lauretti GR, Corrêa SW, Mattos AL. Efficacy of the greater occipital nerve block for cervicogenic headache: comparing classical and subcompartmental techniques. Pain Pract. 2015;15:654-61.
60. Goyal S, Kumar A, Mishra P, et al. Efficacy of interventional treatment strategies for managing patients with cervicogenic headache: a systematic review. Korean J Anesthesiol. 2022;75(1):12-24.
61. Fernandes L, Randall M, Idrovo L. Peripheral nerve blocks for headache disorders Pract Neur. 2021;21:30-5.
62. Santos Lasaosa S, Cuadrado Pérez ML, Guerrero Peral AL, et al. Consensus recommendations for anaesthetic peripheral nerve block. Neurologia. 2017;32(5):316-30.
63. Young WB, Marmura M, Ashkenazi A, et al. Greater occipital nerve and other anesthetic injections for primary headache disorders. Headache. 2008;48:1122-5.
64. Shields KG, Levy MJ, Goadsby PJ. Alopecia and cutaneous atrophy after greater occipital nerve infiltration with corticosteroid. Neurology. 2004;63:2193-4.
65. Lavin PJ, Workman R. Cushing syndrome induced by serial occipital nerve blocks containing corticosteroids. Headache. 2001;41: 902-4.

CHAPTER 17

Hypnic Headache—Do We Know Enough

Vimal Kumar Paliwal, Ajai Kumar Singh

ABSTRACT

Hypnic headache is a rare primary headache characterized by headaches occurring during sleep, usually at night and often at the same time. Most affected individuals are elderly. Headaches may be unilateral or bilateral and may have migrainous or tension-type headache characteristics. A small proportion of patients may report cranial autonomic features, but trigeminal autonomic cephalalgias must be carefully excluded before diagnosing hypnic headache. Another differential diagnosis of hypnic headache is nocturnal hypertension-related headache. Hypertension-related nocturnal headache will respond to control of hypertension. Caffeine is the most effective acute abortive medication, and lithium, caffeine, and indomethacin are effective prophylactic drugs. Spontaneous remissions are known but less common. However, most patients show a favorable response to treatment.

Keywords: Hypnic headache, Alarm-clock headache, Migraine, Cluster headache, Hypertension-related nocturnal headache, Trigeminal autonomic cephalalgias.

INTRODUCTION

Hypnic headache is characterized by diffuse headache occurring at night, at similar times, and awakens the patients from sleep.[1] The headache is usually described in elderly patients. Hypnic headache was first described by Neil H Raskin, a professor of Neurology from San Francisco.[2] He described six patients seen between 1977 and 1986, mostly in their seventh decade of life and having a daily nocturnal diffuse headache with a striking consistency of timing of occurrence of headache. Three patients had a throbbing headache with nausea and none of the patients had cranial autonomic features. Most of the patients responded to lithium after failing to respond to amitriptyline and propranolol, and it was proposed that the headache might be related to the biological clock. Since that time, more than 300 cases have been reported in the form of case reports and case series. The hypnic headache was first adopted by the International Classification of Headache Disorders (ICHD), 2nd edition, under "Other primary headaches."[3] ICHD-3 beta did major modifications in the criterion, and the modified version was as such retained in the ICHD-3 diagnostic criteria.[4]

EPIDEMIOLOGY

Hypnic headache is a rare headache. However, its prevalence in the general population is not known. Among patients with headaches, the prevalence of hypnic headache in different studies have been described as 0.07%, 0.09–0.1%, 0.3–0.6%, and 1.4% in geriatric patients.[5-8] Hypnic headache is more common in females and occurs in people above 50 years of age.[8] Only 5% patients are diagnosed with hypnic headache before they reach the tertiary care.[7] The estimates of prevalence of hypnic headache is available only from the case series. Recent case series report a slightly higher prevalence of hypnic headache possibly because of increasing awareness and recognition of this headache.[9]

CLINICAL FEATURES

The understanding of the clinical characteristics of hypnic headache has evolved over the last decade and that has also resulted in changes in the ICHD since the inclusion of the hypnic headache in ICHD-2.

Age/Sex

Hypnic headache is a disease of the elderly. However, this headache is also reported in young individuals. A majority of patients in recent studies were 60 years or older. The initial report of seven patients by Raskin had six males, but there is a slight female preponderance reported by the recent studies.[8,9] In a recent review of cases, hypnic headache was observed in 7.6% patients before the age of 50 years, and 3 out of 250 adults (1.2%) had hypnic headache below 40 years of age.[8] There might be a minority of childhood hypnic headaches, but the epidemiology of childhood hypnic headache is not known.

Headache Frequency and Duration

The average frequency of headaches is 20.8 ± 9.9.[8] Nearly 65% patients suffered from daily headaches.[10] The duration of headache may range from 15 minutes to 10 hours or more. However, the ICHD-3 considers hypnic headache for a duration of headache attack lasting up to 240 minutes. This is deliberately decided to exclude migraine-like headaches that have the potential to occur in a similar fashion. The headache usually occurs at the same times of night.[7-13] This gave this headache its peculiar name "alarm-clock headache." Some patients reported headache during day-time sleep. Nearly 77% patients reported headache 120–480 minutes after the onset of sleep.[14] The most frequent reported timing of occurrence of headache is between 2 AM and 4 AM. Only minority of patients had headaches before 12 AM. Headache is reported with both nonrapid eye movement (NREM) and rapid eye movement (REM) sleep cycles.[10] Therefore, the initial hypothesis that the hypnic headaches are related to the REM sleep cycles was proven to be untrue. Though most of patients have only one attack per night, a few may have up to 5–6 attacks per night.[8,10,13,14]

Character and Severity

The original case series by Raskin had 3 out of 6 patients with migrainous features.[2] However, in a systemic review of cases, 68.8% patients had dull headache.[9] Throbbing, sharp, stabbing, burning headaches were reported in nearly one-third of the patients. Most patients had moderate headaches. One-third patients reported severe headache and only minority reported mild headaches. Hypnic headaches are not essentially holocranial headaches. One-third of patients may have unilateral headache.[9] Migrainous features such as nausea, vomiting, photophobia, and phonophobia are reported by only small subgroup of patients.

Cranial Autonomic Features

Some studies reported cranial autonomic features in up to 15% of patients. However, the patients did not fulfill the diagnostic criteria for cluster headaches. The trigeminal autonomic features reported were lacrimation, rhinorrhea, ptosis, and nasal congestion.[9] There is a lack of studies focusing on hypnic headaches with cranial autonomic features to suggest any possible relationship with trigeminal autonomic cephalalgias (TACs).

Motor Activities

Most patients with hypnic headache will leave their beds, move around, and perform various types of activities such as roaming, drinking water, and watching television.[7,15] These activities may possibly help in reducing headaches. However, these activities may not reach the level to label them as restlessness as seen in patients with cluster headaches. The motor behavior may differentiate hypnic headache from migraine whereby patients tend to lie motionless during the headache due to the movement-related aggravation of headache in migraine.

Associated Other Headaches

Migraine is the most common comorbid headache seen in one-third of patients with hypnic headaches. Another common comorbid headache is tension-type headache.[10] Nummular headache, hemicrania continua, and cervicogenic headache have also been reported in patients suffering from hypnic headaches.[16,17]

Comorbidities

Several comorbid diseases have been reported in patients with hypnic headaches. In two focused studies that evaluated hypnic headache patients with polysomnography, they found obstructive sleep apnea syndrome in 83% and 73% of patients, respectively.[10,13] The headache was not associated with oxygen desaturation. The high proportion of hypnic headache patients showing obstructive sleep apnea was thought to be mere chance association as hypnic headache and obstructive sleep apnea are common in elderly individuals.[18-21] Arterial hypertension was second most common comorbid illness, and it was postulated that the hypnic headache could be related to nocturnal hypertension. However, there is no conclusive evidence that patients with nocturnal hypertension suffer from hypnic headaches. Other rare comorbid illnesses reported are depression, coronary artery disease, stroke, diabetes mellitus, malignant neoplasms, epilepsy, etc.[14]

DIAGNOSIS

After inclusion of hypnic headache in the ICHD-2, there was considerable modification in the ICHD-3 beta/ICHD-3 **(Table 1)**. ICHD-2 considered hypnic headache to be closer to tension-type headache and required patients to have dull quality headaches. With evolution of knowledge about hypnic headache, it was observed that many hypnic headache patients have migrainous character. Consequently, the criteria A and part of criteria D (requirement of not more than one among nausea, photophobia, and phonophobia) of ICHD-2 was dropped in ICHD-3. The other important change was in the frequency of headache. ICHD-2 required >15 headaches per month to fulfill the diagnostic criteria. However, the mean frequency of headache was later determined to be 20.8 ± 9.9, therefore, the ICHD-3 modified the mandated frequency of headache to 10 per month. The age of onset after 50 years was also dropped from ICHD-2 owing to reports of early onset and childhood onset of hypnic headaches. Another major addition in ICHD-3 was "lack of restlessness" with hypnic attacks as discussed earlier.

PATHOPHYSIOLOGY

The precise mechanism of hypnic headache is not known. The occurrence of headache at night, during sleep, and at the same time each night has intrigued the headache experts. The timing of headache is a feature common between hypnic headache and cluster headache. Since the mechanism of cluster headache involves hypothalamus, the same has been postulated to cause hypnic headache. In a case–control study involving 14 patients with hypnic headache, magnetic resonance imaging (MRI) with voxel-based morphometry was performed to compare volume of various brain areas between cases and age/sex-matched controls.[22] They found gray matter volume loss in posterior hypothalamus in patients with hypnic headache. Additional areas that are associated with modulation of pain signaling such as cingulate cortex, operculum, and frontal and temporal lobe were also found to have decreased volume as compared to controls.[22]

Animal studies have shown that the posterior hypothalamus is involved in sleep regulation and modulation of pain.[23,24] Pain modulation is facilitated by the direct connections between posterior hypothalamus and trigeminal nucleus caudalis via trigeminohypothalamic pathway.[25] There is sufficient evidence for the activation of posterior hypothalamus with acute cluster headache, paroxysmal hemicrania, and short-lasting unilateral neuralgiform headache with conjunctival injection and tearing (SUNCT) and also in patients with hemicrania continua.[26-31] Orexin is a neuropeptide that binds to its receptor in posterior hypothalamus and regulates sleep cycle. Posterior hypothalamic injection of orexin in rats has shown reduced perception of facial pains by reducing the activity of trigeminal nucleus caudalis.[25,32] Other evidence comes from the observations of Sano and colleagues who successfully treated a patient with intractable facial pains by ipsilateral posterior hypothalamotomy.[33] However, the laterality of hypothalamic involvement and its relationship to the side of pain, especially in TACs and bilateral headaches like hypnic headaches, is not clear.

TREATMENT

In the absence of treatment trials, the knowledge about the effective treatment is largely through case reports and case series **(Table 2)**.

■ Acute Abortive Medications

Most patients will have spontaneous resolution of headache and the drugs will not be required. However, many patients will have headaches lasting for hours. The most effective abortive treatment is caffeine and caffeine-containing analgesics. A cup of coffee at the time of headache may be the best choice. The mechanism of action of caffeine is

TABLE 1: Comparison of International Classification of Headache Disorder (ICHD) criteria 2, 3 beta, and 3 for diagnosis of hypnic headache.

ICHD-2	ICHD-3 Beta (2013) and accepted as such in ICHD-3 (2018)
A. Dull headache fulfilling criteria B–D	A. Recurrent headache attacks fulfilling criteria B–E
B. Develops only during sleep and awakens patient	B. Developing only during sleep and causing wakening

C. At least two of the following characteristics:
  1. Occurs >15 times per month
  2. Lasts ≥ 15 minutes after waking
  3. First occurs after age of 50 years
	C. Occurring on ≥10 days per month for >3 months
	D. Lasting ≥15 minutes and for up to 4 hours after waking
	E. No cranial autonomic symptoms or restlessness
	F. Not better accounted for by another ICHD-3 diagnosis

D. No autonomic symptoms and no more than one of nausea, photophobia, or phonophobia.	
E. Not attributed to another disorder	

TABLE 2: Acute abortive medications and prophylactic medicines in order of their efficacy.	
Acute abortive medications	**Prophylactic medications**
• Caffeine • Caffeine-containing analgesics • Triptans • Nonsteroidal anti-inflammatory drugs (NSAIDs) • Oxygen inhalation • Ergotamine derivatives	• Lithium • Caffeine • Indomethacin • Topiramate • Melatonin • NSAIDs • Verapamil • Flunarizine • Beta blockers

precisely known. Caffeine is a cerebral vasodilator and is known to reduce the cerebral neuronal hyperexcitability.[34,35] Other medicines such as aspirin, other nonsteroidal anti-inflammatory drugs (NSAIDs), triptans, oxygen, and ergotamine derivatives have been found to have limited efficacy.[9]

■ Prophylactic Medications

Lithium has been found to be the most efficacious prophylactic drug in most case series. In a systematic review, lithium has been found to be effective in more than 70% of patients with hypnic headache.[9] Other drugs that have been found to be effective are indomethacin, caffeine, topiramate, tricyclic antidepressants, flunarizine, beta blockers, melatonin, verapamil, gabapentin, oxetorone, and prednisolone. There are isolated reports of benefit with botulinum toxin injection, occipital nerve stimulation, and treatment of nocturnal hypertension.[36,37]

CLINICAL OUTCOME

The natural history and clinical outcome of hypnic headache is not precisely known due to the rarity of this headache. Case series have provided limited information about the long-term outcome. With the information available, the hypnic headache seems to be a chronic, long-lasting, and remitting type of headache. Spontaneous remissions are known. Remissions after treatment are also known. In some patients, the headache may remain episodic with widely variable frequency.[9]

KNOWLEDGE GAPS

The knowledge regarding hypnic headache is evolving. Despite its first description nearly half-a-decade ago, much is still to be known about this mysterious headache. Those managing headache clinics believe that hypnic headache is more common than what is shown in studies. It is possibly because of more awareness about this entity that more physicians are diagnosing hypnic headaches. A headache survey or an epidemiological study is required to know the prevalence of hypnic headache in the general population. In view of nocturnal headache, relationship with sleep, possible hypothalamic involvement, and response to indomethacin and lithium, it will be interesting to understand the relationship of hypnic headache with TACs and other primary indomethacin-responsive headaches.

REFERENCES

1. Lanteri-Minet M. Hypnic headache. Headache. 2014;54(9):1556-9.
2. Raskin NH. The hypnic headache syndrome. Headache. 1988;28(8):534-6.
3. Headache Classification Subcommittee of the International Headache Society. The International Classification of Headache Disorders: 2nd edition. Cephalalgia. 2004;24 Suppl 1:9-160.
4. Headache Classification Committee of the International Headache Society (IHS). The International Classification of Headache Disorders, 3rd edition. Cephalalgia. 2018;38(1):1-211.
5. Dodick DW, Mosek AC, Campbell JK. The hypnic ("alarm clock") headache syndrome. Cephalalgia. 1998;18:152-6.
6. Lisotto C, Mainardi F, Maggioni F, et al. Episodic hypnic headache? Cephalalgia. 2004;24:681-5.
7. Donnet A, Lantéri-Minet M. A consecutive series of 22 cases of hypnic headache in France. Cephalalgia. 2009;29(9):928-34.
8. Holle D, Naegel S, Obermann M. Hypnic headache. Cephalalgia. 2013;33(16):1349-57.
9. Liang JF, Wang SJ. Hypnic headache: A review of clinical features, therapeutic options, and outcomes. Cephalalgia. 2014;34(10):795-805.
10. Liang JF, Fuh JL, Yu HY, et al. Clinical features, polysomnography, and outcome in patients with hypnic headache. Cephalalgia. 2008;28:209-15.
11. Silva-Néto RP, Almeida KJ. Hypnic headache: A descriptive study of 25 new cases in Brazil. J Neurol Sci. 2014;338:166-8.
12. Evers S, Rahmann A, Schwaag S, et al. Hypnic headache—the first German cases including polysomnography. Cephalalgia. 2003;23:20-3.
13. Holle D, Wessendorf TE, Zaremba S, et al. Serial polysomnography in hypnic headache. Cephalalgia. 2011;31:286-90.
14. Evers S, Goadsby PJ. Hypnic headache: Clinical features, pathophysiology, and treatment. Neurology. 2003;60:905-9.
15. Holle D, Naegel S, Krebs S, et al. Clinical characteristics and therapeutic options in hypnic headache. Cephalalgia. 2010;30:1435-42.
16. Mulero P, Guerrero-Peral AL, Cortijo E, et al. Hypnic headache: Characteristics of a series of 13 new cases and proposal for modification of the diagnostic criteria. Rev Neurol. 2012;54:129-36.
17. Jiménez-Caballero PE, Gámez-Leyva G, Gómez M, et al. Description of a series of cases of hypnic headache. Differentiation between sexes. Rev Neurol. 2012;54:332-6.
18. Silva-Néto RP, Bernardino SN. Ambulatory blood pressure monitoring in patient with hypnic headache: A case study. Headache. 2013;53:1157-8.
19. Cugini P, Granata M, Strano S, et al. Nocturnal headache-hypertension syndrome: A chronobiologic disorder. Chronobiol Int. 1992;9:310-3.

20. Caminero AB, Martín J, del Río MS. Secondary hypnic headache or symptomatic nocturnal hypertension? Two case reports. Cephalalgia. 2010;30:1137-9.
21. Gil-Gouveia R, Goadsby PJ. Secondary "hypnic headache." J Neurol. 2007;254:646-54.
22. Holle D, Naegel S, Krebs S, et al. Hypothalamic gray matter volume loss in hypnic headache. Ann Neurol. 2011;69(3):533-9.
23. Moore RY. Circadian rhythms: Basic neurobiology and clinical applications. Annu Rev Med. 1997;48:253-66.
24. Montagna P. Hypothalamus, sleep, and headaches. Neurol Sci. 2006;27(suppl 2):S138-43.
25. Malick A, Strassman RM, Burstein R. Trigeminohypothalamic and reticulohypothalamic tract neurons in the upper cervical spinal cord and caudal medulla of the rat. J Neurophysiol. 2000;84:2078-112.
26. May A, Bahra A, Büchel C, et al. Hypothalamic activation in cluster headache attacks. Lancet. 1998;352:275-8.
27. Matharu MS, Cohen AS, Frackowiak RSJ, et al. Posterior hypothalamic activation in paroxysmal hemicrania. Ann Neurol. 2006;59:535-45.
28. May A, Bahra A, Büchel C, et al. Functional magnetic resonance imaging in spontaneous attacks of SUNCT: Short-lasting neuralgiform headache with conjunctival injection and tearing. Ann Neurol. 1999;46:791-4.
29. Sprenger T, Valet M, Platzer S, et al. SUNCT: Bilateral hypothalamic activation during headache attacks and resolving of symptoms after trigeminal decompression. Pain. 2005;113:422-6.
30. Cohen AS, Matharu MS, Kalisch R, et al. Functional MRI in SUNCT shows differential hypothalamic activation with increasing pain. Cephalalgia. 2004;24:1098-9.
31. Matharu MS, Cohen AS, McGonigle DJ, et al. Posterior hypothalamic and brainstem activation in hemicrania continua. Headache. 2004;44:747-61.
32. de Lecea L, Kilduff TS, Peyron C, et al. The hypocretins: Hypothalamus-specific peptides with neuroexcitatory activity. Proc Natl Acad Sci U S A. 1998;95:322-7.
33. Sano K, Sekino H, Hashimoto I, et al. Posteromedial hypothalamotomy in the treatment of tractable pain. Confin Neurol. 1975;37:285-90.
34. Mathew RJ, Wilson WH. Caffeine consumption, withdrawal, and cerebral blood flow. Headache. 1985;25:305-9.
35. Holle D, Obermann M. Hypnic headache and caffeine. Expert Rev Neurother. 2012;12:1125-32.
36. Marziniak M, Voss J, Evers S. Hypnic headache successfully treated with botulinum toxin type A. Cephalalgia. 2007;27:1082-4.
37. Son BC, Yang SH, Hong JT, et al. Occipital nerve stimulation for medically refractory hypnic headache. Neuromodulation. 2012;15:381-6.

Diagnosis and Management of Idiopathic Intracranial Hypertension: An Update

Debaleena Mukherjee, Adreesh Mukherjee

ABSTRACT

Idiopathic intracranial hypertension (IIH) is a condition characterized by headache, papilledema, visual symptoms, and elevated cerebrospinal fluid opening pressure in the absence of a definitive etiology or intracranial mass. In this chapter, the authors have described the clinical clues, emphasizing upon the heterogeneous headache phenotypes in IIH including migraine, tension-type headache, and medication overuse headache. The putative mechanisms behind this entity have been elaborated. Obesity has been considered the strongest link. Authors have suggested that IIH is a neurometabolic disease, laying grounds for newer therapeutic targets. However, increasing recognition of intracranial venous hypertension as the core pathophysiology has led to the proposal of "chronic intracranial venous hypertension syndrome" as a more appropriate nomenclature. The diagnostic modalities have been detailed with focus on magnetic resonance/computed tomography (MR/CT) venography of brain vessels along with manometry to identify venous sinus stenosis and document trans-stenotic pressure gradient. Optical coherence tomography (OCT) is rapidly becoming an essential tool in the diagnosis and monitoring of papilledema in IIH. In addition to older pharmacological therapies including acetazolamide and topiramate, newer upcoming agents include glucagon-like peptide 1 (GLP-1) agonist and 11-beta-hydroxysteroid dehydrogenase inhibitor. The role of newer techniques such as venous sinus stenting warrant future robust studies.

Keywords: CIVHS, Headache, IIH, Management, MRI, OCT, Pathophysiology.

INTRODUCTION

Idiopathic intracranial hypertension (IIH) is a disorder of increased intracranial pressure (ICP) in the absence of a mass lesion or a definite identifiable cause.[1,2] Quincke in 1890s attributed these cases to increased cerebrospinal fluid (CSF) production, coining it "meningitis serosa." Nonne in 1904 renamed it "pseudotumor cerebri" as the cases mimicked the presence of intracranial mass. Though Foley described it as "benign intracranial hypertension," the occurrence of severe visual impairment contradicted its benign nature.[3] Recently, some authors have proposed "chronic intracranial venous hypertension syndrome" (CIVHS) as a more inclusive terminology, recognizing intracranial venous hypertension as the root cause for raised ICP.[4] The changing nosology is perhaps indicative of our still evolving understanding of the pathophysiology.

EPIDEMIOLOGY

The estimated incidence of IIH in the general population is 0.03–2.36 per 100,000.[5,6] It is typically known to occur in obese women in childbearing age groups.[1,6] Adult women are more likely to develop IIH than men.[1,6] The incidence rises in those with a body mass index (BMI) higher than 30 kg/m².[5,6] IIH in women is associated with a twofold increased risk of cardiovascular diseases, while men have a greater risk of vision loss and obstructive sleep apnea (OSA).[1,7] Worldwide, IIH is more common in UK, Italy, Israel, and the USA, with a relatively lower incidence in

Asia.[1] The incidence of IIH in childhood is lesser (0.5 per 100,000). It occurs mainly after puberty but is also reported in prepubertal age groups. Three main patterns identified include a young subgroup who are not overweight, a second early adolescent subgroup that is overweight or obese, and a late adolescent group that is mostly obese.[1,3,8]

CLINICAL FEATURES

Headache dominates the clinical presentation (90%), the heterogeneous phenotypes of which often mimic primary headache disorders including migraine and tension-type headache (TTH).[9] They mostly occur daily with increasing frequency and severity. Often described as throbbing or pressure-like, they may be generalized or localized to the frontal or retro-orbital region, and aggravated by Valsalva maneuver. Nausea, vomiting, photophobia, phonophobia, and worsening on exertion are reported. Several patients describe a continuous or daily headache and may develop medication overuse headache. Migrainous headaches often persist post resolution of raised ICP, which raises the question whether increased ICP is contributory to the headache or is it a pressure-induced exacerbation of preexisting migraine. Thus, the International Headache Society criteria for IIH has not included resolution of headache following ICP reduction as essential.[1,3,9,10]

Visual symptoms are commonly encountered in the form of blurring, unilateral/bilateral transient visual obscurations (TVO) with posture change (graying/blacking out of vision lasting <1 minute), horizontal binocular diplopia, and altered visual fields (enlarged blind spot, loss of nasal visual field, and generalized field constriction). TVO result from edema and transient ischemia of the optic nerve. Diplopia results from unilateral/bilateral sixth nerve palsy due to traction on the nerve in about 20% of the patients. The seventh cranial nerve involvement is rare.[1-3]

Pulsatile tinnitus (unilateral/bilateral) is present in more than half, resulting from turbulence in the stenosis in venous sinuses. Other symptoms include dizziness, nausea, vomiting, lethargy, and back and neck pain.[1,3,6,10]

On physical examination, papilledema, a cardinal feature of IIH, is a harbinger of impending visual impairment secondary to optic atrophy. It is usually bilaterally present, but may be unilateral in 4%, and even absent in few (<5%) of the cases.[3,11,12] **Table 1** summarizes the clinical features of IIH.

PATHOPHYSIOLOGY

While the pathophysiology remains to be confirmed, the most debated mechanisms include:[1-3]
- Cerebrospinal fluid dysregulation—increased CSF production/decreased CSF resorption

TABLE 1: Summary of clinical features in idiopathic intracranial hypertension.[2,6]

Idiopathic intracranial hypertension symptoms	Frequency (%)
Headache	76–94
Visual obscuration	68–72
Pulsatile tinnitus	52–61
Back pain	53
Dizziness	52
Neck pain	42
Blurred vision	32
Cognitive disturbance	20
Radicular pain	19
Diplopia	18

- Increased cerebral blood flow/altered venous hemodynamics
- Role of obesity and hormonal dysregulation

Cerebrospinal Fluid Dysregulation

Cerebrospinal fluid is secreted by the choroid plexus into the ventricles from where it flows into the subarachnoid spaces and then into the venous sinuses via arachnoid granulations. The movement of sodium from the blood into the ventricles creates an osmotic gradient for CSF flow regulated by Na^+–K^+-dependent adenosine triphosphatase (ATPase). Targeted inhibition of this decreases CSF production. Although the role of aquaporin 1 (AQP1) expression, obesity, and raised ICP has been explored in animal studies, human studies are lacking. Impaired drainage of CSF is another cause of IIH, possibly due to microthrombi, alterations in arachnoid granulations, and intracranial lymphatics.[1,2]

Altered Venous Hemodynamics

Dandy suggested alterations in vasomotor control and sudden increases in intracranial blood volume. In 1959, Sahs reported evidence of both intracellular and extracellular edema in brain biopsies of patients with IIH, suggesting that IIH resulted from cerebral edema. Raichle, in 1978, highlighted an abnormality in the cerebral microvasculature using tracer techniques, suggesting increased cerebral blood volume led to raised ICP which decreased cerebral venous outflow. Around 1951, venography studies by Ray and Dunbar had revealed obstruction in superior sagittal sinus and dominant transverse sinus. In 1970, Johnston proposed that increased pressure in the dural venous sinuses led to a decreased CSF-dural venous sinus gradient and consequent impaired CSF absorption. In 1995, venous hypertension was documented in the sagittal

TABLE 2: Proposed diagnostic criteria for CIVHS.[4]					
		Proposed diagnostic criteria			
CIVHS type	Cause	Venous sinus stenosis	ICP (cmH$_2$O)	SSSP (mm Hg)	CVP (mm Hg)
1	Craniocervical origin (venous sinus stenosis mediated)	Present	≥25	≥18	<12
2	Central origin (elevated CVP mediated)	Absent	≥25	≥18	≥12
3	Mixed (both elevated CVP and venous sinus stenosis mediated)	Present	≥25	≥18	≥12
4	Postvenous sinus thrombosis	Either	≥25	≥18	Any
(CIVHS: chronic intracranial venous hypertension syndrome; CVP: central venous pressure; ICP: intracranial pressure; SSSP: superior sagittal sinus pressure)					

sinus and transverse sinus using cerebral venography and manometry in IIH.[3]

Thus, recent times have witnessed a paradigm shift, recognizing intracranial venous hypertension as the critical pathophysiological cause of IIH, leading to increased ICP and CSF opening pressure. Recent authors have proposed CIVHS as a more inclusive nomenclature,[4] and have suggested a classification scheme to stratify patients according to etiology of venous hypertension **(Table 2)**. However, debates continue whether the venous sinus stenosis commonly found in IIH is a cause or a consequence.

■ Obesity and Hormonal Dysregulation

Obesity: It appears to have the strongest association with IIH. Recently, authors have emphasized on the contributory role of hormonal dysregulation and metabolic neuroendocrine axis in IIH, which may serve as potential therapeutic targets. Increased weight gain by 5–15% was observed in the year preceding IIH.[2,6] Recurrence of IIH following symptom resolution was seen with 6% weight gain.[1] Moreover, the markers of inflammation observed in obesity were present in the CSF of IIH patients, such as chemokine (C-C motif) ligand 2. Some studies also showed raised CSF leptin levels.[2] Some authors suggest that increased intra-abdominal pressure in obesity elevates the diaphragm, increasing right atrial pressure, which is transmitted to the central venous system, leading to venous hypertension. However, arguments remain that obesity alone without a significant venous sinus stenosis is unlikely to produce a CSF opening pressure >25 cmH$_2$O.[3,13]

Polycystic ovarian syndrome (PCOS): 64% of patients with IIH have PCOS, which is common in childbearing age groups, and 44% of the affected women are obese.[2]

Role of glucagon-like peptide 1 (GLP-1): It is an incretin, which inhibits Na$^+$/H$^+$ exchanger in proximal renal tubular cells causing natriuresis. Choroid plexus also expresses GLP-1 receptor and shares a similar functionality to proximal renal tubule. Thus, GLP-1 agonist (exendin-4) can reduce the activity of Na$^+$–K$^+$ ATPase, modulate CSF production, and lead to ICP reduction.[14]

Role of glucocorticoids: 11 beta-hydroxysteroid dehydrogenase type 1, which serves as an intracellular enzyme, converting inactive cortisone to active cortisol is also expressed in choroid plexus epithelial cell. A global decline in its activity occurs with weight loss and correlates with reduction in ICP, which has future therapeutic implications.[15]

Role of androgens: Serum testosterone and 5-alpha reductase have been found to be higher in those with IIH compared to age- and BMI-matched controls. Women with IIH also showed a pattern of androgen excess with increased serum testosterone and increased CSF testosterone and androstenedione distinct from that observed in PCOS and simple obesity. The choroid plexus expresses androgen receptor and androgen-activating enzyme. Testosterone increases Na$^+$–K$^+$ ATPase activity, which increases CSF production, thus becoming a potential therapeutic target.[16]

EVALUATION

■ Step 1: Systemic and Neurological Assessment

Thorough assessment of history and clinical examination including blood pressure is important. It is essential to exclude secondary causes and associated conditions **(Box 1)**. Cranial nerve abnormalities must be noted. Involvement of cranial nerves aside the sixth cranial nerve should be considered a red flag sign for an alternative diagnosis.

■ Step 2: Ophthalmological Assessment

All patients should be immediately assessed for papilledema and impending threat to vision. Visual acuity, pupillary examination, intraocular pressure, and perimetry and dilated fundus examination must be performed. Optical coherence tomography (OCT) is rapidly becoming a useful technique in the assessment of IIH. Newer techniques to examine the optic nerve head include wide field imaging for high-resolution image capture through an undilated pupil along with a magnification tool.[10]

> **BOX 1: Associations of idiopathic intracranial hypertension.**[2,6,10]
>
> *Iatrogenic causes*:
> - *Antibiotics*: Tetracycline, minocycline, doxycycline, nitrofurantoin, sulfonamides, and nalidixic acid
> - *Hormonal factors*: Thyroxine, growth hormones, and tamoxifen
> - Excess vitamin A and retinoids
> - *Other drugs*: Corticosteroids, lithium, and cyclosporine
>
> *Associated conditions*:
> - Anemia
> - *Respiratory disorders*: Obstructive sleep apnea, COPD, and hypercapnia
> - Renal failure
> - *Obstructions to venous drainage*: Cerebral venous sinus thrombosis, jugular venous sinus thrombosis, superior vena cava syndrome, increased right atrial pressure, and thrombophilia
> - *Endocrinological disorders*: Addison's disease, adrenal insufficiency, Cushing's disease, hypoparathyroidism, hypothyroidism, and hyperthyroidism
> - *Syndromic*: Down syndrome, Turner syndrome, and Craniosynostosis
> - *Autoimmune conditions*: Systemic lupus erythematosus (SLE) and Sjögren's syndrome
> - Systemic, CNS, and middle ear and mastoid infections
>
> (CNS: central nervous system; COPD: chronic obstructive pulmonary disease)

Role of Optical Coherence Tomography

- *Assessment and monitoring of papilledema*: Papilledema causes thickening of the retinal nerve fiber layer (RNFL), which directly corresponds to the CSF opening pressure. Techniques quantifying the elevation and volume of the disc itself in papilledema may be better than conventional peripapillary RNFL (pRNFL) scans. Treatment of IIH with acetazolamide, weight loss, or ventriculoperitoneal (VP) shunt causes improvement in OCT measures of disc height, volume, and pRNFL.[17]
- *Deformation of peripapillary retinae*: Measurement of deformation of the deeper layers of neural retina (peripapillary retinal pigment epithelium and Bowman's membrane) toward the vitreous corresponds to the inward deformation of the posterior sclera on magnetic resonance imaging (MRI). The degree of deformation corresponds to lumbar puncture (LP) opening pressure and improves with therapy.[17]
- *Diagnosis of pseudopapilledema*: OCT can differentiate tilted discs, crowded hypermetropic discs, and buried disc drusen from true papilledema. OCT uses enhanced depth imaging to examine structures as deep as the lamina cribrosa to detect even very small drusen.
- *Macular ganglion cell layer* (mGCL) *imaging in IIH*: A challenging issue in monitoring IIH-related papilledema is to differentiate a reduction in the degree of disc or pRNFL swelling due to improvement in edema and decreasing ICP from the loss of RNFL fibers due to optic atrophy. Macular OCT imaging is extremely helpful in this situation. Early thinning of the mGCL before frank thinning of the pRNFL indicates disc damage.[17] Absence of thinning or no progression of thinning of the mGCL in a patient with chronic papilledema despite medical therapy suggests that the optic nerve is not losing axons at an abnormal rate.

■ Step 3: Radiological Assessment

Role of MRI Brain and Orbit and MR Venography

As per consensus guidelines, an MRI must be done within 24 hours.[6] If unavailable, urgent CT brain followed by an MRI is recommended. It is an indispensable tool in the evaluation of IIH, which is essential for ruling out structural lesions (such as venous sinus thrombosis, mass lesions, vascular malformations, and hydrocephalus) and identifying the tell-tale though often subtle signs of IIH **(Figs. 1A to F)**.[3,6,10]

- *Empty sella*: Observed in 76–85% with a sensitivity and specificity of 80–88% and 76–92%, respectively, reduction of midsagittal height of the pituitary gland is considered highly suggestive of IIH. Chronically increased ICP may cause herniation of an arachnocele through the diaphragmatic sellae. Consequent flattening of the pituitary gland leads to concavity of its superior aspect.[3,17]
- *Distension of perioptic subarachnoid space*: Observed in 95% with a sensitivity of 72–80% and specificity of 96%, and results from chronically increased CSF pressure transmitted to the perioptic subarachnoid space. Diffusion tensor imaging (DTI) can detect microstructural changes in the optic nerve that reverse after ICP normalization. DTI of the optic disc also shows abnormal values of fractional anisotropy in patients with IIH.[3,17]
- *Posterior flattening of globe*: Although observed in 43–71% and less sensitive (28–43%), it has a high specificity (100%), especially with perioptic space distension. In severe cases, protrusion of the optic nerve head may be observed, which is the imaging equivalent of papilledema.[3]
- *Optic nerve tortuosity*: Vertical kinking is more specific than horizontal kinking. Observed in 40–62%, it has a low sensitivity (40%) but higher specificity (91%).[3]
- *Transverse sinus stenosis (TSS)*: Unilateral or bilateral TSS is commonly observed in IIH (65–90%). With increasing recognition of venous hypertension and stenosis of sinuses, cerebral angiography (contrast enhanced MR and CT venography) and venous manometry are becoming indispensable in evaluation of IIH.[3,13]

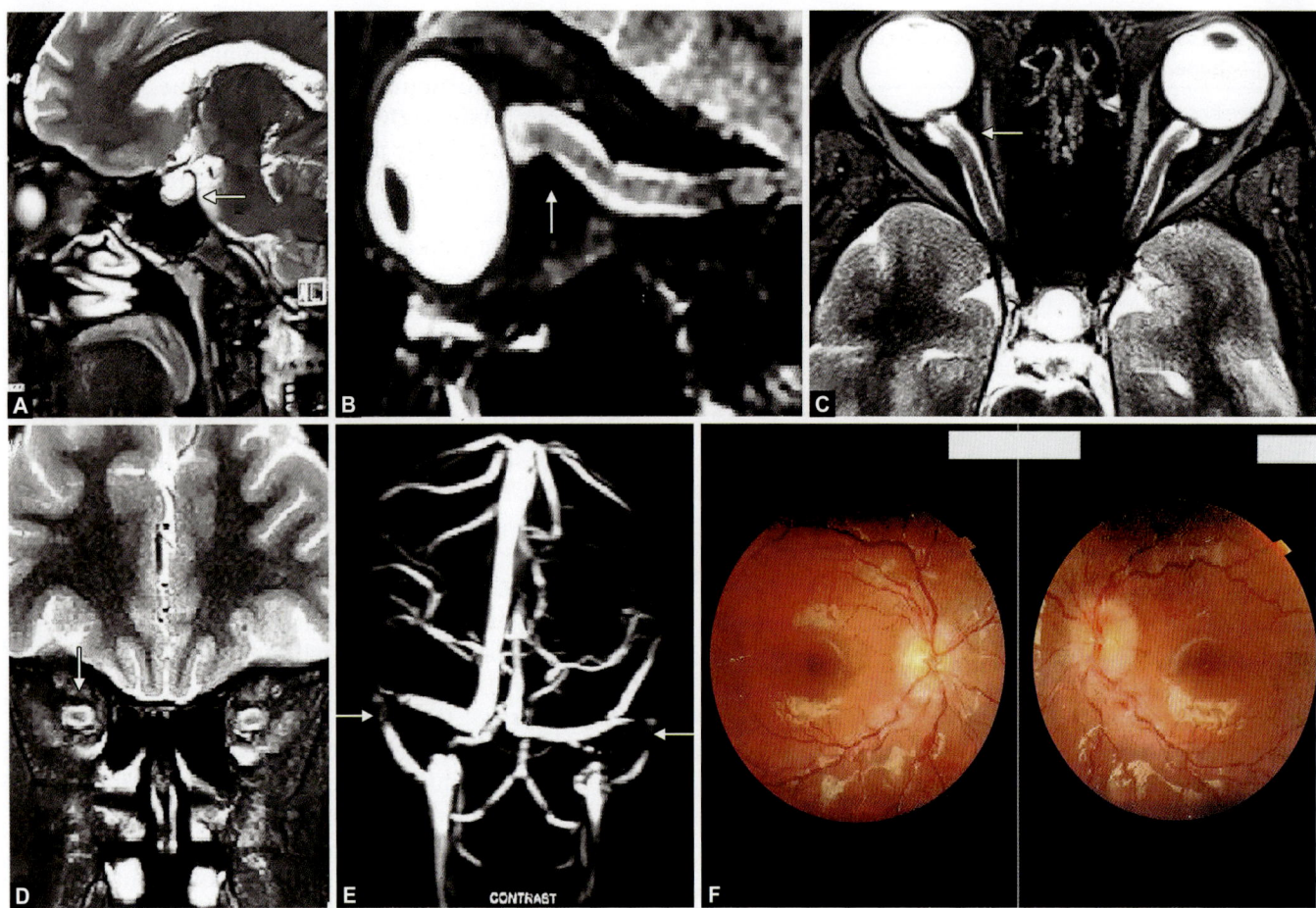

FIGS. 1A TO F: Magnetic resonance imaging of brain T2-weighted images showing: (A) Sagittal view showing partially empty sella; (B) Sagittal view of optic nerve showing vertical optic nerve tortuosity and flattening of posterior aspect of globe; (C) Axial view of bilateral optic nerves showing optic nerve tortuosity with flattening of posterior aspect of globe; (D) Coronal view showing perioptic disc space distension; (E) Magnetic resonance venography showing bilateral transverse sinus stenosis; and (F) Fundoscopy in a patient of idiopathic intracranial hypertension (IIH) with bilateral papilledema.

- *Other findings*: These include spontaneous encephaloceles, meningoceles, prominent Meckel's cave, and other enlarged CSF spaces.[3]

Step 4: Lumbar Puncture

Following imaging, patients should undergo LP to check the CSF opening pressure. This should be done in lateral decubitus position with pressure level documented when patient is relaxed and the CSF level has settled. In addition, a routine assessment of cell count, glucose, and protein is done to exclude secondary causes. As CSF pressure may vary, a normal opening pressure in a background of high suspicion warrants a second assessment or continuous monitoring.

DIAGNOSTIC CRITERIA

The first criteria were summarized by Dandy in 1937. Following the introduction of CT, it was revised in 1985 and called the Modified Dandy Criteria. In the recent revision of the criteria by Friedman in 2013, he emphasized that pseudotumor cerebri syndrome (PTCS) is a more inclusive terminology including primary and secondary PTCS and further classified the patients as with and without papilledema.[18] Friedman classified IIH as subset of primary PTCS. Fargen proposed a new nomenclature CIVHS and suggested changes in the diagnostic criteria in which the diagnosis requires opening pressure on LP ≥25 cmH$_2$O and an elevated superior sagittal sinus pressure ≥18 mm Hg in the absence of mass lesion **(Tables 2 and 3)**.[4]

MANAGEMENT

Management includes:
- Treatment of underlying cause
- Prevention of visual impairment
- Management of headache

TABLE 3: Idiopathic intracranial hypertension diagnostic criteria.	
IIH diagnostic criteria*[18]	A. Papilledema
	B. Normal neurological examination (except sixth cranial nerve palsy)
	C. Neuroimaging: Normal brain parenchyma (no hydrocephalus, mass, structural lesion, or meningeal enhancement) on MRI, with and without gadolinium, for typical patients (female and obese), and MRI, with and without gadolinium, and MR venography for others; if MRI is unavailable or contraindicated, contrast-enhanced CT may be used. Venous thrombosis must be excluded in all
	D. Normal CSF constituents
	E. Elevated lumbar puncture opening pressure [≥250 mm CSF in adults and ≥280 mm CSF in children (250 mm CSF if the child is not sedated and not obese)] in a properly performed lumbar puncture
IIH without papilledema (IIHWOP)*[18]	1. Presence of criteria B–E for IIH plus
	2. Unilateral or bilateral sixth cranial nerve palsy
Suggestion of possible IIHWOP*[18]	1. Presence of criteria B–E for IIH plus

	2. Three neuroimaging findings suggestive of raised ICP:
	  a. Empty sella
	  b. Flattening of posterior aspect of globe
	  c. Distension of perioptic subarachnoid space ± tortuous optic nerve
	  d. Transverse venous sinus stenosis

Headache attributed to IIH according to ICHD-3[19]	A. New headache or a significant worsening of a preexisting headache, fulfilling criterion C
	B. Both of the following:
	  a. Idiopathic intracranial hypertension (IIH) has been diagnosed
	  b. Cerebrospinal fluid (CSF) pressure exceeds 250 mm CSF (or 280 mm CSF in obese children)
	C. Either or both of the following:
	  a. Headache has developed or significantly worsened in temporal relation to the IIH or led to its discovery
	  b. Headache is accompanied by either or both of the following:
	    i. Pulsatile tinnitus
	    ii. Papilledema
	D. Not better accounted for by another ICHD-3 diagnosis

Important definitions[6]	*Malignant/Fulminant IIH*: Patients fulfilling the criteria for IIH with: • Precipitous decline in vision within 4 weeks of symptoms onset or diagnosis of IIH • Severe papilledema (≥Frisen grade 3) • Substantial visual field or visual acuity loss • And/or transient visual obscurations ≥30/month
	Typical IIH: Classically described for female patients in childbearing age group with BMI ≥30 kg/m²
	Atypical IIH: Described for patients who are not females, do not belong to childbearing age group, or have a BMI <30 kg/m²
	IIH in ocular remission: Patients diagnosed with IIH in whom the papilledema has resolved. Their vision is not at risk; however, they may be suffering from headache

*The criteria originally mentioned Pseudotumor cerebri syndrome.
(BMI: body mass index; CSF: cerebrospinal fluid, CT: computed tomography; ICHD-3: International Classification of Headache Disorders, 3rd edition: ICP: intracranial pressure; IIH: idiopathic intracranial hypertension; MRI: magnetic resonance imaging)

■ Treatment of Underlying Cause

Obesity is strongly linked with IIH, and weight loss constitutes an essential disease-modifying therapy **(Flowchart 1)**.[6,10] It reduces intra-abdominal pressure and consequently central venous pressure (CVP). It also reduces incidence of OSA and nocturnal ICP elevation that provokes venous sinus stenosis feedback loops. Weight management should be advised to all patients with a BMI ≥30 kg/m².[6] While the target of weight loss is debated, 3–15% weight loss is advised for remission.[6,20] In a prospective cohort trial in IIH, very low-calorie diet (425 kcal/day) resulted in 15% weight loss along with reduction in ICP, headache, and papilledema and stabilization of visual fields.[21] Low sodium diet weight reduction program should be recommended to all obese patients.

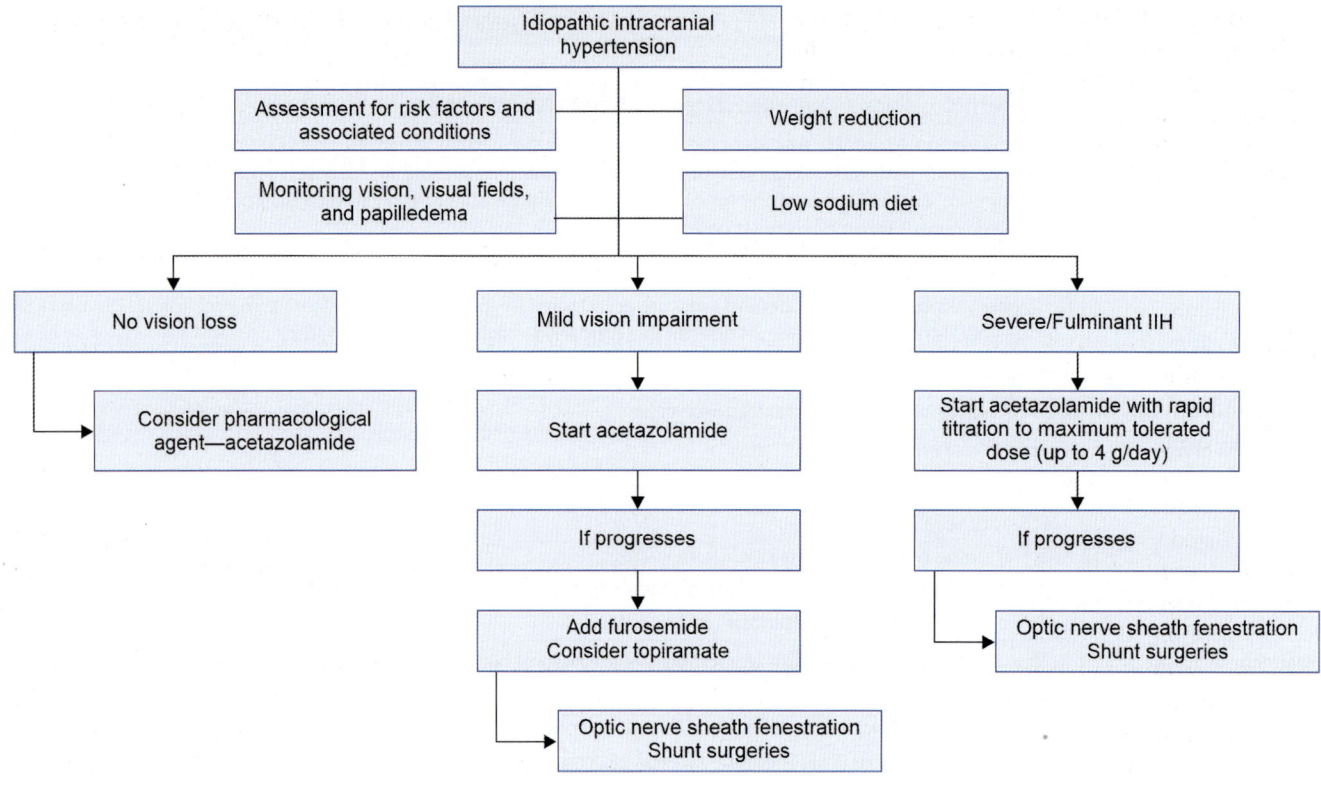

FLOWCHART 1: Algorithm for management of idiopathic intracranial hypertension (IIH).

Role of bariatric surgery: With increasing incidence of obesity, bariatric surgery has emerged as an effective technique for substantial weight loss in the morbidly obese (15–30% weight loss over 15–20 years depending on procedure).[1] It causes reduction in headache, visual complaints, tinnitus, and papilledema. Further studies are warranted to compare its efficacy with standard care for IIH and establish IIH as an indication for bariatric surgery.[22]

Prevention of Visual Impairment

About 5–15% of patients are at risk of severe permanent vision loss. Important identifiers include:
- Frisen grade 3–5 papilledema
- Significant vision loss at presentation (higher risk)
- TVO (intermediate risk)
- Patients who develop such symptoms despite therapy
- Male gender
- Younger age or age of onset at puberty
- Comorbidities—anemia, hypertension, recent weight gain, and more severe obesity
- Higher CSF opening pressure
- MRI parameters do not appear as significant predictors

Pharmacological Measures
- *Carbonic anhydrase inhibitors (decrease CSF production)*: Evidence in favor of acetazolamide is based on few randomized controlled trials (RCTs) and observational studies. In Idiopathic Intracranial Hypertension Treatment Trial (IIHTT), in mild vision loss, acetazolamide with a low sodium weight reduction diet demonstrated modest improvement at 6 months in CSF pressure, visual field (perimetric mean deviation), vision-related quality of life, papilledema, and weight, compared to diet and placebo, but did not show benefit in visual acuity and symptomatic headache.[20] In the pilot study by Ball et al., while 44% were judged to be in remission at the end of trial, adverse effects due to acetazolamide and poor drug compliance were a limitation.[23] A long-term follow-up study showed that while recurrence is not reported while on therapy, an overall recurrence rate of 38% has been observed over 6.2 years.[24] The commonly used starting dose for acetazolamide is 500 mg twice daily, with uptitration to a maximal 2–4 g daily dose. In children, the recommended starting dose is 25 mg/kg/day to a maximum of 100 mg/kg/day or 2 g/day. The known adverse effects include allergic reaction, teratogenicity, nausea, vomiting, oral paresthesia, metallic taste and dyselectrolytemia, metabolic acidosis, and kidney stones.[3] IIHTT found monitoring of electrolytes not necessary if this is the only diuretic used, however, clinical discretion is essential.

Topiramate, another carbonic anhydrase inhibitor, showed similar efficacy as acetazolamide in symptom relief and visual field improvement.[25] Common side effects include paresthesia, cognitive impairment, and teratogenicity, and caution is advised for those with prior depression. Recently, a study assessing the efficacy of drugs lowering ICP in rats demonstrated that both subcutaneous and oral administration of topiramate significantly lower ICP in comparison to acetazolamide, furosemide, amiloride, and octreotide.[26]

- *Adjunctive therapies—loop diuretics (decrease CVP)*: Furosemide 20-40 mg/day in adults or 1-2 mg/kg/day in children can be used in persistent visual worsening despite acetazolamide. A case series showed that use of acetazolamide together with loop diuretics decreased CSF pressure and papilledema within 1 week and normalized it by 6 weeks.[27]
- *Future therapies*:
  o *11 beta-hydroxysteroid dehydrogenase type 1 inhibitor*: AZD4017 (phase II multicenter, randomized, double-blind, placebo-controlled trial) was compared to placebo in IIH. The drug was well tolerated and inhibited the enzyme activity, and reduction in serum cortisol:cortisone, correlated with decreased ICP. Assessment of mean change in LP opening pressure showed significant reduction in AZD4017 group.[28]
  o *Glucagon-like peptide 1 receptor agonist (exenatide)*: A randomized, double-blind, placebo-controlled phase 2 trial demonstrated reduction in ICP in short- and long-term measurements and headache frequency.[29]

Urgent Temporizing Measures

In patients with fulminant IIH, urgent therapy is required to preserve vision. This includes pharmacological therapy (prompt initiation and rapid uptitration of acetazolamide) and surgical interventions. In the interim while awaiting surgery, the following temporizing measures can be considered:

- *Glucocorticoids*: Short course IV glucocorticoids [methylprednisolone 250 mg intravenous (IV) qid for 5 days] followed by oral taper along with acetazolamide may be considered. Long-term use of steroids must be avoided to prevent weight gain and rebound increase in ICP.[30]
- *Serial LP/lumbar drainage*: This provides short duration of mild benefit for 6 hours. Furthermore, with post-LP exacerbation of headache being commonly reported in nearly 64% and severe exacerbations in 30% along with 47% being extremely anxious regarding future LPs, this is not routinely recommended by consensus guidelines.[31,32]

Interventions for Severe/Refractory Disease

These are considered for patients with:
- Failure or intolerance to maximum medical therapy
- Progressive visual loss (worsening visual field defect despite therapy/loss of visual acuity due to papilledema and not due to macular edema/choroidal folds)
- Intractable headache (which is not due to migraine, medication overuse headache, caffeine overuse, or non-IIH related)

Optic nerve sheath fenestration (ONSF): Most observations are based on case series, which demonstrated that visual acuity stabilized/improved in 94% and visual fields stabilized in 88%.[33] It also helps reduce headache. A less severe and shorter duration of vision loss is associated with a better outcome. During this procedure, a medial orbital approach is adopted, the optic nerve sheath is identified, and a window is created to allow CSF to enter into the orbital space. Persistence of raised ICP is a major disadvantage. Adverse effects have been noted in 40-45%, which are mostly transient and nondisabling including temporary diplopia and efferent pupillary dysfunction. Vision loss has been reported in 11%, which may be permanent in 1.5-2.6%. Relapses have been known to occur in 7-32% within months or years.[3,34,35]

Cerebrospinal fluid shunting: CSF diversion procedures include VP, lumboperitoneal, and rarely ventriculoatrial shunts. VP shunts are placed using neuronavigation and adjustable valves to reduce low-pressure headaches. It reduces papilledema in 78.9%, prevents visual deterioration in 66.8%, and reduces headache in 69.8%.[36] VP shunt is preferred over lumboperitoneal shunt due to lower shunt failures and revision rates. Efficacy as reported based on uncontrolled observation studies include relief of headache, diplopia, papilledema, and vision loss. Outcomes are mixed, while stabilization/remission of vision has been reported in most patients, it has worsened in about 10%. The reduction in headache may not be a sustained outcome and may recur. CSF diversion is not recommended for treatment of isolated headache symptoms as headache may persist in 68% at 6 months and 79% at 2 years along with high revision rates.[10] Adverse effects include shunt failure in 50% requiring revision shunts in 10-38%, shunt infections, pain abdomen, overdrainage of CSF, and low-pressure headaches. Rarely tonsillar herniation, syrinx, subarachnoid hemorrhage, and subdural hemorrhage may occur.[6,36]

Venous sinus stenting (VSS): While CSF diversion procedures help reduce ICP by decreasing extramural sinus compression and aggravation of venous sinus stenosis, it may recur with shunt failure. VSS attempts to reinforce the venous wall and prevent extramural compression, breaking the positive feedback loop. Based on reviews and case series, VSS is still a novel treatment option for patients with documented trans-stenotic pressure gradient of at least 8 mm Hg.[13] Nicholson et al. reported an improvement in headache, tinnitus, and papilledema in approximately 80%, 90%, and 94%, respectively.[37] VSS seemed more durable for visual symptoms than headache. There is insufficient evidence to support venous stenting to treat isolated headache. Fargen proposed that in CIVHS type 1, stenting of offending stenosis is likely to be more beneficial than weight loss and loop diuretics as CVP is normal. Conversely in CIVHS type 2, therapy should be targeted toward CVP reduction, and surgical options such as CSF diversion, ONSF, and bariatric surgery may provide benefit. CIVHS type 3 will require both stenting as well as treatment of systemic venous congestion. For CIVHS type 4, stenting may be required if stenosis is present.[4] While Nicholson et al. reported a recurrence rate of 12.4%, Garner reported 54.3%.[37,38] Adverse effects of this technique include short-lived ipsilateral headache, intracranial hemorrhage, retroperitoneal bleed, contrast reaction, restenosis, stent migration and thrombosis, and femoral pseudoaneurysms. Patients undergoing VSS require anticoagulation, starting prior to the procedure, which is maintained for 6 months or lifelong.[1] While increasing procedural volumes are being reported, robust RCTs are still lacking to establish a definitive role of VSS in IIH.[39]

Management of Headache

- *Acute management*: Short-term NSAIDs/paracetamol may be used in the weeks following diagnosis. Indomethacin, with its ICP-reducing effect, may be helpful, but opioids must be avoided. There is a dearth of evidence regarding the use of greater occipital nerve blocks. Currently, CSF diversion surgeries and VSS are not recommended for management of headache alone.
- *Long-term management*: The pattern of headache may change, and the phenotype must be assessed and treated accordingly—migraine, TTH, medication overuse headache, and headache attributed to low CSF pressure/iatrogenic Chiari secondary to CSF shunting.

It is essential to diagnose and avoid medication overuse headache. For migraine, it is important to note that beta blockers, flunarizine, low doses of valproate, and tricyclic antidepressant may lead to increased weight gain and defeat the purpose. Topiramate may thus help. If topiramate is not tolerated, zonisamide may be tried.

MANAGEMENT OF IDIOPATHIC INTRACRANIAL HYPERTENSION IN PREGNANCY

With limited evidence with regards to acetazolamide in pregnancy and evidence of teratogenicity in rodents, it requires a risk–benefit assessment. Overall, there are no recommendations for acetazolamide in pregnancy with IIH. Topiramate should not be used during pregnancy. In IIH with immediate risk of vision loss, temporizing measures including serial LP should be considered till permanent CSF diversion or ONSF can be executed.

CONCLUSION

Epidemiological trend in IIH is witnessing a rising incidence in both women and men, albeit more in women, in concordance with increasing worldwide obesity. It has been proposed that IIH is a neurometabolic disease, and identifying markers of hormonal dysregulation has future therapeutic implications. A paradigm shift in the understanding of IIH lies in the recognition of intracranial venous hypertension as the major mechanism of raised ICP (CIVHS). Management of IIH consists of appropriate pharmacological and surgical treatment modalities along with weight reduction. In the background of venous hypertension and documented trans-stenotic pressure gradient, VSS is a potential therapeutic option. However, more robust studies are required before it is established as a first-line therapy.

ACKNOWLEDGMENTS

The authors would like to thank Subhadeep Mandal and Samya Sengupta for their help regarding the MRI images of IIH.

REFERENCES

1. Virdee J, Larcombe S, Vijay V, et al. Reviewing the Recent Developments in Idiopathic Intracranial Hypertension. Ophthalmol Ther. 2020;9:767-81.
2. Markey KA, Mollan SP, Jensen RH, et al. Understanding idiopathic intracranial hypertension: Mechanisms, management, and future directions. Lancet Neurol. 2016;15:78-91.
3. Rehder D. Idiopathic Intracranial Hypertension: Review of Clinical Syndrome, Imaging Findings, and Treatment. Curr Probl Diagn Radiol. 2020;49:205-14.
4. Fargen KM. Idiopathic intracranial hypertension is not idiopathic: Proposal for a new nomenclature and patient classification. J Neurointerv Surg. 2020;12:110-4.
5. McCluskey G, Doherty-Allan R, McCarron P, et al. Meta-analysis and systematic review of population-based epidemiological studies in idiopathic intracranial hypertension. Eur J Neurol. 2018;25:1218-27.
6. Mollan SP, Davies B, Silver NC, et al. Review: Idiopathic intracranial hypertension: Consensus guidelines on management. J Neurol Neurosurg Psychiatry. 2018;89:1088-100.

7. Adderley NJ, Subramanian A, Nirantharakumar K, et al. Association Between Idiopathic Intracranial Hypertension and Risk of Cardiovascular Diseases in Women in the United Kingdom. JAMA Neurol. 2019;76:1088-98.
8. Sheldon CA, Paley GL, Xiao R, et al. Pediatric Idiopathic Intracranial Hypertension: Age, Gender, and Anthropometric Features at Diagnosis in a Large, Retrospective, Multisite Cohort. Ophthalmology. 2016;123:2424-31.
9. Mollan SP, Hoffmann J, Sinclair AJ. Advances in the understanding of headache in idiopathic intracranial hypertension. Curr Opin Neurol. 2019;32(1):92-8.
10. Hoffmann J, Mollan SP, Paemeleire K, et al. European Headache Federation guideline on idiopathic intracranial hypertension. J Headache Pain. 2018;19(1):93.
11. Banerjee M, Aalok SP, Vibha D. Unilateral papilledema in idiopathic intracranial hypertension: A rare entity. Eur J Ophthalmol. 2020;1120672120969041.
12. Favoni V, Pierangeli G, Toni F, et al. Idiopathic Intracranial Hypertension Without Papilledema (IIHWOP) in Chronic Refractory Headache. Front Neurol. 2018;9:503.
13. Townsend RK, Fargen KM. Intracranial Venous Hypertension and Venous Sinus Stenting in the Modern Management of Idiopathic Intracranial Hypertension. Life (Basel). 2021;11(6):508.
14. Botfield HF, Uldall MS, Westgate CSJ, et al. A glucagon-like peptide-1 receptor agonist reduces intracranial pressure in a rat model of hydrocephalus. Sci Transl Med. 2017;9(404):eaan0972.
15. Sinclair AJ, Onyimba CU, Khosla P, et al. Corticosteroids, 11beta-hydroxysteroid dehydrogenase isozymes and the rabbit choroid plexus. J Neuroendocrinol. 2007;19(8):614-20.
16. O'Reilly MW, Westgate CS, Hornby C, et al. A unique androgen excess signature in idiopathic intracranial hypertension is linked to cerebrospinal fluid dynamics. JCI Insight. 2019;4(6):e125348.
17. Moreno-Ajona D, McHugh JA, Hoffmann J. An Update on Imaging in Idiopathic Intracranial Hypertension. Front Neurol. 2020;11:453.
18. Friedman DI, Liu GT, Digre KB. Revised diagnostic criteria for the pseudotumor cerebri syndrome in adults and children. Neurology. 2013;81(13):1159-65.
19. Headache Classification Committee of the International Headache Society (IHS) The International Classification of Headache Disorders, 3rd edition. Cephalalgia. 2018;38:1-211.
20. Michael M, McDermott MP, Kieburtz KD, et al.; NORDIC Idiopathic Intracranial Hypertension Study Group Writing Committee. Effect of Acetazolamide on Visual Function in Patients With Idiopathic Intracranial Hypertension and Mild Visual Loss. JAMA. 2014;311(16):1641-51.
21. Sinclair AJ, Burdon MA, Nightingale PG, et al. Low energy diet and intracranial pressure in women with idiopathic intracranial hypertension: Prospective cohort study. BMJ. 2010;341:c2701.
22. Sun WYL, Switzer NJ, Dang JT, et al. Idiopathic intracranial hypertension and bariatric surgery: A systematic review. Can J Surg. 2020;63:E123-8.
23. Ball AK, Howman A, Wheatley K, et al. A randomised controlled trial of treatment for idiopathic intracranial hypertension. J Neurol. 2011;258(5):874-81.
24. Kesler A, Hadayer A, Goldhammer Y, et al. Idiopathic intracranial hypertension: Risk of recurrences. Neurology. 2004;63(9):1737-9.
25. Celebisoy N, Gökçay F, Sirin H, et al. Treatment of idiopathic intracranial hypertension: topiramate vs. acetazolamide, an open-label study. Acta Neurol Scand. 2007;116(5):322-7.
26. Scotton WJ, Botfield HF, Westgate CS, et al. Topiramate is more effective than acetazolamide at lowering intracranial pressure. Cephalalgia. 2019;39(2):209-18.
27. Schoeman JF. Childhood pseudotumor cerebri: Clinical and intracranial pressure response to acetazolamide and furosemide treatment in a case series. J Child Neurol. 1994;9(2):130-4.
28. Markey K, Mitchell J, Botfield H, et al. 11β-Hydroxysteroid dehydrogenase type 1 inhibition in idiopathic intracranial hypertension: A double-blind randomized controlled trial. Brain Commun. 2020;2(1):fcz050.
29. Mitchell JL, Lyons HS, Walker JK, et al. The effect of GLP-1RA exenatide on idiopathic intracranial hypertension: A randomized clinical trial. Brain. 2023;146(5):1821-30.
30. Liu GT, Glaser JS, Schatz NJ. High-dose methylprednisolone and acetazolamide for visual loss in pseudotumor cerebri. Am J Ophthalmol. 1994;118(1):88-96.
31. Yiangou A, Mitchell J, Markey KA, et al. Therapeutic lumbar puncture for headache in idiopathic intracranial hypertension: Minimal gain, is it worth the pain? Cephalalgia. 2019;39(2):245-53.
32. Scotton WJ, Mollan SP, Walters T, et al. Characterising the patient experience of diagnostic lumbar puncture in idiopathic intracranial hypertension: A cross-sectional online survey. BMJ Open. 2018;8(5):e020445.
33. Banta JT, Farris BK. Pseudotumor cerebri and optic nerve sheath decompression. Ophthalmology. 2000;107(10):1907-12.
34. Gilbert AL, Chwalisz B, Mallery R. Complications of Optic Nerve Sheath Fenestration as a Treatment for Idiopathic Intracranial Hypertension. Semin Ophthalmol. 2018;33(1):36-41.
35. Plotnik JL, Kosmorsky GS. Operative complications of optic nerve sheath decompression. Ophthalmology. 1993;100(5):683-90.
36. Kalyvas A, Neromyliotis E, Koutsarnakis C, et al. A systematic review of surgical treatments of idiopathic intracranial hypertension (IIH). Neurosurg Rev. 2021;44(2):773-92.
37. Nicholson P, Brinjikji W, Radovanovic I, et al. Venous sinus stenting for idiopathic intracranial hypertension: A systematic review and meta-analysis. J Neurointerv Surg. 2019;11(4):380-5.
38. Garner RM, Aldridge JB, Wolfe SQ, et al. Quality of life, need for retreatment, and the re-equilibration phenomenon after venous sinus stenting for idiopathic intracranial hypertension. J Neurointerv Surg. 2021;13(1):79-85.
39. Fargen KM. Venous stenting for idiopathic intracranial hypertension: Lessons learned from a high-volume practice. J Neurointerv Surg. 2022;14(6):528-32.

CHAPTER 19

Spontaneous Intracranial Hypotension

Satish Khadilkar, Mehul Desai, Darshan Pandya, Kanchana Pillai, Sonali Shah, Chandrashekhar Deopujari

ABSTRACT

Spontaneous intracranial hypotension (SIH) is a condition resulting from leakage of cerebrospinal fluid (CSF) through a dural defect. The classical presentation is with an orthostatic headache. MRI brain usually shows diffuse pachymeningeal enhancement and sagging of the brain. Investigations such as computed tomography/magnetic resonance (CT/MR) myelography can help locate the site of the leak. A proportion of patients improve with conservative treatment, but others may require interventions such as an epidural blood patch, epidural glue application, or surgical repair at the site of the leak. In this chapter, we elaborate on the etiology, clinical features, diagnostic modalities, and management options for patients with SIH.

Keywords: Spontaneous intracranial hypotension, Secondary headache, Orthostatic headache, Dural tear, Cerebrospinal fluid leak, Myelogram, Epidural blood patch.

INTRODUCTION

Spontaneous intracranial hypotension (SIH) is a secondary headache disorder wherein a leak occurs within the dura at the spinal level. It is different from cranial or sinonasal cerebrospinal fluid (CSF) leaks. It was first described by Georges Schaltenbrand, a neurologist in Wurzburg, Germany, in 1938, who named it "hypoliquorrhea." It is associated with low CSF pressure (<60 mm CSF) and/or evidence of a CSF leak on imaging.[1] Although better recognized now than in the past, particularly with the advent of newer imaging modalities, the awareness of this condition is still limited. Atypical or refractory symptoms and often normal initial findings are reasons for delayed diagnosis or misdiagnosis. SIH is a misnomer, as most patients have a preceding event, an extracranial pathology, and not all patients have low CSF pressure.

DEMOGRAPHICS

There is a paucity of large-scale prospective studies for SIH demographics. The estimated annual incidence is 5 per 100,000.[2] The condition is more common in females (F:M = 2:1) and typically occurs in the third to fifth decade, with an average age of onset being 40–45 years.[3]

ETIOLOGY

Spontaneous spinal CSF leaks cause SIH. The exact cause of the leak remains unknown in the majority of patients and is presumed to be multifactorial. Underlying fragility of the spinal meninges has been suggested. A history of a traumatic event can be elicited in about one-third of patients, suggesting mechanical factors as well.[1] Inherited connective tissue disorders can play a role in developing CSF leaks, as dura is also connective tissue. There have been some case reports of familial SIH affecting first-degree relatives of index cases of SIH.[3,4] The predisposing factors are enumerated in **Table 1**, and the types of CSF leaks are described in **Flowchart 1**.[5]

PATHOPHYSIOLOGY

Essentially, a low CSF volume, low CSF pressure, and low compliance of spinal dura are significant factors in the pathophysiology of SIH. CSF hypovolemia is more critical

Spontaneous Intracranial Hypotension

TABLE 1: Predisposing factors for the CSF leak.[2]	
Connective tissue disorders	• Marfan syndrome • Ehler–Danlos syndrome type 2 • Autosomal dominant polycystic kidney disease are the three most common associated disorders • Excessive joint hypermobility • Personal or family history of arterial dissections or aneurysms • Secondary to unrecognized intracranial hypertension
Spine disorders—osseous spinal pathology	• Most commonly degenerative disc disease—cervical spine • Calcified herniated discs • Osteophytes—sharp areas which can pierce the dura • Occasionally, congenital bony spurs • Dural abnormalities: Dural holes or rents, meningeal diverticula, or even absence of dura • CSF venous fistula
Surgery	• Previous spine surgery • Lumbar puncture • Nerve root avulsions or tears • Previous spinal or epidural anesthesia • Bariatric surgery
Trauma—even a mild trauma	• Whiplash injury • Lifting heavy objects or sometimes turning or twisting can be sufficient for spinal CSF leak

(CSF: cerebrospinal fluid)

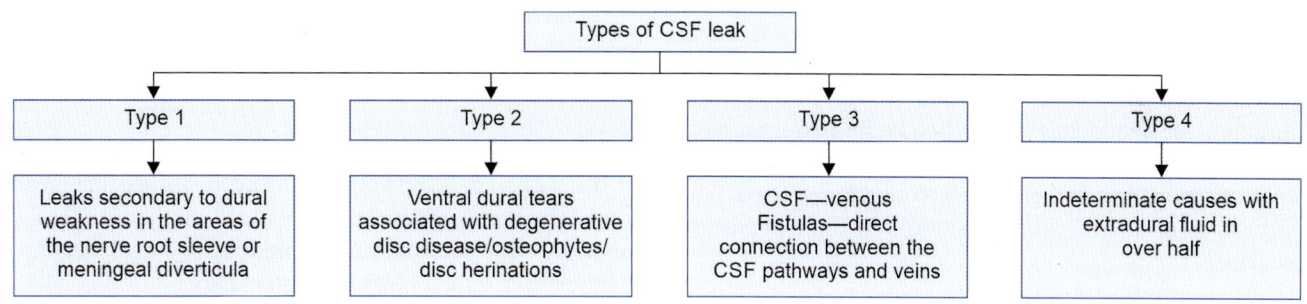

FLOWCHART 1: Types of CSF leaks.[6]
(CSF: cerebrospinal fluid)

than CSF hypotension, as classical features can occur in the absence of demonstrable lowering of the CSF pressure.[7]

There are two proposed mechanisms for SIH:[8]
1. *Monro-Kellie doctrine*: CSF volume, blood volume, and brain volume remain constant at a given time. In SIH, CSF volume reduces, but arterial blood and brain volume remain the same. So, an excess of volume is compensated by venous blood, and the venous blood volume increases which leads to dilatation of intracranial venous structures.[9,10]
2. *Hydrostatic indifference point mechanism*: A zero-pressure point is usually located in the upper cervical spine, where CSF pressure changes from positive to negative relative to the atmospheric pressure. CSF pressure will be the same in the upright and supine positions. In people with SIH, this zero-pressure point moves downward, leading to a negative intracranial pressure relative to the lower spine. It leads to increased CSF expulsion in the upright position with possible venous dilation, causing orthostatic headaches. The pressure difference equalizes in the supine position with minor CSF leak and headache. This hydrostatic indifference point highlights the change in lumbar compliance in the presence of SIH. Conversely, cranial CSF leaks are not associated with orthostatic headaches.[11-13]

CLINICAL FEATURES

Spontaneous intracranial hypotension is suspected in patients with orthostatic or postural headaches, a headache that worsens on coughing, laughing, and the Valsalva maneuver. Orthostatic headache is the most common and

TABLE 2: Uncommon presentations.[18-20]	
Vertigo	Ataxia
Blurred vision; diplopia	Cognitive and behavioral changes
Hiccups	Ocular motor nerve palsies
Dysgeusia	Parkinsonism
Transient visual obscuration	Other movement disorders
Bimelic paralysis	Subdural hemorrhage[21]

prototypical manifestation. It can occur within seconds to minutes of assuming an upright position but can also be delayed. The headache improves or resolves after lying down, usually within 30 minutes.[2,12] The patient often feels much better early in the morning. Headache is generally holocephalic and diffuse but may be localized to one region of the head or is asymmetric. The quality of headache can vary from pounding, throbbing, or pressure sensations. The onset of headache in the majority is gradual or subacute. A sudden presentation with a thunderclap headache is a rare occurrence. The severity of headaches varies from mild to severe, which is resistant to analgesics. The exact cause of headaches is unknown. It may be related to the downward displacement of the brain due to loss of CSF buoyancy, causing traction of pain-sensitive structures.[14] Compensatory dilatation of the pain-sensitive intracranial venous structures may also play a role. An orthostatic headache can become less prominent or even disappear over time. Rarely, the reverse pattern may occur. Some patients have no postural component of headaches. Other headache patterns, such as exertional headaches, headaches at the end of the day, or even paradoxical headaches, are infrequently reported. One should think of SIH in patients with a new daily persistent headache.[15-17]

Other common symptoms are posterior neck pain or stiffness, nausea, and vomiting. Besides these common clinical presentations, some patients present with unusual clinical features, resulting in diagnostic difficulties. These are listed in **Table 2**. Up to 25% of patients may have echoing sounds in the ear, tinnitus, and a disturbed sense of balance, resulting from the transmission of abnormal CSF pressure to the perilymph of the cochlea and vestibular apparatus. Cranial nerve palsies are attributed to the traction of intracranial structures secondary to the caudal displacement of the brain. Complications such as subdural hematoma (SDH), uncal herniation, sinus thrombosis, brainstem ischemia, and Duret hemorrhage can occur, which can be potentially life-threatening.

DIAGNOSIS AND DIFFERENTIAL DIAGNOSIS

Diagnosis of SIH is based on an amalgamation of a detailed headache history, clinical features, and imaging findings. As a result of it being an uncommon cause of headache and low

> **BOX 1: Diagnostic criteria for SIH as per ICHD-3.[22]**
>
> Developed in temporal relation to a low CSF pressure or leak, or led to the discovery of low CSF pressure or leak, or either or both of the following:
>
> 1. CSF pressure <60 mm CSF
> 2. Evidence of CSF leak on neuroimaging
> 3. And not better accounted for by another ICHD-3 diagnosis
>
> (CSF: cerebrospinal fluid; ICHD-3: International Classification of Headache Disorders 3; SIH: spontaneous intracranial hypotension)

> **BOX 2: Differential diagnosis of SIH.**
>
> - Postural orthostatic tachycardia syndrome—orthostatic headache without associated leakage of CSF
> - Orthostatic hypotension
> - Chiari I malformation—cerebellar tonsils inferiorly pointed with absent midbrain descent
> - Cervicogenic headache—headache with neck pain worsening with cervical motion, relieved with medication
> - Craniocervical instability
> - Subdural fluid collections—usually unilateral
> - Conditions with dural thickening—IgG4-related disease, neurosarcoidosis, tuberculosis, autoimmune diseases, infection
>
> (CSF: cerebrospinal fluid; IgG4: immunoglobulin G4; SIH: spontaneous intracranial hypotension)

index of suspicion on the part of the clinician, the diagnosis of SIH is often delayed for months. By the time a diagnosis is made, the headache has often evolved into a chronic daily headache. The International Headache Society has defined diagnostic criteria for SIH as given in **Box 1**.[1]

The condition is pathogenetically separated from post lumbar puncture headache and postoperative CSF loss.[23] The differential diagnoses are given in **Box 2**. As can be seen from **Table 2**, when patients present with an uncommon set of clinical features, the differential diagnosis would be much broader.

IMAGING MODALITIES

Cranial Magnetic Resonance Imaging

The most important investigation in the diagnosis of SIH is craniospinal magnetic resonance imaging (MRI). The majority of findings of SIH on MRI is related to low CSF volume. The most sensitive MRI finding is diffuse pachymeningeal contrast enhancement **(Fig. 1)**, which may be mistaken for meningitis in the presence of headache and vomiting. Other findings suggestive of SIH include the following:

- Unilateral or bilateral subdural collections (hygromas more often than hematomas) **(Fig. 2)**

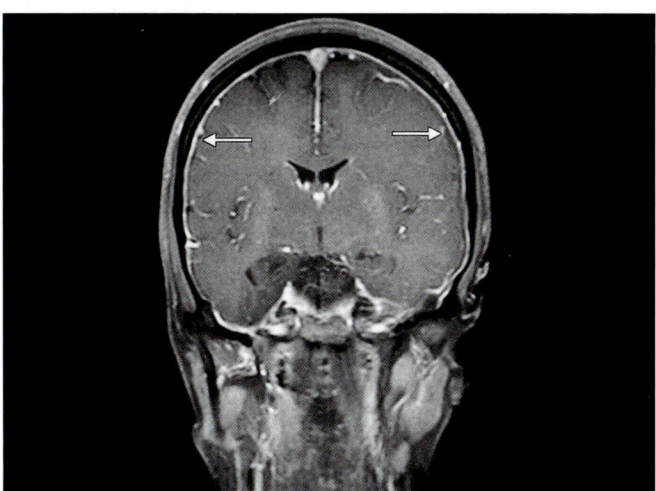

FIG. 1: Coronal postcontrast T1W image with diffuse pachymeningeal enhancement along the cerebral convexities.
Courtesy: Radiology Department, Bombay Hospital Institute of Medical Sciences, Mumbai, Maharashtra.

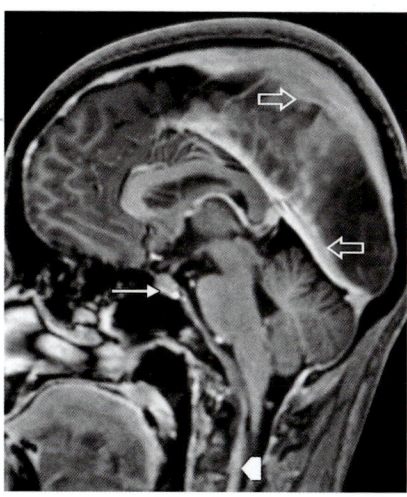

FIG. 3: Sagittal postcontrast T1W image with hyperemia of the pituitary gland (closed arrow), engorgement of the superior sagittal sinus and straight venous sinuses (open arrows), and pachymeningeal enhancement (lower arrowhead).
Courtesy: Radiology Department, Bombay Hospital Institute of Medical Sciences, Mumbai, Maharashtra.

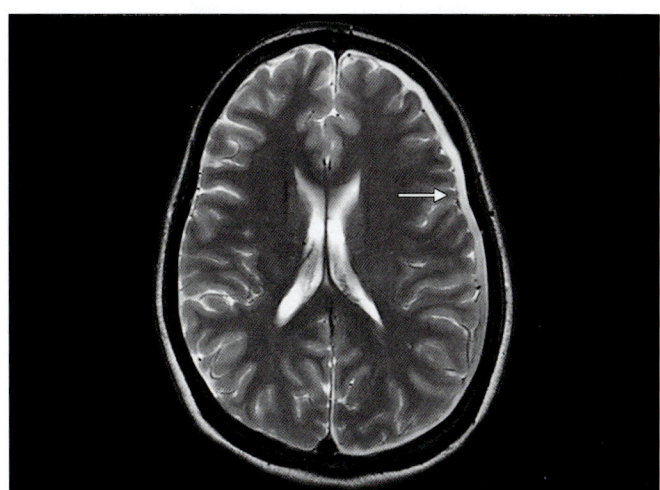

FIG. 2: Axial T2W MRI image of brain revealing thin left-sided subdural hematoma (closed arrow).
Courtesy: Radiology Department, Bombay Hospital Institute of Medical Sciences, Mumbai, Maharashtra.

- Venous engorgement with distension of the major venous sinuses, appearing rounded on cross-section images. Distension of the transverse sinus is described when there is a convexity of its inferior border, which is a reliable sign. The straight sinus can also be similarly evaluated **(Fig. 3)**.
- Hyperemia of the pituitary gland appearing globular, enlarged, and enhancing **(Fig. 3)**
- Sagging of the brain with reduced mamillopontine distance (<5.5 mm) and downward displacement of cerebellar tonsils

Although such findings are present in most patients, imaging can still be normal in SIH, especially in cases with a prolonged duration of CSF leak.[15,24,25]

Spinal Imaging

Magnetic Resonance Imaging Spine

- MRI spine is the first step toward detection of the CSF leak and ascertaining the site of the leak. It is very helpful in detecting indirect signs of CSF leak and for developing a systematic approach for localizing and possibly managing the site of CSF leak.[24]
- A common finding in the spine is the detection of the extradural collections over a long segment [spinal longitudinal extradural collection (SLEC)], likely due to dural tears, commonly along the ventral aspect **(Fig. 4A)**. This finding can be subtle but confirmed on axial images **(Fig. 4B)**. SIH without spinal collection usually has tears laterally as a CSF-venous fistula.
- MRI of the whole spine helps us to stratify patients with suspected SIH into positive/negative for spinal longitudinal extradural collections, which helps in deciding the preferred positioning of subsequent myelography.
- Other findings are similar to brain MRI which are noted in the form of engorged and dilated spinal epidural venous plexi **(Fig. 5)** and enhancement of spinal dura. Detection of spinal meningeal diverticula is noted in a minority of patients, which is likely the site of the leak.[25]

A computed tomography (CT) scan of the spine can also show spinal longitudinal extradural collection, as shown in **Figure 6**.

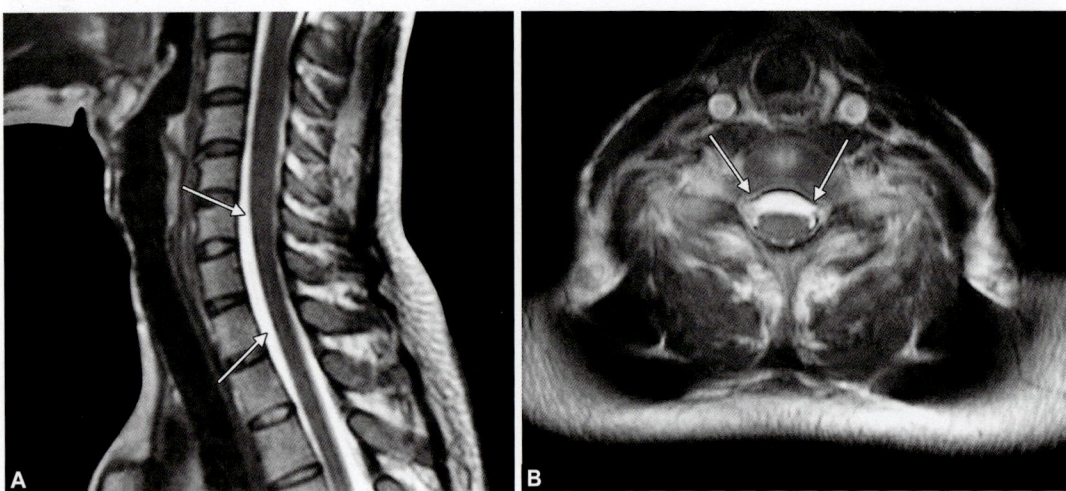

FIGS. 4A AND B: (A) Sagittal image and (B) axial image revealing cervicodorsal spinal fluid collections in the anterior epidural region (closed arrows).
Courtesy: Radiology Department, Bombay Hospital Institute of Medical Sciences, Mumbai, Maharashtra.

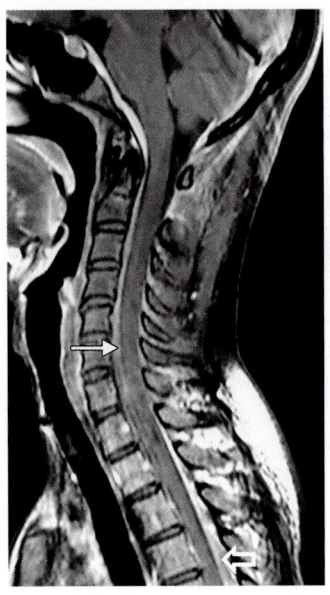

FIG. 5: Sagittal postcontrast T1W image revealing spinal pachymeningeal enhancement (closed arrow) and posterior epidural venous engorgement (open arrow).
Courtesy: Radiology Department, Bombay Hospital Institute of Medical Sciences, Mumbai, Maharashtra.

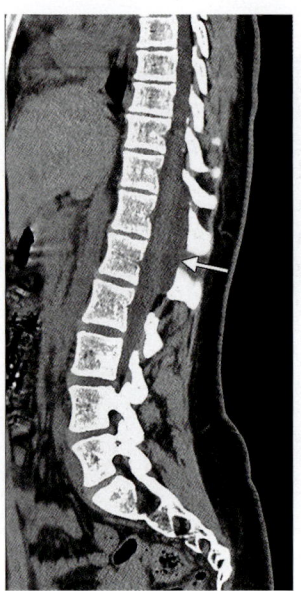

FIG. 6: Sagittal plain CT spine revealing focal widening of the dorsolumbar spinal canal with fluid collection in the posterior epidural region (closed arrow).
Courtesy: Radiology Department, Bombay Hospital Institute of Medical Sciences, Mumbai, Maharashtra.

■ Myelography

In cases where there is a need to find the site of a CSF leak (SIH refractory to epidural blood patch), digital subtraction/CT/MRI myelography can be used to detect the site of the leak, depending on the institute's preference, expertise, and availability **(Figs. 7A and B)**. Digital subtraction myelography (DSM) is used in various institutes and performed in different positions; in SLEC-positive SIH, DSM is performed in a prone position which easily detects ventral dural tear, whereas in a patient without spinal collection, DSM is performed in a lateral decubitus position to detect lateral tears/CSF-venous fistulas.[24,26]

While standard CT myelography (CTM) is better at detecting slow CSF leaks, dynamic CTM is superior in identifying fast leaks. Despite being a complex procedure, gadolinium-based enhanced magnetic resonance imaging (GdMRI) is very good at localizing spinal CSF leaks. As per

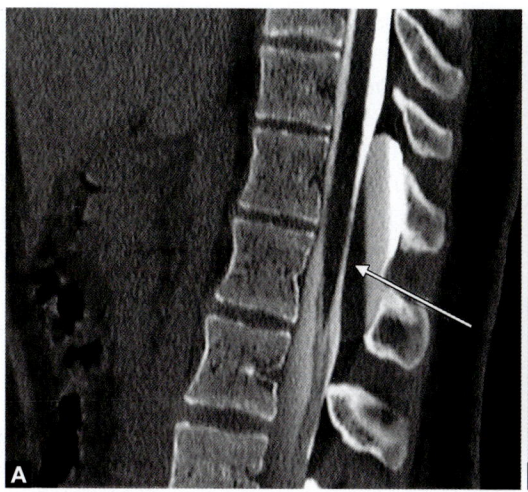 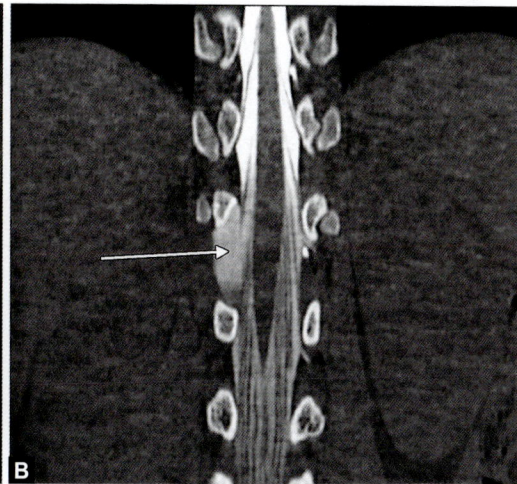

FIGS. 7A AND B: CT myelography (A) sagittal and (B) coronal images of the same patient exhibiting a right lateral dural tear and cerebrospinal fluid (CSF) leak into localized dorsolateral epidural fluid collection (closed arrows).
Courtesy: Radiology Department, Bombay Hospital Institute of Medical Sciences, Mumbai, Maharashtra.

a study, it is significantly better than CTM in detecting slow CSF leaks.

■ Radioisotope Cisternography

Cisternography can help detect CSF leaks in patients with suspected SIH, but it is not a very sensitive procedure. The usage of cisternography has largely been replaced by CT or MR myelography. The exact site of spinal CSF leak can be identified in most but not all patients with SIH. Those whose exact location of CSF leak cannot be identified likely fall into the category of the intermittent leak or cases beyond the detection by currently available modalities.

MANAGEMENT

Symptoms of SIH often resolve spontaneously in the minority of patients, and no further treatment is usually required. In one of the studies of eight patients of SIH analyzed who received conservative management, only three out of eight patients totally recovered immediately after conservative management; two patients recovered after 6–8 months, and three continued to have persistent mild headaches.[27]

■ Medical Management

In patients with mild SIH, conservative therapeutic options should be considered. Strict bed rest is advisable as it reduces pressure at the site of CSF leakage. Adequate oral and IV hydration is necessary. Caffeine is helpful in CSF hypovolemia as it causes arterial constriction and subsequent reduced cranial blood flow and reduced venous engorgement. Medications such as nonsteroidal anti-inflammatory agents are beneficial for pain relief. Theophylline can be considered to reduce the severity of headaches. The role of steroids in the management of SIH remains controversial.

■ Surgical Management

Surgical intervention is indicated in patients with SIH after a fair trial of conservative therapy has been tried. Occasionally, an acute presentation with neuro deficit, either in sensorium or focal motor deficits, due to the development of secondary complications such as subdural hemorrhage may require early intervention in these patients. A meta-analysis of 17 studies with 748 patients has shown a success rate in up to 28% of patients.[9,15]

Epidural blood patch remains the most common and efficacious treatment for this condition, either at the site if the leak has been identified (targeted) or a blind lumbar injection if the site of the leak is not clear. The success of the patch treatment is 64% in a meta-analysis of 1,758 patients comprising 33 studies. The blind lumbar procedure is usually done first in most patients to avoid the risk associated with higher levels. Targeted and nontargeted therapies have shown approximately similar success rates. However, some studies show a greater clinical improvement (80%) in targeted blood patches compared to 52% in nontargeted blood patch patients. 10–20 cc of autologous blood is usually injected. Over 50% of patients require a second treatment, while some may require four to six patches for sustained relief.[1,28,29]

Patients with persistent symptoms may need further investigations if the site of the leak is undetermined and endovascular intervention and surgical repair at the site of the leak if well identified. Further studies to locate the location of the leak include noninvasive as well as invasive (gadolinium intrathecal injection) myelography, CT intrathecal contrast myelography in the prone and supine positions, and DSM. The treatment may be in the form of epidural glue application, surgical repair at the site of the leak, or endovascular interruption of CSF-venous fistula if identified. Epidural fibrin glue has been recently reported in a few patients. Interventional treatment has been successfully employed in rare cases of CSF-venous fistulae.

Surgery for a dural defect may be simple suturing or applying a fascial graft and rarely muscle. Simple suturing is usually impossible except in ectatic dura near a root sleeve. Fascia lata or dorsolumbar fascia is usually preferred for repair. This is either sutured or overlaid on the dural defect and held in position with glue.[15]

Two representative case vignettes are narrated below, emphasizing some important clinical points.

Case 1. A 35-year-old businessman developed neck pain while lying on a sofa 2 years before the presentation. He received a vigorous neck massage for the pain, which led to the aggravation of the pain. The pain persisted despite analgesics and a cervical collar. The pain spread to the head, became generalized, and was worse when sitting or standing. MRI scan with venography showed thrombosis of the superior sagittal and sigmoid sinuses and small bilateral subdural collections. He was treated with low molecular weight heparin in a therapeutic dose followed by oral anticoagulants and aspirin. Two days later, he developed a severe orthostatic headache and required readmission. MRI scan with venography showed no improvement. Over the next 2 days, the headache became continuous and unbearable. Subdural hemorrhage was drained, and the patient was provided adequate bed rest and hydration. His thrombophilia workup was negative. Symptoms were relieved after 1 month of conservative treatment, but a tiny thin SDH remained after 1 month.

Thus, neck manipulation can lead to a CSF leak.[30] But if SDH develops, the characteristics of the headache change, and the original features become obscure. Venous sinus thrombosis is known in patients with SIH.

Case 2. A 51-year-old male complained of insidious onset, gradually progressive weakness of the left upper limb for 3 years and similar weakness of the right upper limb for 2 years. He had no lower limb symptoms, sensory complaints, or sphincter disturbance. On examination, it was a pure lower motor neuron (LMN) syndrome involving C5–T1 segments. The creatine phosphokinase (CPK) level was 184. Electromyography was suggestive of anterior horn cell involvement. Retrospectively, he had a fall and pain in the neck 3.5 years ago. He developed orthostatic headaches and had to lie in bed for 15 days. The headache gradually settled, but the shoulder weakness developed subsequently. Thus, SIH can rarely manifest as bilateral upper limb weakness, which can prove challenging to diagnose. Chronic CSF leak can lead to weakness and atrophy of upper extremities due to extensive extradural fluid collection leading to stretching of cervical nerve roots.

REFERENCES

1. Wang SJ. Spontaneous Intracranial Hypotension. Continuum (Minneap Minn). 2021;27(3):746-66.
2. Practical Neurology. (2020). Spontaneous Intracranial Hypotension. [online] Available from https://practicalneurology.com/articles/2020-may/spontaneous-intracranial-hypotension-1 [Last accessed June, 2023].
3. Rando TA, Fishman RA. Spontaneous intracranial hypotension: report of two cases and review of the literature. Neurology. 1992;42(3 Pt 1):481-7.
4. Larrosa D, Vázquez JL, Mateo I, et al. [Familial spontaneous intracranial hypotension]. Neurologia. 2009;24(7):485-7.
5. Schievink WI, Maya MM, Moser F, et al. Multiple spinal CSF leaks in spontaneous intracranial hypotension: Do they exist? Neurol Clin Pract. 2021;11(5):e691-7.
6. Upadhyaya P, Ailani J. A review of spontaneous intracranial hypotension. Curr Neurol Neurosci Rep. 2019;19(5):22.
7. Ferrante E, Savino A, Sances G, et al. Spontaneous intracranial hypotension syndrome: Report of twelve cases. Headache. 2004;44(6):615-22.
8. Goldberg J, Häni L, Jesse CM, et al. Spontaneous intracranial hypotension without CSF leakage—concept of a pathological cranial to spinal fluid shift. Front Neurol. 2021;12:760081.
9. Kranz PG, Gray L, Malinzak MD, et al. Spontaneous intracranial hypotension: pathogenesis, diagnosis, and treatment. Neuroimaging Clin N Am. 2019;29(4):581-94.
10. Ferrante E, Trimboli M, Rubino F. Spontaneous intracranial hypotension: review and expert opinion. Acta Neurol Belg. 2020;120(1):9-18.
11. Garza I, Mokri B. Cerebrospinal Fluid (CSF) Pressure change and headaches. Encyclopedia of the Neurological Sciences. 2014: 712-7.
12. Spampinato MV. Spontaneous intracranial hypotension. In: Rumboldt Z, Castillo M, Huang B, et al. (Eds). Brain Imaging with MRI and CT: An Image Pattern Approach. Cambridge: Cambridge University Press; 2010. pp. 75-6.
13. Mokri B. Spontaneous cerebrospinal fluid leaks: From intracranial hypotension to cerebrospinal fluid hypovolemia--evolution of a concept. Mayo Clin Proc. 1999;74(11):1113-23.
14. Schievink WI, Meyer FB, Atkinson JLD, et al. Spontaneous spinal cerebrospinal fluid leaks and intracranial hypotension. J Neurosurg. 1996;84(4):598-605.
15. D'Antona L, Jaime Merchan MA, Vassiliou A, et al. Clinical presentation, investigation findings, and treatment outcomes of spontaneous intracranial hypotension syndrome: a systematic review and meta-analysis. JAMA Neurol. 2021;78(3):329-37.
16. Mamlouk MD, Shen PY, Sedrak MF. Spontaneous intracranial hypotension in the critical patient. J Intensive Care Med. 2022;37(5):618-24.
17. Shukla D, Sadashiva N, Saini J, et al. Spontaneous intracranial hypotension - a dilemma. Neurol India. 2021;69(8):S456-62.

18. Kranz PG, Gray L, Amrhein TJ. Spontaneous intracranial hypotension: 10 myths and misperceptions. Headache. 2018;58(7):948-59.
19. Bond KM, Benson JC, Cutsforth-Gregory JK, et al. Spontaneous intracranial hypotension: atypical radiologic appearances, imaging mimickers, and clinical look-alikes. AJNR Am J Neuroradiol. 2020;41(8):1339-47.
20. Hong M, Shah G V, Adams KM, et al. Spontaneous intracranial hypotension causing reversible frontotemporal dementia. Neurology. 2002;58(8):1285-7.
21. Capizzano AA, Lai L, Kim J, et al. Atypical presentations of intracranial hypotension: Comparison with classic spontaneous intracranial hypotension. AJNR Am J Neuroradiol. 2016;37(7):1256-61.
22. Schievink WI, Dodick DW, Mokri B, et al. Diagnostic criteria for headache due to spontaneous intracranial hypotension: a perspective. Headache. 2011;51(9):1442-4.
23. Schievink WI. Misdiagnosis of spontaneous intracranial hypotension. Arch Neurol. 2003;60(12):1713-8.
24. Chazen JL, Talbott JF, Lantos JE, et al. MR myelography for identification of spinal CSF leak in spontaneous intracranial hypotension. AJNR Am J Neuroradiol. 2014;35(10):2007-12.
25. Rabin BM, Roychowdhury S, Meyer JR, et al. Spontaneous intracranial hypotension: Spinal MR findings. AJNR Am J Neuroradiol. 1998;19(6):1034-9.
26. Mamlouk MD, Ochi RP, Jun P, et al. Decubitus CT myelography for CSF-venous fistulas: A procedural approach. AJNR Am J Neuroradiol. 2021;42(1):32-6.
27. Kong DS, Park K, Nam DH, et al. Clinical features and long-term results of spontaneous intracranial hypotension. Neurosurgery. 2005;57(1):91-6.
28. Beck J, Raabe A, Schievink WI, et al. Posterior approach and spinal cord release for 360° repair of dural defects in spontaneous intracranial hypotension. Neurosurgery. 2019;84(6):E345-51.
29. Luetzen N, Dovi-Akue P, Fung C, et al. Spontaneous intracranial hypotension: diagnostic and therapeutic workup. Neuroradiology. 2021;63(11):1765-72.
30. Schievink WI, Maya MM. Cerebral venous thrombosis in spontaneous intracranial hypotension. Headache. 2008;48(10):1511-9.

CHAPTER 20

Vestibular Migraine

Meenakshisundaram U, Sreenivas Meenakshisundaram

ABSTRACT

Vestibular migraine (VM) is a complex neurological disorder characterized by recurrent episodes of vertigo and migrainous symptoms. It represents a significant burden on the quality of life for affected individuals, causing debilitating symptoms and functional limitations. This chapter provides a comprehensive review of VM, encompassing its epidemiology, pathophysiology, clinical manifestations, diagnostic criteria, and treatment options. Recent advancements in research over the past 5 years have shed light on various aspects of this condition, contributing to a better understanding and improved management.

Keywords: Dizziness, Migraine, Vestibular, Nystagmus, Vertigo.

INTRODUCTION

Vestibular migraine (VM) is a subtype of migraine headache characterized by the presence of vestibular symptoms during migraine attacks. It is estimated to affect approximately 1–3% of the general population, making it a prevalent disorder with substantial impact.[1] The term VM was first used in 1917 by Blenheim and reintroduced by Dietrich and Brandt in 1999. This was rebranded as Migrainous Vertigo by Neuhauser in 2010, when diagnostic criteria for the same were defined as well. There was some contention from the scientific community, but with increasing support, it has been recognized as a diagnostic entity, despite ongoing disputes over pathophysiology and treatment.[1] Previously, vertigo occurring in episodes of migraine was attributed to basilar migraine or recurrent vertigo of childhood. However, not all of these patients fulfilled the criteria for either condition, suggesting the possibility of a separate entity.

In 2012, the first diagnostic criteria were described by Lempert et al.[2] This established the usage of the term "vestibular migraine." Prior to this, multiple terms had been used. This has been updated in 2021 by the same team.

Over the past 5 years, research efforts have focused on unraveling the underlying mechanisms of VM, refining diagnostic criteria, and exploring novel treatment modalities. This article aims to provide an updated overview of VM based on the latest scientific evidence.

EPIDEMIOLOGY AND CLINICAL MANIFESTATIONS

Epidemiological studies are scarce for VM worldwide. Studies in the USA have shown a prevalence of around 2.7% in adults, which made up around 23.4% of all respondents with dizziness. Studies have also indicated a female predominance, varying from 1.5 to 5 times, and an association with a family history of migraine. VM has been suggested to be the most prevalent neurological cause of recurrent episodic dizziness, accounting for 7% of all dizziness and 9% of all migraine. However, this still remains an underdiagnosed condition. An autosomal dominant pattern of inheritance has been suggested with incomplete penetration in males, although the gene has not yet been identified.[3,4]

The onset of vestibular symptoms often occurs during the fourth and fifth decades of life, coinciding with the peak incidence of migraine. In addition to vertigo, patients commonly experience migrainous headache, photophobia, phonophobia, and visual disturbances. Recent studies have highlighted the heterogeneity of clinical presentations, including nonvertiginous symptoms such as dizziness, unsteadiness, and postural instability.[5]

The symptomatology can vary from patient to patient, with spontaneous rotational vertigo being the most common, followed by positional vertigo, head movement intolerance, and vertigo induced by moving objects. Many patients might also complain about headache around the same time of the vertiginous symptoms, but it may precede or follow the headache as well. Other auditory symptoms such as auditory fullness, tinnitus, or hearing disturbance have been described in around a third of patients with VM.[5,6]

The attack duration varies from seconds to days, but the diagnostic criteria require an attack lasting at least 5 minutes.

CLINICAL EXAMINATION

During an acute attack, vestibular eye signs are seen in upto 70% of patients. There may be spontaneous or positional nystagmus, which is of a central type in 50%, peripheral type in 15%, and mixed in the rest.

Interictally, eye examination is usually normal, although central oculomotor abnormalities can occur in a small proportion of patients. These findings include gaze-induced nystagmus, saccadic pursuit, central positional nystagmus, and dysmetric/slow saccades. The most common finding reported is central positional nystagmus. The chance of an abnormal oculomotor finding on examination increases over time with increasing total number of attacks.[5,6]

PATHOPHYSIOLOGY

The pathophysiology of VM involves intricate interactions between the trigeminal vascular system, cortical spreading depression, and the vestibular system. Neuroimaging studies utilizing functional magnetic resonance imaging (fMRI) have demonstrated altered connectivity patterns and cortical excitability in patients with VM. One theory suggests that there is parallel activation of the vestibular system and the cranial nociceptive system. Trigeminal and vestibular ganglion cells share neurochemical properties and express similar serotonin and capsaicin receptors.

Functional imaging during VM attacks has shown activation of the posterior and anterior insula, orbitofrontal cortex, and the cingulate gyrus, which are usually associated with pain perception. Increased activity in bilateral ventroanterior thalami has been demonstrated in patients with VM, with the activity correlating with the frequency of the attacks.

Studies have demonstrated reciprocal innervation between the trigeminal and vestibular system. One theory suggests that migraine reduces the threshold for cross stimulation between these systems. In a patient with migraine, stimulation of the trigeminal nerve led to nystagmus. Such communications can lead to motion sensitivity and reduced perceptual thresholds of dynamic head movements.

Genetic factors, ion channelopathies, and dysfunction of the serotonin and calcitonin gene-related peptide (CGRP) systems have also been implicated in the pathogenesis of this condition. This theory has gained traction since migraine and vertigo have been described together in the same condition such as familial hemiplegic migraine and episodic ataxia type 2. However, a single gene has not been found to be associated with VM.

Thus, the most likely pathophysiology underlying VM has been described to be increased connectivity between the vestibular and trigeminal systems at multiple levels from the peripheral to the thalamic and cortical.[5-7]

DIAGNOSTIC CRITERIA

The diagnostic criteria for VM have evolved over time to improve accuracy and facilitate clinical decision-making. The Bárány Society first described diagnostic criteria in 2012 and this was included in the International Classification of Headache Disorders (ICHD) in 2013. The International Headache Society (IHS) and the Bárány Society have formulated consensus diagnostic criteria that incorporate the typical vestibular symptoms and their temporal relationship with migrainous headache in 2021, which is an update on the previous guidelines. Diagnostic tools such as the Headache-Associated Vertigo Questionnaire (HAVQ) and the Vestibular Migraine Diagnostic Index (VMDI) have been developed and validated to aid in the clinical evaluation of patients.[8]

The currently used criteria classify VM as either definite or probable. These are defined in **Boxes 1 and 2**, respectively. The different vestibular symptoms, which are considered to fulfill these criteria, are mentioned in **Box 3**.[8,9]

BOX 1: ICHD diagnostic criteria for vestibular migraine.

A. At least five episodes with vestibular symptoms of moderate or severe intensity, lasting 5 minutes to 72 hours
B. Current or previous history of migraine with or without aura according to the International Classification of Headache Disorders (ICHD-3)
C. One or more migraine features with at least 50% of the vestibular episodes:
   a. Headache with at least two of the following characteristics: One-sided location, pulsating quality, moderate or severe pain intensity, and aggravation by routine physical activity
   b. Photophobia and phonophobia
   c. Visual aura
D. Not better accounted for by another vestibular or ICHD diagnosis

> **BOX 2: ICHD diagnostic criteria for probable vestibular migraine.**
>
> A. At least five episodes with vestibular symptoms of moderate or severe intensity, lasting 5 minutes to 72 hours
> B. Only one of the criteria B and C for vestibular migraine is fulfilled (migraine history or migraine features during the episode)
> C. Not better accounted for by another vestibular or ICHD diagnosis
>
> (ICHD: International Classification of Headache Disorders)

> **BOX 3: Vestibular symptoms reported in vestibular migraine.**
>
> - Spontaneous vertigo—either internal (self-spinning sensation) or external (environment spinning sensation)
> - Positional vertigo
> - Visually-induced vertigo—can be complex or large visual stimulus-induced
> - Head motion-induced vertigo
> - Head motion-induced dizziness with nausea, where dizziness is described as disturbed spatial orientation[8,9]

DIFFERENTIAL DIAGNOSIS

Distinguishing VM from other vestibular disorders and migraine subtypes is crucial for appropriate management. Due to the nonspecificity of the symptoms, there is a high chance of misdiagnosis.

The most significant differentials to be considered are:

- *Ménière's disease*: It is a disorder of the inner ear characterized by recurrent episodes of vertigo, hearing loss, tinnitus (ringing in the ears), and a feeling of fullness in the affected ear. It can sometimes be challenging to differentiate Ménière's disease from VM due to overlapping symptoms, but careful evaluation of clinical history and diagnostic tests can help distinguish between the two conditions.
- *Benign paroxysmal positional vertigo (BPPV)*: It is a common vestibular disorder, characterized by brief episodes of vertigo and triggered by specific head movements. It occurs due to the displacement of calcium carbonate crystals (otoconia) within the inner ear. Unlike VM, BPPV typically does not involve headache or other migraine-related symptoms.
- *Vestibular paroxysmia*: It is a rare condition characterized by recurrent short-lasting episodes of vertigo or dizziness. It is caused by neurovascular compression of the eighth cranial nerve (vestibulocochlear nerve). Diagnostic tests such as MRI and response to antiepileptic medications can help differentiate vestibular paroxysmia from VM.
- *Vestibular schwannoma (acoustic neuroma)*: Vestibular schwannoma is a benign tumor that develops on the vestibular nerve, which connects the inner ear to the brain. It can cause symptoms such as hearing loss, tinnitus, imbalance, and episodes of vertigo. Imaging studies, such as MRI, can help identify the presence of a vestibular schwannoma.
- *Central nervous system (CNS) disorders*: Certain CNS disorders, such as multiple sclerosis (MS), stroke, and cerebellar degeneration, can present with symptoms similar to VM. Clinical evaluation, imaging studies, and sometimes cerebrospinal fluid analysis are necessary to differentiate these conditions from VM.
- *Medication-induced vertigo*: Some medications can cause vertigo or dizziness as a side effect. For example, certain antibiotics, anticonvulsants, and antihypertensive drugs may induce vestibular symptoms. A careful review of the patient's medication history is important in considering medication-induced vertigo as a potential differential diagnosis.

The common differentials and the differentiating factors are given in **Table 1**.

TABLE 1: Differential diagnosis of vestibular migraine.

Diagnosis	Clinical features	Differentiation from VM
Ménière's disease	Episodes of vertigo, hearing loss, and tinnitus	Overlapping symptoms with VM, but careful evaluation of clinical history and diagnostic tests can help distinguish between the two conditions
Benign paroxysmal positional vertigo (BPPV)	Brief episodes of vertigo triggered by specific head movements	BPPV typically does not involve headache or other migraine-related symptoms
Vestibular paroxysmia	Recurrent short-lasting episodes of vertigo or dizziness, caused by neuromuscular compression of VIII CN	Magnetic resonance imaging (MRI) and response to antiepileptic medications can help differentiate vestibular paroxysmia from vestibular migraine
Central nervous system (CNS) disorders	Multiple sclerosis (MS), stroke, and cerebellar degeneration can present with symptoms similar to vestibular migraine	Clinical evaluation, imaging studies, and sometimes cerebrospinal fluid analysis are necessary to differentiate
Medication-induced vertigo	Certain antibiotics, anticonvulsants, and antihypertensive drugs may induce vestibular symptoms	A careful review of the patient's medication history is important

(VM: vestibular migraine; CN: cranial nerve)

Recent studies have highlighted the value of clinical examination, vestibular function testing, and neuroimaging in the differential diagnoses of these conditions.[5,10]

INVESTIGATION

Peripheral vestibular dysfunction has been demonstrated on testing in patients with VM. Cervical vestibular evoked myogenic potential testing has shown saccular dysfunction, while some studies have shown utricular dysfunction in ocular vestibular evoked myogenic potential testing, in patients with VM. However, these findings have not been reproduced consistently in multiple studies and continue to be debated.

MANAGEMENT STRATEGIES

The management of VM involves both acute symptomatic treatment and preventive strategies. However, there are no existing treatment guidelines.

Acute treatment options include abortive medications such as triptans and nonsteroidal anti-inflammatory drugs (NSAIDs). Zolmitriptan and rizatriptan have been shown to be efficacious in aborting attacks. However, it is still unclear if they work by the same mechanism as migraine abortion or by antinausea effects and antimotion sickness improving the dizziness.

Preventive therapies encompass pharmacological agents, lifestyle modifications, and complementary approaches. Trigger avoidance has been effective, especially when avoiding dietary triggers. Data for efficacy of nutraceuticals such as magnesium, riboflavin, and coenzyme Q10 are currently lacking for VM. Common pharmacological agents used in migraine have shown efficacy in VM as well. These have shown to reduce the frequency, duration, and intensity of the vertigo episodes.

The maximum efficacy has been demonstrated with beta blockers, with the least effect being demonstrated with calcium channel blockers. Sodium valproate has reduced the frequency of migraine attacks but has not shown effect on vertigo or dizziness.

Vestibular rehabilitation has been offered as add-on therapy in a few patients. A study including VM and vestibular impairment patients demonstrated similar efficacy over 6 months in both groups, regardless of use of antimigraine prophylactic. This is yet to be replicated in a controlled study.

Recent research has explored the efficacy of novel preventive treatments, including CGRP monoclonal antibodies, antiepileptic drugs, and vestibular rehabilitation therapy.[5,10,11]

PROGNOSIS AND FUTURE DIRECTIONS

The long-term prognosis of VM varies among individuals, with some experiencing episodic symptoms, while others develop chronic vestibular dysfunction. Further research is needed to identify reliable biomarkers, refine treatment algorithms, and develop personalized therapeutic interventions. Technological advancements, such as virtual reality and wearable devices, hold promise in improving diagnosis, monitoring, and treatment outcomes in VM.

CONCLUSION

Vestibular migraine remains a challenging condition with significant impact on affected individuals. Recent advancements in research have contributed to a deeper understanding of its epidemiology, pathophysiology, clinical manifestations, diagnostic criteria, and treatment options. By incorporating the latest scientific insights into clinical practice, healthcare professionals can provide better management and improve the quality of life for patients with VM.

REFERENCES

1. Neuhauser HK, Lempert T. Vestibular migraine. Neurol Clin. 2009;27(2):379-91.
2. Lempert T, Olesen J, Furman J, et al. Vestibular migraine: Diagnostic criteria. Consensus document of the Bárány Society and the International Headache Society. J Vestib Res. 2012;22(4):167-72.
3. Vukovic V, Plavec D, Galinovic I, et al. Prevalence of vertigo, dizziness, and migrainous vertigo in patients with migraine. Headache. 2007;47(10):1427-35.
4. Radtke A, Neuhauser H. Epidemiology of vestibular migraine: A systematic review and meta-analysis. J Neurol. 2019;266(3):555-72.
5. von Brevern M, Lempert T. Vestibular migraine. In Handb Clin Neurol. 2016;137:301-16.
6. Furman JM, Marcus DA, Balaban CD. Vestibular migraine: Clinical aspects and pathophysiology. Lancet Neurol. 2013;12(7):706-15.
7. Huang R, Zhou L, Lin L, et al. The association between vestibular migraine and benign paroxysmal positional vertigo: A systematic review and meta-analysis. Front Neurol. 2021;12:656689.
8. Lempert T, Olesen J, Furman J, et al. Vestibular migraine: Diagnostic criteria. Consensus document of the Bárány Society and the International Headache Society. J Vestib Res. 2021;31(4):289-96.
9. von Brevern M. Diagnostic criteria for vestibular migraine. Cephalalgia. 2018;38(5):769-74.
10. Teggi R, Colombo B, Albera R, et al. Clinical features, familial history, and migraine precursors in patients with definite vestibular migraine: The VM-Phenotypes projects. Headache. 2018;58(4):534-44.
11. von Brevern M, Radtke A. Treatment of Vestibular Migraine. Curr Treat Options Neurol. 2022;24(1):1-15.

CHAPTER 21

Neuromodulation in Headache Disorders

Sumit Singh, Archana Sharma

ABSTRACT

Headache disorders are very common globally and have a profound impact on the quality of life of patients. Neuromodulation offers a promising approach in the management of headache disorders, providing new treatment modalities for individuals suffering from debilitating headaches, and involves the targeted modulation of neural activity to alleviate pain and restore normal functioning. Neuromodulation techniques can be invasive and noninvasive, each offering different approaches to headache management **(Table 1)**.

Centrally invasive techniques are deep brain stimulation (DBS), spinal cord stimulation (SCS), and transcortical motor stimulation, where electrodes are implanted in specific areas of the brain, cervical spinal cord, and motor cortex involved in pain processing. Peripheral approaches are occipital nerve stimulation (ONS) and sphenopalatine ganglion stimulation (SPGS), which involve the placement of electrodes near the occipital nerves and sphenopalatine ganglion **(Table 2)**. Noninvasive neuromodulation techniques do not require surgical intervention and are generally considered safer and more accessible. Centrally noninvasive techniques are transcranial magnetic stimulation (TMS) and transcranial direct current stimulation (tDCS). Peripheral approaches are external trigeminal nerve stimulation, transcutaneous vagal nerve stimulation, and remote electric stimulation.

The choice between invasive and noninvasive neuromodulation depends on the severity of the headache disorder, individual patient characteristics, and the potential risks and benefits associated with each approach. As our understanding of the brain advances and technology improves, neuromodulation may offer new hope for individuals living with chronic and debilitating headaches. The present communication aims to highlight the role of neuromodulation in headache disorders according to the available evidence.

Keywords: Neuromodulation, Migraine, Cluster headache, Neuralgia, Stimulation.

TABLE 1: Overview of relevant neuromodulating procedures in the treatment of headache.		
	Noninvasive	**Invasive**
Peripheral	• Trigeminal nerve stimulation • Noninvasive vagal nerve stimulation • Remote electric neuromodulation	• Occipital nerve stimulation • Sphenopalatine ganglion stimulation
Central	• Transcranial magnetic stimulation • Transcranial direct current stimulation	• Deep brain stimulation • Spinal cord stimulation • Transcortical neuromodulation

TABLE 2: Invasive neuromodulation.			
Method	For	Evidence for	Side effects observed
Deep brain stimulation	Cluster headache	Case studies and randomized controlled trial (RCT)	Appetite change, bradycardia, diplopia/other vision changes, euphoria, nausea, intracerebral hemorrhage, hardware infection, transient loss of consciousness, and skin infection/hardware malfunction
Occipital nerve stimulation	Chronic cluster headache	Positive case series and clinical trials	Battery replacement, lead migration, infection, pain/numbness, and intra-abdominal at battery site
	Chronic migraine	RCTs	
	Occipital neuralgia	Case series	
Sphenopalatine ganglion stimulation	Cluster headache	RCTs	Infection, lead migration, lead misplacement, need for surgical revision, and sensory disturbances
Transcortical neuromodulation	Various headaches	Case series	Surgical complications, seizures, and cognitive difficulties

INTRODUCTION

Headache disorders, being the most common neurological problem, pose a great dilemma to the healthcare providers in terms of management. Literature reveals that almost half of the adult population has suffered with headaches at least once within the last year. Recurrent and severe headaches are not only associated with discomfort due to pain but also hamper the quality of life, social interaction, and add to the financial burden. Only a minority of people, however, are accurately diagnosed with the type of headache and managed adequately. Headaches can be characterized into primary and secondary headache disorders based on the etiology. Primary headaches include migraine, tension-type headache, and trigeminal autonomic cephalalgias (TACs). Secondary headaches are because of a long list of other conditions known to cause headaches. The pathophysiology of many of these headaches is not understood completely. Pain in headache disorders is because of a complex interplay of central and peripheral nervous system, which provides the substrates for pain. Systemic medications are already aboard to provide symptomatic relief in the acute settings as well as prophylaxis of various headache disorders. Sensory blockades and ablative procedures are also part of the pain management algorithms but still underused. "Neuromodulation" is an evolving modality for management of pain and the associated features of headache disorders and is defined as "the process of inhibition, stimulation, modification, regulation, or therapeutic altercation of brain activity electrically or chemically, in the central, peripheral, or autonomic nervous systems."[1] It works on neurons and modulates their activity in both invasive and noninvasive ways to reduce the pain and other features.

THEORETICAL MECHANISMS OF NEUROMODULATION

Physiological brain is largely an insensate structure; however, the pain sensitive craniocervical structures are the meninges, pial, dural, and extracranial blood vessels. These structures have peripheral nociceptors, which process and transmit pain within trigeminal, vagus, or glossopharyngeal cranial nerves and the upper cervical cranial roots. A complex neuroanatomic relationship exists between these peripheral nociceptive neurons in the head and neck, the brainstem [trigeminocervical complex (TCC)], subcortical relay centers (thalamus), and higher order processing centers of the cerebral cortex. Sensations over the anterior part of head and face are supplied via the trigeminal nerve and posterior aspect of the head via upper cervical nerves. Nociceptive signals from these areas are processed in the TCC. Activity of the TCC is also modulated by projections from periaqueductal gray matter, nucleus raphe magnus, rostral ventral medulla, hypothalamus as well as descending cortical inhibitory pathways. The second order neurons exit from TCC and transmit the nociceptive information to the thalamus and further to the cortex via the third order neurons. Another important pathway is trigeminal autonomic reflex, which plays an important role in pathogenesis of TACs. Most of the pain-carrying nerve fibers are pseudounipolar neurons, which carry nociceptive signals from blood vessels on the same side, explaining the unilateral distribution of pain in various TACs and migraine. Superior salivatory nucleus of pons plays a pivotal role in the cranial parasympathetic outflow via sphenopalatine ganglion (SPG) and is modulated by trigeminal nerve fibers (**Fig. 1**).[2] All these structures are being utilized

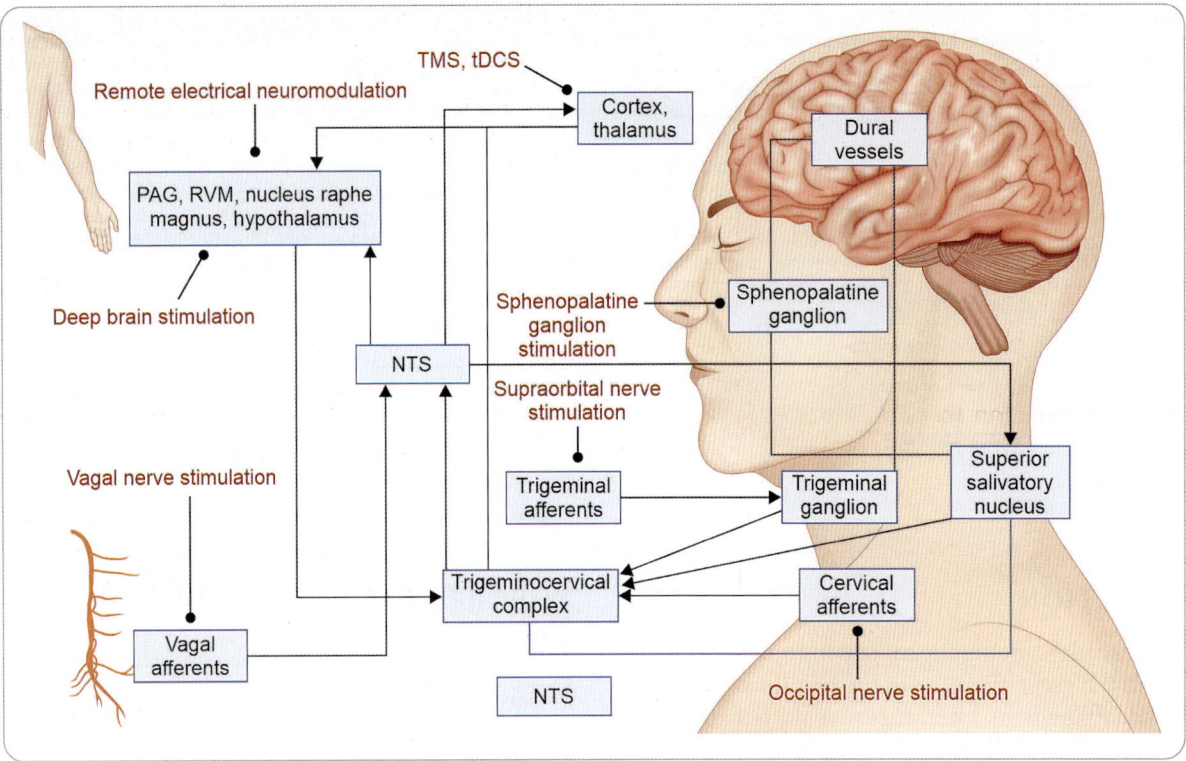

FIG. 1: Invasive and noninvasive as well as peripheral and central methods of neuromodulation with their active agents.
(NTS: nucleus tractus solitarius; PAG: periaqueductal gray matter; RVM: rostral ventral medulla; tDCS: transcranial direct current stimulation; TMS: transcranial magnetic stimulation)
Source: BioRender.com

to modulate the chemical or electrical signaling in the nociceptive pathways via continuous or intermittent stimulation/inhibition using both invasive and noninvasive methods. In the present communication, we will attempt to explain the methods of neuromodulation with their possible mechanisms of action, safety profiles, and possible adequate usage in an evidence-based manner.

▪ Invasive Peripheral Neuromodulation

Invasive peripheral neuromodulatory techniques include occipital nerve stimulation (ONS) and sphenopalatine ganglion stimulation (SPGS).

Occipital Nerve Stimulation

Trigeminocervical complex consists of afferents from trigeminalis-caudalis nucleus and from greater occipital nerve (GON). The modulation of GON therefore indirectly modifies the pain-producing mechanisms. It is postulated that ONS alters the central as well as peripheral nociceptive mechanisms. The occipital nerve stimulator consists of four to eight electrodes that are placed extracranially at the level of occiput overlying greater and lesser occipital nerves connected to a pulse generator by a subcutaneous lead and implanted on the chest wall. A handheld device is used to program the generator. A trial of neurostimulation is given for at least 2 weeks and if there is >50% reduction in the pain, then only the permanent device is implanted. ONS efficacy has been demonstrated in prevention of medication refractory primary headaches.

Migraine

A systematic review and meta-analysis of four randomized controlled trials (RCTs) by Cadalso et al. demonstrated that primary endpoint of pain freedom could not be achieved, but secondary endpoints, i.e., attack frequency, reduction in headache days per month, and responder rates were achieved.[3] RELIEF, an open-labelled multicenter study, also showed reduction in pain relief and headache disability.[4] Burst ONS was studied by Garcia-Ortega et al. in which significant reduction in the headache days was observed.[5]

Cluster Headache

There are no RCTs in refractory chronic cluster headaches (CHs) using ONS as a treatment modality; however, a meta-analysis of eight case series was published by Cadalso et al., which included 96 patients of chronic CH.[3] It was observed that responder rate was variable, but there were reduction headache days per month and few of chronic headaches were converted into episodic ones. ICON is a randomized, double-blinded multicenter study that is currently investigating prevention of CH using ONS.[6]

Occipital Neuralgia

A systematic review published in 2015 by Sweet et al. observed that reduction in pain relief was achieved in 50–85% of the patients where GON stimulation was used for occipital neuralgias.[7] Evidence for management of occipital neuralgias using ONS has been limited to case reports and series only. Unfortunately, ONS is not Food and Drug Administration (FDA) approved for any indication in headache and therefore, this invasive modality is reserved for patients with refractory chronic headaches.

Sphenopalatine Ganglion Stimulation

Sphenopalatine ganglion located in the pterygopalatine fossa is a relay center in the trigeminal autonomic reflex and is thought to play an important role in the pathophysiology of TACs. Neuromodulation of the SPG allows modification of this reflex with resultant reduction in frequency and intensity of headaches. A microstimulator device called "Pulsante" comprising of an integral lead containing six electrodes and a device body housing the electronic circuitry is implanted in the upper jaw and its position is checked radiologically. A handheld remote, which emits radio waves, can be used to induce the device and generate controlled impulses in variable frequencies, which can cause depletion of the parasympathetic neurotransmitters or can act via feedback mechanisms in centrally mediated headache mechanisms.[8] This technique has been widely studied for acute and preventive therapy of CHs and migraines.

Cluster Headaches

Evidence for effectiveness of SPGS comes from Pathway CH-1, Pathway CH-2, and Pathway R1 studies.[9] Pathway CH-1 study was conducted in 33 patients for aborting attacks of CH. Primary endpoint of >50% efficacy in aborting an attack was observed and secondary endpoints were also achieved in the form of reduction in frequency of headaches. The patients received either full, subthreshold, or sham stimulation.[10] Pathway CH-2 study evaluated the long-term results of these patients to evaluate the preventive role of SPGS in CH.[11] To conclude, SPGS can be used as a viable option to treat refractory chronic CHs with tolerable side effects.

Migraine

There is lack of promising evidence for effectiveness of SPGS in migraine headaches. However, Schoenen et al. prospectively studied the efficacy of SPGS in 11 patients with chronic migraine, 9 with medication overuse headaches, and 2 with episodic migraine. The results were conflicting and inconclusive.[12]

■ Invasive Central Neuromodulation

Invasive central neuromodulation includes spinal cord, transcortical, and deep brain stimulation (DBS) of hypothalamus and thalamus.

Spinal Cord Stimulation

In spinal cord stimulation (SCS), stimulating electrodes and leads are applied in the epidural space on dorsal aspect of the cervical spinal cord from C1 to C4 via vertebral laminectomy. Leads displacement, cerebrospinal fluid (CSF) leak, and local infections are the potential side effects. Finnern et al. published a systematic review of 16 studies comprising 107 patients on the role of cervical SCS in treating intractable headache disorders, such as refractory migraine, trigeminal neuropathy, CH, cervicogenic headache, occipital neuralgia, post-traumatic headache, short-lasting unilateral neuralgiform headache with conjunctival injection and tearing (SUNCT), poststroke headache, and tension-type headaches. It was found that cervical SCS is associated with reduction in pain intensity in migraine, CH, and the frequency of migraine headaches.[13] Owing to the limited data and invasive nature of this procedure, it has not been FDA approved for management of any chronic headache.

Deep Brain Stimulation

Deep brain stimulation has been tried in hypothalamus and thalamus for variable indications.

Hypothalamus

Observation of hypothalamic activation during an attack of CH forms the basis of trials using hypothalamic DBS in CHs. Stimulating electrodes via frontal burr hole surgery are placed in posterior hypothalamus using a combination of magnetic resonance imaging (MRI), stereotactic frame, and neuronavigation guidance. The pulse generator is then placed in infraclavicular area or periumbilical area via subcutaneous tunneling for further stimulation.[8] Other targets for stimulation are the ventral tegmental area, the lateral wall of third ventricle, and floating electrodes that stimulate the nearby area of third ventricle. The side effects include lead migration, incorrect placement of electrodes, infection, and intracranial hemorrhage apart from diplopia, dizziness, seizures, thirst and transient ischemic attacks, anxiety, and syncope as rare side effects.

A meta-analysis was published by Nowacki et al. in 2019 to study the various targets of hypothalamic DBS. Around more than 100 cases have been published in the literature for hypothalamic DBS in refractory chronic CH and majority of them showed >50% responder rates. The attack frequency and headache intensity were also decreased.[14] DBS is ineffective in bilateral CH.

Thalamus

Thalamic DBS is still in an experimental state for headache management. In 2003, Green et al. performed DBS of the contralateral periventricular gray (PVG) area and ventroposterior nucleus of thalamus in a patient of postherpetic trigeminal neuralgia, where the patient remained pain free for 6 months.[15] Boccard et al. conducted

DBS of PVG, ventral posterolateral (VPL), or both the targets (dual stimulation) in 197 patients over 12 years for various etiologies such as 9 with phantom limb pain, 7 brachial plexopathies, 31 post-stroke patients, 15 atypical head and facial pain, 13 with spinal cord pathologies, and 10 miscellaneous pathologies.[16] 30% or more improvement was observed in various pain scales for almost 2 years. However, there is a lot of heterogeneity in these diseases, targets, procedures, and follow-up periods in the reported case series. Hence, a conclusion cannot be drawn and FDA does not approve thalamic DBS for headache.

Transcortical Neuromodulation

Transcortical neuromodulation method is used to treat secondary trigeminal neuropathies due to multiple sclerosis or trauma, atypical facial pain, deafferentiated pain, or central neuropathic pain. Similar to ONS, four electrodes are placed after locating the area of facial pain using functional MRI (fMRI). These are then connected to an impulse generator placed in infraclavicular area via subcutaneous tunneling.[17] Eight case series have been published so far reporting the efficacy of transcortical neuromodulation in abovementioned refractory painful condition with promising results. The side effects observed were surgical complications, seizures, and cognitive alterations.[17-24]

■ Noninvasive Peripheral Neuromodulation

Noninvasive techniques, which are used to treat headaches, are noninvasive vagus nerve stimulation, transcranial magnetic stimulation (TMS), peripheral electrical stimulation, and external trigeminal nerve stimulation (eTNS) **(Table 3)**.

External Trigeminal Nerve Stimulation

Supratrochlear and supraorbital branches of the trigeminal nerve, stimulated transcutaneously by external wearable devices, have been found to be useful in the acute and preventive treatment of migraine in several studies.

Migraine

Two RCTs and several case series have evaluated the role of transcutaneous devices in the management of episodic and chronic migraine. Prevention of Migraine using Cefaly (PREMICE) study involved patients with episodic migraine, subjected to 20 minutes of external neuromodulation daily. Reduction of the headache frequency as well as pain intensity was observed in most patients.[25] Acute migraine therapy with external trigeminal neurostimulation (ACME) was conducted in patients with chronic migraine and similar results were obtained.[26] Magis et al. conducted a survey of 2,313 patients with headache using Cefaly device and showed good tolerability and safety for the device except for mild paresthesia and local pain.[27] Reed et al. showed simultaneous stimulation of occipital nerve and supraorbital nerves are more efficacious than single stimulation for migraine.[28]

Transcutaneous Vagal Nerve Stimulation

After successful trials in epilepsy, vagal nerve stimulation (VNS) is being tried in headache disorders. Both invasive and noninvasive techniques have been developed and are in use. Noninvasive VNS has a benefit of being devoid of implant-related complications such as asystole, bradycardia, lead displacement, migration, or infections. In noninvasive VNS, auricular branches or cervical branches are externally stimulated by use of a portable device, which emits

TABLE 3: Noninvasive neuromodulation devices for treatment of headache disorders.					
Mode	Device/Manufacturer	FDA approved	Migraine indication	CH indication	Side effects
nVNS	gammaCore/electroCore	Yes	Acute treatment in adults	Acute treatment and adjunctive preventive treatment for adults	Local pain and paresthesias
TMS	sTMSMini/eNeura	Yes	Acute and preventive treatment in adults and adolescents >age 12 years		Discomfort
eTNS	Multiple/Cefaly	Yes	Acute and preventive treatment of migraine in adults aged 18 years and up		Paresthesias, local pain, skin problems, and facial swelling
REN	Nerivio Migra/Theranica	Yes	Acute treatment in adults aged 18 years and up		Local reactions and discomfort

(CH: cluster headache; eTNS: external trigeminal nerve stimulation; FDA: Food and Drug Administration; nVNS: noninvasive vagal nerve stimulation; REN: remote electrical neuromodulation; TMS: transcranial magnetic stimulation)

transcutaneous pulsating low voltage electric signals. VNS is thought to reduce cortical spreading depression, inhibit parasympathetic pathways, and act on TCC. Noninvasive VNS is best avoided in patients with vagus nerve lesions and pacemakers.

Migraine

Noninvasive VNS has been evaluated in both for acute and preventive management of migraine. The PRESTO (Prospective Study of nVNS for the Acute Treatment of Migraine) trial compared VNS versus sham stimulation for acute symptomatic treatment of migraine. 12% patients in the treatment group versus 4% in the sham group reported pain freedom at 30 minutes post procedure.[29] EVENT and PREMIUM studies were done to understand the role of VNS in preventive treatment of migraine. In both these studies, stimulation was given twice for 90 seconds every 8 hourly and it showed significant reduction in headache days and pain intensity. Side effects observed were dizziness, neck pain, and face pulling or twitching.[30,31] gammaCore is a FDA-approved device for acute treatment of adult migraineurs.

Cluster Headache

Noninvasive VNS has been tried in both acute symptomatic treatment and preventive treatment of CH. ACT 1 and ACT 2 trials included patients with episodic and chronic CH and it was observed that only patients with episodic CH were benefitted with VNS.[32,33] In the PREVA (Prevention and Acute Treatment of Chronic Cluster Headache) trial, patients were randomized to receive standard treatment versus standard treatment plus VNS. A significant reduction was observed in the number of weekly attacks and usage of symptomatic medications in the latter group.[34] FDA has approved VNS for acute treatment of CH and as adjunctive preventive treatment of CHs.

Remote Electrical Stimulation (Peripheral Electrical Neuromodulation)

In this technique, a nonpainful electric current is generated via an impulse generator and electrodes are placed in upper arm. It acts via central gate control theory of pain and stimulates the inhibitory pain pathways. Nerivio Migra is a commercially available device that is FDA approved for use in episodic migraine and chronic migraine after better outcomes were noted in two double-blinded, sham-controlled trials.

■ Noninvasive Central Neuromodulation

Transcranial magnetic stimulation and transcranial direct current stimulation (tDCS) are the two noninvasive neuromodulation methods with favorable results in headache management and involve direct excitatory stimulation of the motor cortex.

Transcranial Magnetic Stimulation

Transcranial magnetic stimulation is a noninvasive painless and a portable system in which multiple high intensity magnetic pulses are delivered to the motor area of brain. A magnetic coil is placed on the head with a stimulator attached to it, which generates electric pulses. The changing electric current within the coil induces a magnetic field, which generates inverted electric charge in the brain. Both single pulse and repeated TMS have been used to treat headache disorders. In migraine, TMS modulates the electric activity in the thalamus and cortex and thus controls aura and pain. TMS has been tried in both acute and preventive treatment of migraine. In acute treatment, a multicenter controlled trial evaluated 82 patients using sham stimulation and single pulse TMS. Two magnetic pulses were given 30 seconds apart and it was observed that giving pulse TMS at the onset of aura reduces the pain within 2 hours. However, the results were not statistically significant. In the ESPOUSE (eNeura SpringTMS Post-Market Observational US Study of Migraine) and PREMICE studies, patients with episodic migraine were given active single pulse TMS versus sham stimulation with similar results.[35] Two systematic reviews on repetitive TMS showed that high-frequency repetitive TMS over the motor cortex area can be used as effective migraine treatment. This neuromodulation technique cannot be used in patients with metal plates, cranial defects, or pacemakers.

Transcranial Direct Current Stimulation

Transcranial direct current stimulation is another noninvasive neuromodulation technique, which is currently gaining its space in headache management. tDCS modulates the resting membrane potential of the neurons in a particular area. In this a weak current is delivered via sponge electrodes to selected targets via a battery-driven stimulator. This modulation depends upon the stimulation property of the cathode and anode and eventually leads to depolarization and hyperpolarization of the stimulated area, respectively. Occipital cortex, dorsolateral prefrontal cortex, primary motor cortex, and primary sensory cortex are the various targets under evaluation currently; however, most of the studies have heterogeneity of stimulation duration, cortical targets, stimulation sides, and reference electrodes and therefore inconclusive.

PERIPHERAL NERVE BLOCKS

Peripheral nerve blocks have been utilized in the management of craniofacial neuralgias and headaches with the rationale for inducing local anesthesia by blocking the afferent pain sensations. Various targets such as SPG, stellate ganglion, and greater or lesser occipital nerve blocks using local anesthetics and often steroids singularly or in combination have been tried. These have additional effect of phenomenon of convergence and hence blocks pain sensations from anatomic regions outside the area of supply. GON block is used widely and is diagnostic, prognostic, and therapeutic in occipital neuralgias and cervicogenic headaches and migraine. SPG blocks are effective in management of CHs, refractory migraines, postdural puncture headaches, postherpetic neuralgias, and hemicrania continua intolerant to indomethacin.

CONCLUSION

Recent era has witnessed a paradigm shift in headache treatment options with the emerging neuromodulation techniques. Noninvasive neuromodulation techniques owing to pain-free, hassle-free usage of portable devices have gained more interest and hence more growing data on its investigation in primary and secondary headache disorders. Invasive neuromodulation techniques are surgically challenging and related complications make them lower at the table in choice. Promising literature data has paved a way for these neuromodulation techniques to have brighter future in headache medicine. However, FDA has approved four noninvasive neuromodulation devices, i.e., external TNS (eTNS), TMS, remote electrical neuromodulation (REN), and noninvasive VNS (nVNS) for acute or preventive management of headache. Noninvasive techniques can be considered when patients are refractory to noninvasive options and medical management as well.

The abovementioned neuromodulation techniques are useful to a person who is intolerant to oral medication, has serious side effects, or has contraindications to oral medications. A person cannot be put directly on these techniques and are not used as first line of management of headache disorders. The aforementioned techniques and the evidence support the utility of neuromodulatory techniques and offer a glimmer of hope for patients who are refractory to the debilitating headaches. However, in view of the heterogeneity of the results and no unanimous standard protocols, these studies need to be interpreted with caution. Additional research is still needed to define the most appropriate choice of neuromodulation, most appropriate targets, and standardized protocols for the treatment of headache disorders.

REFERENCES

1. Krames ES, Hunter Peckham P, Rezai A, et al. What is neuromodulation? In: Krames ES, Hunter Peckham P, Rezai A (Eds). Neuromodulation. Academic Press; 2009. pp. 3-8.
2. da Silva Freitas T, de Monaco BA, Golovac S (Eds). Neuromodulation Techniques for Pain Treatment. A Step-by-Step Guide to Interventional Procedures and Managing Complications. Switzerland: Springer Science and Business Media LLC; 2022.
3. Cadalso RT, Daugherty J, Holmes C, et al. Efficacy of electrical stimulation of the occipital nerve in intractable primary headache disorders: A systematic review with meta-analyses. J Oral Facial Pain Headache. 2018;32:40-52.
4. Ashkan K, Sokratous G, Gobel H, et al. Peripheral nerve stimulation registry for intractable migraine headache (RELIEF): A real-life perspective on the utility of occipital nerve stimulation for chronic migraine. Acta Neurochir (Wien). 2020;162(12):3201-11.
5. Garcia-Ortega R, Edwards T, Moir L, et al. Burst occipital nerve stimulation for chronic migraine and chronic cluster headache. Neuromodulation. 2019;22(5):638-44.
6. Wilbrink LA, Teernstra OP, Haan J, et al. Occipital nerve stimulation in medically intractable, chronic cluster headache. The ICON study: Rationale and protocol of a randomised trial. Cephalalgia. 2013;33:1238-47.
7. Sweet JA, Mitchell LS, Narouze S, et al. Occipital nerve stimulation for the treatment of patients with medically refractory occipital neuralgia: Congress of neurological surgeons systematic review and evidence-based guideline. Neurosurgery. 2015;77:332-41.
8. Belvís R, Irimia P, Seijo-Fernández F, et al. Neuromodulación en cefaleas y neuralgias craneofaciales: Guía de la Sociedad Española de Neurología y de la Sociedad Española de Neurocirugía. Neurología. 2021;36:61-79.
9. Barloese MCJ, Jurgens TP, May A, et al. Cluster headache attack remission with sphenopalatine ganglion stimulation: Experiences in chronic cluster headache patients through 24 months. J Headache Pain. 2016;17:67.
10. Jurgens TP, Barloese M, May A, et al. Long-term effectiveness of sphenopalatine ganglion stimulation for cluster headache. Cephalalgia. 2017;37:423-34.
11. Jurgens TP, Schoenen J, Rostgaard J, et al. Stimulation of the sphenopalatine ganglion in intractable clúster headache: Expert consensus on patient selection and standards of care. Cephalalgia. 2014;34:1100-10.
12. Schoenen J. Sphenopalatine ganglion stimulation in neurovascular headaches. Prog Neurol Surg. 2015;29:106-16.
13. Finnern MT, D'Souza RS, Jin MY, et al. Cervical Spinal Cord Stimulation for the Treatment of Headache Disorders: A Systematic Review. Neuromodulation. 2022:S1094-7159(22)01369-1.
14. Nowacki A, Moir L, Owen SL, et al. Deep brain stimulation of chronic cluster headaches: Posterior hypothalamus, ventral tegmentum, and beyond. Cephalalgia. 2019;39(9):1111-20.
15. Green AL, Nandi D, Armstrong G, et al. Postherpetic trigeminal neuralgia treated with deep brain stimulation. J Clin Neurosci. 2003;10:512-4.
16. Boccard SG, Pereira EA, Moir L, et al. Long-term outcomes of deep brain stimulation for neuropathic pain. Neurosurgery. 2013;72:221-30.
17. Brown JA, Pilitsis JG. Motor cortex stimulation for central and neuropathic facial pain: A prospective study of 10 patients and observations of enhanced sensory and motor function during stimulation. Neurosurgery. 2005;56:290-7.
18. Fontaine D, Hamani C, Lozano A. Efficacy and safety of motor còrtex stimulation for chronic neuropathic pain: Critical review of the literature. J Neurosurg. 2009;110:251-6.
19. Thomas L, Bledsoe JM, Stead M, et al. Motor cortex and deep brain stimulation for the treatment of intractable neuropathic face pain. Curr Neurol Neurosci Rep. 2009;9:120-6.
20. Raslan AM, Nasseri M, Bahgat D, et al. Motor còrtex stimulation for trigeminal neuropathic or deafferentation pain: An institutional case series experience. Stereotact Funct Neurosurg. 2011;89:83-8.

21. Kolodziej MA, Hellwig D, Nimsky C, et al. Treatment of central deafferentation and trigeminal neuropathic pain by motor cortex stimulation: Report of a series of 20 patients. J Neurol Surg A Cent Eur Neurosurg. 2016;77:52-8.
22. Meyerson BA, Lindblom U, Linderoth B, et al. Motor cortex stimulation as treatment of trigeminal neuropathic pain. Acta Neurochir. 1993;58:150-3.
23. Ebel H, Rust D, Tronnier V, et al. Chronic precentral stimulation in trigeminal neuropathic pain. Acta Neurochir. 1996;138:1300-6.
24. Nguyen JP, Keravel Y, Feve A, et al. Treatment of deafferentation pain by chronic stimulation of the motor cortex: Report of a series of 20 cases. Acta Neurochir. 1997;68:54-60.
25. Schoenen J, Vandersmissen B, Jeangette S, et al. Migraine prevention with a supraorbital transcutaneous stimulator: A randomized controlled trial. Neurology. 2013;80:697-704.
26. Chou DE, Yugrakh MS, Winegarner D, et al. Acute migraine therapy with external trigeminal neurostimulation (ACME): A randomized controlled trial. Cephalalgia. 2019;39:3-14.
27. Magis D, Sava S, d'Elia TS, et al. Safety and patients' satisfaction of transcutaneous supraorbital neurostimulation (tSNS) with the Cefaly® device in headache treatment: A survey of 2,313 headache sufferers in the general population. J Headache Pain. 2013;14:95.
28. Reed KL, Black SB, Banta CJ 2nd, et al. Combined occipital and supraorbital neurostimulation for the treatment of chronic migraine headaches: Initial experience. Cephalalgia. 2010;30:260-71.
29. Tassorelli C, Grazzi L, de Tommaso M, et al. Noninvasive vagus nerve stimulation as acute therapy for migraine: The randomized PRESTO study. Neurology. 2018;91:e364-73.
30. Silberstein SD, Calhoun AH, Lipton RB, et al. Chronic migraine headache prevention with noninvasive vagus nerve stimulation: The EVENT study. Neurology. 2016;87:529-38.
31. Diener HC, Goadsby PJ, Ashina M, et al. Noninvasive vagus nerve stimulation (nVNS) for the preventive treatment of episodic migraine: The multicentre, double-blind, randomised, sham-controlled PREMIUM trial. Cephalalgia. 2019;39:1475-87.
32. Silberstein SD, Mechtler LL, Kudrow DB, et al.; ACT1 Study Group. Noninvasive vagus nerve stimulation for the acute treatment of cluster headache: Findings from the randomized, double-blind, sham-controlled ACT1 study. Headache. 2016;56:1317-32.
33. Goadsby PJ, de Coo IF, Silver N, et al.; ACT2 Study Group. Noninvasive vagus nerve stimulation for the acute treatment of episodic and chronic cluster headache: A randomized, double-blind, sham-controlled ACT2 study. Cephalalgia. 2018;38:959-69.
34. Gaul C, Diener HC, Silver N, et al.; PREVA Study Group Noninvasive vagus nerve stimulation for PREVention and acute treatment of chronic cluster headache (PREVA): A randomised controlled study. Cephalalgia. 2016;36:534-46.
35. Starling AJ, Tepper SJ, Marmura MJ, et al. A multicenter, prospective, single arm, open label, observational study of sTMS for migraine prevention (ESPOUSE Study). Cephalalgia. 2018;38:1038-48.

Index

Page numbers followed by *b* refer to box, *f* refer to figure, *fc* refer to flowchart, and *t* refer to table.

A

Abortive therapies 121
Acemetacin 123
Acetazolamide 28, 120
Acetyl salicylic acid 119
Acetylcholine 84
Acupuncture 130
Acute abortive medications 149, 150, 150*t*
Acute migraine 72, 76*t*, 135
   attacks 73
   management of 72, 135*t*
   medications for 79*t*
   therapy 178
   treatment 72, 138
      classes of 73
Addison's disease 155
Adenosine triphosphate 134
Adrenal insufficiency 155
Allodynia 83, 134
Alopecia 144
Alpha-1 antitrypsin deficiency 17
Amitriptyline 125
Amphetamine 2, 11
Androgens, role of 154
Anemia 155
Anesthesia
   allergy, local 144
   epidural 163
Aneurysm 21, 163
   dissecting 16
Angiitis, primary 12*f*
   diagnosis of 10*f*
Angiography 1
Antibiotics 155
Anticoagulation therapy 144
Antidepressants 22
   tricyclic 92
Antiepileptic drugs 119, 120
Antinuclear antibody, low-titers of 10
Antiphospholipid antibody syndrome 11
Antiplatelet therapy 144
Antithrombotic prophylaxis, efficacy of 32
Antithrombotic therapy 19
Anti-tumor necrosis factor alpha
      inhibitors 10
Aortic root dilation 17
Aquaporin, role of 153
Arachnoid granulation 26
Arterial dissections 16, 163
Arterial spin labelling 57, 58
Arterial wall 36
Arteriolar vasodilators 50
Arteriovenous fistula 59
   secondary dural 29
Aspergillosis 11
Aspirin 19, 119, 123
Ataxia 164
Atkins diet, modified 113
Atogepant 75, 76, 78
Atrial myxoma 11
Attacks, acute 111
Auditory aura 85
Aura
   persistent 82
   phase, symptoms during 85
Auriculotemporal nerve 143
Autoimmune diseases 164

B

Back pain 153
Bacteria 11
Balloon
   thromboplasty 31*f*
   use of 61
Barbiturates 90
Bariatric surgery 163
   role of 158
Basal ganglia 84
   bilateral 31*f*
Behçet's disease 11
Bernasconi-Cassinari artery 55
Beta-blockers 150
Betamethasone 142
Bilirubin oxidation products 46
Bimelic paralysis 164
Binding studies 73
Biobehavior therapy 99
Biopsy 9
Blind spots 83
Blood
   based biomarkers 10
   pressure 2

Blurred vision 153, 164
Body mass index 152, 157
Bony spurs, congenital 163
Borden classification 55, 55*t*
Botulinum toxin 93*t*, 119, 130
Brain
   atrophy 41
   functions, abnormal 128
   imaging 38
   MRI, role of 155
   tissue oxygen 48
Brainstem
   aura 82, 83
   ischemia 164
Bupivacaine 138, 142
   maximum dose of 142

C

Cadasil 37*fc*
   pathogenesis of 35*fc*
   proposed for 39*t*
Caffeine 150
   overuse 90
Calcified herniated discs 163
Calcitonin gene-related peptide 72, 73,
      79, 84, 97-99, 103, 107, 110, 130, 133,
      134, 171
Calcium channel
   antagonists, intra-arterial
      administration of 50
   blockers 119
Candesartan 92
Carbamazepine 119, 120
   lamotrigine 119
Carbonic anhydrase inhibitor 158, 159
Cardiovascular diseases 86
Carotico-cavernous fistulas, used for
      indirect 62
Carotid artery, external 58, 62
Catecholamine secreting tumors 2
Catheter angiography 48
Cavernous sinus 56, 57
Celecoxib 119, 123
Central nervous system 2, 10*f*, 12*f*, 22, 37,
      73, 79, 106, 128, 134, 155
   disorders 172

primary 23
   angiitis of 9, 14
   vasculitis of 21
vasculitis 11
   secondary 9, 11*t*
Central oculomotor abnormalities 171
Central venous pressure 154, 157
Cerebellar artery
   posterior inferior 55
   superior 55
Cerebellar degeneration 172
Cerebellar hemorrhage 67
Cerebellar tonsils 164
Cerebral aneurysm 17, 46
Cerebral angiography 155
Cerebral artery 12*f*
   anterior 4, 5, 48, 55
   middle 4, 5, 48
   posterior 4, 55
Cerebral autosomal
   dominant arteriopathy 34, 36, 37, 41-43
   recessive arteriopathy 37
Cerebral blood flow 48
Cerebral convexities 165*f*
Cerebral cortex 84*f*
Cerebral ischemia 46, 49
   delayed 46, 47, 51
   risk of delayed 47*t*
Cerebral micro dialysis 48
Cerebral microbleeds 41
Cerebral microdialysis 48
Cerebral sinus venous thrombosis 26
   treatment 27
Cerebral vasculitis 10*f*
Cerebral vasospasm 46, 47
   management of 51*fc*
Cerebral vein 26, 29, 32
   chronic 30*f*
   pathogenesis of 26
   therapy in 28*f*
   thrombosis of internal 30
Cerebral venous thrombosis 21, 23, 26, 28, 32, 69
   anticoagulation for 28
   chronic 30*f*
   hereditary causes of 26
Cerebrospinal fluid 2, 12, 22, 23, 28, 37, 57, 152, 153, 157, 162-164, 167*f*, 177
   absorption 26
   dysregulation 153
   flow 49
   leak 162
   shunting 159
   types of 163*fc*
Cervical
   ganglia 84*f*
   motion 164
   spine 163
Cervical artery dissection 16, 17, 17*t*, 19, 19*t*, 21
   pathogenesis of 17*f*

Cervicodorsal spinal fluid collections 166*f*
Chemical angioplasty intra-arterial calcium channel antagonists 50
Chiari malformation 164
Cholecystokinin 84
Chronic cluster headache 98, 104, 106, 111
   acute treatment of 113
Chronic headache 127*t*
   subtype 127
Chronic intracranial venous hypertension syndrome 152, 154
Chronic migraine 82, 89-91, 93*t*, 95*t*, 96, 97*t*, 98-100, 127, 133, 136, 138
   diagnostic criteria of 89
   management of 90, 100
   pharmacological treatment of 91
Chronic obstructive pulmonary disease 155
Chronic venous congestion 56*f*
Churg–Strauss syndrome 11
Cingulate cortex 84
Cisternography 167
Cluster attacks, acute treatment of 105
Cluster headache 103, 104, 110, 111*t*, 116-118, 118*f*, 133, 134, 139, 142, 143, 147, 178
   acute treatment of 113
   chronic 98, 104, 106, 111
   classification of 104*t*
   episodic 98, 104, 106, 111
   management of 103
   refractory chronic 176
   transitional treatment of 139
   treatment for 105*t*
Cluster period 106
Cocaine 2, 11
Coccidioidomycosis 11
Coenzyme Q10 173
Cogan's syndrome 11
Cognard classification 55, 55*t*
Cognitive behavioral therapy 99, 130
Cognitive impairment 38, 42
Competitive angiogram 58
Computed tomography 56, 157
   angiogram 47
   angiography 51
Connective tissue 17
   diseases 11
   disorders 163
Continuous electroencephalography 51
Conventional digital subtraction angiogram 9
Coronavirus disease 2019 32
   infection-related cerebral vein 32
   vaccination 32
Cortical vein 27*f*, 57*f*
   right frontal 59*f*
   thrombosis 26
Cortical venous
   drainage 55, 56
   reflux 54, 55, 58*f*

Corticosteroids 10, 108
Coughing, severe 17
Cranial autonomic
   features 148
   symptoms 83, 118, 119, 121
Cranial fossa, anterior 56, 59
Cranial magnetic resonance imaging 164
Cranial nerve 172
   palsies 61
Craniocervical dissection 16
Craniosynostosis 155
Craniotomy 144
C-reactive protein, elevated levels of 10
Creatine phosphokinase 168
Cryoglobulinemia 11
Crystalloids 49
Cushing's disease 155
Cutaneous atrophy 144
Cyclic guanosine monophosphate 50
Cyclic vomiting syndrome 86
Cyclooxygenase-2 119
   inhibitors 119
Cyclophosphamide 10, 14

D

Dandy criteria, modified 156
Davidoff and Schechter artery 55
Daytime somnolence, excessive 126
Death 56
Decompressive surgery 28
Deep brain stimulation 111, 112, 119, 177
Deep cerebral venous thrombosis 26, 31*f*
Dementia 38, 42
Dermatomyositis 11
Dexamethasone 142
Diclofenac 119
Diffusion tensor imaging 155
Diffusion-weighted imaging 5
Digital subtraction angiogram 4, 5, 47, 48
Dihydroergotamine 120
Diplopia 153, 164
Ditans 72-74
   adverse effects 74
   efficacy 74
Divalproex sodium 92
Dizziness 153
Dopamine 84
Dorsolumbar spinal canal 166*f*
Down syndrome 155
Doxycycline 155
Draining vein, status of 59
Duloxetine 119
Dural arterial feeder 55
Dural arteriovenous fistula 55, 56*f*, 57*f*, 58, 59, 61-63
   high-grade 56
   primary 29
Dural arteriovenous malformations 54
Dural sinus 27*f*
   drainage, direction of 59
   thrombosis 26, 28*f*, 29, 29*f*, 30*f*, 32

Dural tear 162
   right lateral 167f
Duret hemorrhage 164
Dysgeusia 164

E

Eales disease 11
Ectatic cortical veins 59f
Ehler–Danlos syndrome 163
Electrical neuromodulation 180
Electromyography 129
Embolization 54
Empty sella 155
Encephalopathy 10
   acute reversible 38
Endocrinological disorders 155
Endothelial nitric oxide, loss of 46
Endothelin, overproduction of 46
Endovascular therapies 31
Enzyme-linked immunosorbent assay 32
Epidural blood patch 162, 167
Epidural region, posterior 166f
Epidural venous engorgement, posterior 166f
Epilepsy 178
Epileptiform discharges 48
Epinephrine 11
Episodic migraine, high-frequency 143
Episodic syndromes 82, 86
Episodic tension-type headache 125, 129
Eptinezumab 97
Erenumab 97
Ergot alkaloids 22
Ergotamine 150
   derivatives 107, 150
Euvolemia 49
Exenatide 159
Exercise, regulation of 130
Extensive cortical venous reflux 61f
Extracellular domain 35

F

Falcine artery, anterior 55
Fibromuscular dysplasia 17
Fibrosis 36
Fisher score, modified 47t
Fistula 56
   complete exclusion of 61f
   complete obliteration of 62f
   drainage of 58f
   without cortical venous drainage 55
Fluid-attenuated inversion recovery 2, 41, 57
Flunarizine 91, 119, 150
Fogarty balloon thromboplasty, modified 31f
Foggy vision 83

Foramen magnum 56
Fremanezumab 97
French Headache Society 100
Fungi 11

G

Gabapentin 106, 110, 119, 120, 123
Gadolinium-based enhanced magnetic resonance imaging 166
Galcanezumab 97, 106
Gamma-aminobutyric acid 109
Gamma-knife radiosurgery 63
Gastrointestinal disturbance, recurrent 82
Gastrointestinal symptoms 83
Genetic stroke syndrome 34
Gepants 72, 75
   adverse effects of 78t
Giant cell arteritis 11, 21
Glasgow coma scale 47
Gliovascular unit, impairment of 36
Global Burden of Disease 81, 126
Glucagon-like peptide
   receptor agonist 159
   role of 154
Glucocorticoids 159
   role of 154
Granular osmiophilic material 35, 40
Greater occipital nerve 95, 120, 133, 134, 136, 138, 141f, 143, 144, 176
   block 89, 94, 95t, 106, 108, 135, 140, 142t
      injections 144t
      use of 143fc
Growth hormone 155

H

Head pain 129
Headache 21, 34, 65, 66, 66b, 68, 69b, 90, 121, 133, 148, 152, 153, 164
   alarm-clock 147
   associated vertigo questionnaire 171
   attacks, severe 103
   cervicogenic 133, 135, 140, 148, 164
   characteristics 68
   chronic 127t
   cluster 103, 104, 110, 111t, 116-118, 118f, 133, 134, 139, 142, 143, 147, 178
   diagnostic criteria for 67b, 69b
   duration of 67
   episode 126
   exacerbations of 122
   frequency 89, 148
   hypnic 147-149
   impact test 93, 136
   intractable 159
   management of 156, 160
   medication overuse 89, 129, 136, 138, 143

   number of 127
   phenotypes 22
   prevalence of 66t
   preventive management of 180
   primary 72, 140, 147
   secondary 129, 140, 162
   treatment of 174t
Headache disorder 104t, 133, 135, 142, 143t, 174, 175
   classification of 141f, 149t, 157, 164
   international classification of 103, 116, 126, 140, 147, 157, 171, 172
   primary 81
   secondary 162
   treatment of 178t
Headache phase 83
   symptoms during 85
Hearing loss 172
Hematoma 16, 164
   intramural 16
Hemicrania 122t
   continua 116-119, 121-123, 148
      classification of 122
      secondary 122
Hemochromatosis, hereditary 17
Hemodynamic augmentation 49
Hemoglobin optimization 50
Hemorrhage 61
   aneurysmal subarachnoid 46, 51
   cortical subarachnoid 2f
   intracerebral 21, 66, 67, 67b
   intracranial 56
   intraventricular 47
   ischemic 21
Hemorrhagic infarction 28
Henoch–Schönlein purpura 11
Heparins 32
Hiccups 164
High-flow oxygen therapy 105, 107
Histoplasma 11
Hodgkin's lymphomas 11
Hormonal alterations 83
Hormonal dysregulation 153, 154
Hormone, antidiuretic 84
Human immunodeficiency virus 11
Hydrostatic indifference point mechanism 163
Hygromas 164
Hypercapnia 155
Hyperemia 165
Hyperhomocysteinemia 17
Hypertension 1, 2f
   benign intracranial 29, 30f, 152
   chronic venous 57, 57f
   intracranial 163
Hyperthyroidism 155
Hypnic headache 147-149
   diagnosis of 149t
Hypoliquorrhea 162
Hypoparathyroidism 155

Hypoperfusion 18
Hypothalamic activation, observation of 177
Hypothalamic deep brain stimulation 120
Hypothalamus 177
   lateral 134
     paraventricular nucleus of 134
   posterior 111
Hypothyroidism 155

I

Ibuprofen 119, 123
Idiopathic intracranial hypertension 152, 153*t*, 156*f*, 157, 157*t*
   diagnosis of 152
   management of 152, 158*fc*, 160
   symptoms 153
   treatment trial 158
Immune thrombotic thrombocytopenia, vaccine-induced 32
Immunoglobulin 164
   G 98
Immunosuppression 32
Indomethacin 116, 119, 150
Infection 11, 164
   spread of 31
Inferior obliquus capitis muscle 95
Inflammatory peptides 72
Interleukin-1 47
Internal carotid artery 4, 18, 58, 61
Internal cerebral artery 55
Intra-arterial therapies 6
Intracranial arteriovenous malformations 54
Intracranial atherosclerotic disease 9
Intracranial dissections 16
Intracranial dural arteriovenous fistula 54
Intracranial hemorrhage, substantial risk of 56
Intracranial pressure 57, 152, 154, 157
   reducing raised 28
Intrathecal therapies 49
Intravascular lymphoma 11
Intravenous immunoglobulin, high-dose 32
Invasive central neuromodulation 177
Invasive neuromodulation 175*t*
Ipsilateral cranial autonomic
   signs 103
   symptoms 103
Ischemic stroke, symptoms of 67
Isolated cortical vein thrombosis 30, 30*f*

J

Joint hypermobility, excessive 163
Jugular venous sinus thrombosis 155

K

Kawasaki disease 11
Ketoprofen 119
Kidney stones 158

L

Lactic acidosis 10, 37
Lacunar lesions 40
Lacunar lesions site 40
Lamotrigine 120
Language 83
Large venous infarcts, pathogenesis of 27*f*
Lasmiditan 74, 79
Lesser occipital nerve 112, 134, 143
Leukoencephalopathy 34, 36, 37, 41, 68
Lidocaine 130, 142
   maximum dose 142
   patches 119
Listeria 11
Lithium 106, 108, 109, 120, 150
Local muscle tension, action of 93
Loop diuretics 159
Lower motor neuron 168
Lower segment cesarean section 5
Low-grade dural arteriovenous fistulae 55
Lumbar puncture 156, 163
Lumen stenosis, progressive 36
Lyme disease 11
Lysergic acid diethylamide 22

M

Macular ganglion cell layer 155
Magnesium 173
Magnetic resonance angiography 5, 57
Magnetic resonance imaging 4, 5, 57, 149, 157, 165
Malaria 11
Marfan syndrome 17, 163
Mastoid
   infection 155
   process 136
Medial dural tentorial branch 55
Melatonin 106, 108, 109, 119, 123, 150
Ménière's disease 172
Meningeal artery
   middle 58, 62
   posterior 55
Meningeal diverticula 163
Meninges penetrate 94
Meningitis 21
   serosa 152
Meningocortical biopsy 10*f*, 13
Methylprednisolone 95, 142
Methysergide 120
Mexiletine 119
Microvascular decompression 111, 119
Middle ear infection 155
Migraine 10, 36, 38, 42, 81, 82, 86, 87, 87*t*, 96, 126, 134, 134*f*, 142, 143*fc*, 147, 148
   abdominal 86
   acute 72, 76*t*, 135
   aura-triggered seizure 82
   chronic 82, 89-91, 93*t*, 95*t*, 96, 97*t*, 98-100, 127, 133, 136, 138
   chronification 90, 100
   classification of 82*b*
   complications of 82
   confusional 86
   criteria for 90
   episodic 89, 98, 99, 138
   familial hemiplegic 82
   headache, subtype of 170
   hemiplegic 82, 86
   non-headache symptoms of 84*t*, 87
   number of episodes of 127
   pathology 73
   pathophysiology of 73
   phases of 83*t*
   physical function impact diary 99
   postdrome 85
   prevention of 78*t*, 178
   preventive treatment in 99*fc*, 136
   probable 82
   side-locked 122, 122*t*
   symptomatology, pathophysiology of 84*f*
   treatment for 137*t*
   variants 86, 86*t*
Migraine disability assessment 99
   scale 136
   score 74
   test 138
Migrainous infarction 82
Milrinone 50
Minocycline 155
Mirtazapine 130
Mitochondrial encephalomyopathy 10, 37
Mitochondrial inheritance 37
Mixed connective tissue disease 11
Molecular pathology 36
Monoamine oxidase inhibitors 107
Monoclonal antibody 98*t*, 103, 110, 133
Monogenic hereditary small vessel disease 34
Monro–Kellie doctrine 163
Monthly headache days 138
Mood changes 85
Movement disorders 164
Moyamoya disease 9, 17
Mucormycosis 11
Multigene panel 41
Multiple cranial nerve blocks 139
Multiple sclerosis 172
Multiple thrombosed cortical veins 30*f*
Muscle relaxants 130
Mycoplasma 11

Myelography 166
Myocardial infarction 106, 107
Myofascial trigger points 127

N

Nalidixic acid 155
Naproxen 119, 123
Nasal decongestants 21
Nausea 149, 153
Near-infrared spectroscopy 48
Neck
   discomfort 84
   muscle areas 93
   pain 153
      worsening 164
   stiffness 83
Neoplasms 11
Nerve 38
   blocks 94
   root avulsions 163
Nerve stimulation
   device, transcutaneous vagal 98
   transcutaneous
      electrical 130
      supraorbital 98
      vagal 98, 178
Neural crest group 54
Neuralgias 140
Neurochemical systems 84t
Neurocysticercosis 11
Neurogenic locus notch homolog protein 3 40
Neuroimaging 12f
Neurological diseases 86
Neuroma, acoustic 172
Neuromodulation 89, 98, 111t, 174, 174t, 175, 176f
   theoretical mechanisms of 175
Neuropeptide Y 84
Neuroprotective mechanisms 49
Neuropsychiatric symptoms 38
Neurosarcoidosis 164
Nicardipine 46, 49, 50, 119
   microparticles 49
Nitric oxide synthase 84
   inhibitors 131
Nitrofurantoin 155
N-methyl-D-aspartate 109
   receptor 130
Nociceptive flexion 128
Nocturnal headache, hypertension-related 147
Non-headache symptoms 83t
   differential diagnosis of 87t
   management of 87
Nonhemorrhagic neurological deficits 56
Non-Hodgkin lymphomas 11
Noninvasive central neuromodulation 179
Noninvasive neuromodulation devices 178t, 180

Noninvasive peripheral neuromodulation 178
Noninvasive vagus nerve stimulation 111, 120, 178
Nonpharmacological therapies 98
Nonrapid eye movement 148
Nonsteroidal anti-inflammatory drugs 119, 129, 135, 136, 150, 173
Non-vitamin K antagonist, safety of 32
Noradrenaline 84
Norepinephrine reuptake inhibitors 2
Normal saline 136
Nortriptyline 91
Nucleus tractus solitaries 176
Numerical pain rating scale 136
Numerical rating scale 95
Nummular headache 148

O

Obesity 154, 157
   role of 153
Obstructive sleep apnea 152, 155
Occipital cortex 29
Occipital nerve
   blocks, role of greater 133
   innervation 133
   stimulation 111, 112, 119, 120, 176
Occipital neuralgia 133, 140
Occipital protuberance 136
Ocular motor nerve palsies 164
Olfactory branches 55
Oligoclonal bands 37
Onabotulinum toxin A 99
Open skull defect 144
Ophthalmic artery 61f
Ophthalmic vein, superior 57
Opioids 90
   endogenous 130
Optic nerve
   bilateral 156f
   sheath fenestration 159
   tortuosity 155, 156f
Optical coherence tomography 152, 154
   role of 155
   vision using 29
Oral anticoagulants 32
Oral contraceptives 21
Oral steroids 105
Orbitofrontal hematoma, right 61f
Orthostatic
   headache 162, 164
   hypotension 164
Osmophobia 83, 134
Osseous spinal pathology 163
Osteogenesis imperfecta 17
Osteophytes 163
Otoconia 172
Oxcarbazepine 119
Oxygen 150
   inhalation 150

P

Pain
   local 144
   mild-moderate background 118f
   scale score 136
Papaverine 50
Papilledema 57f, 155
   assessment of 155
   bilateral 156f
   monitoring of 155
Parasites 11
Parenchymal lesions 28
Parkinsonism 164
Paroxysmal disorders 86
Paroxysmal hemicrania 116-119
   classification of 119
   pathophysiology of 123
   secondary 119
Partially empty sella 156f
Periaqueductal gray 84, 134
   matter 176
Pericallosal branches 55
Pericranial tenderness 127
Perioptic subarachnoid space, distension of 155
Peripapillary retinae, deformation of 155
Peripartum period 1, 3
Peripheral electrical
   neuromodulation 179
   stimulation 178, 78t
Peripheral nerve 144
   block 119, 120, 133, 134f, 140, 141f, 143t, 144, 179
Peripheral vascular disease 106
Peripheral vasoconstriction 50
Peripheral vestibular dysfunction 173
Periventricular gray 177
Permissive hypertension 49
Petrosal sinus, inferior 61
Pharmacological treatment 91
Pharmacotherapy, acute 129
Phonophobia 68, 83, 134, 149, 153
Photophobia 83, 134, 149, 153
Physical therapy 130
Physiological brain 175
Pial-dural connections 55t
Piriform cortex 134
Piroxicam 119, 123
   derivatives 119
Pituitary adenylate cyclase-activating peptide 84
Pituitary apoplexy 24
Pituitary gland, hyperemia of 165f
Polyarteritis nodosa 11
Polycystic kidney disease, autosomal dominant 17, 163
Polycystic ovarian syndrome 154
Positron emission tomography 48, 123
Postdrome, symptoms during 82, 85
Postdural puncture headache 140

Posterior reversible leukoencephalopathy syndrome 3
Postpartum
 period 17
 state 2
Postural orthostatic tachycardia syndrome 164
Postvenous sinus thrombosis 154
Preeclampsia symptoms 38
Pregabalin 119
Pregnancy 2, 17, 144
 complications 38
Preimplantation genetic testing 43
Prenatal testing 43
Pressure pain threshold 138
Proinflammatory cytokine release 93
Prophylactic medications, consumption of 94
Prophylactic medicines 150, 150t
Prophylaxis 48
Propranolol 91, 91t, 92
Pseudopapilledema, diagnosis of 155
Pseudotumor cerebri 152
Psychiatric
 comorbidities 126
 disturbances 38
 illness 86
Pulsatile tinnitus 153

R

Radicular pain 153
Radiofrequency lesioning 111
Radioisotope cisternography 167
Radiosurgery 111
Randomized controlled trial 91, 107, 111, 139, 176
Rapid eye movement 148
Reactive oxygen species 35
Refractory disease 159
Refractory vasospasm 50
Regular neurological monitoring 48
Remote electrical
 neuromodulation 178
 stimulation 179
Renal failure 155
Respiratory disorders 155
Reticulum, endoplasmic 35
Retinal migraine 82
Retinal nerve fiber layer 155
Retinoids 155
Reversible cerebral vasoconstriction syndrome 1, 2, 4-6, 17, 21, 22
 diagnostic criteria of 2b
 precipitating factors for 2b
Rheumatoid arthritis 11
Rho-kinase inhibitor 50
Riboflavin 173
Rickettsia 11
Rimegepant 75, 77-79

Rituximab 10, 32
Rizatriptan 173
Rofecoxib 119, 123
Roller coaster rides 17
Rostroventral medulla 176, 84f
Ruptured intracranial aneurysm 21

S

Saccular intracranial aneurysm 65
Salivatory nucleus, superior 134
Sarcoidosis 11
Seizures 3, 10, 38
 prevention of 28
 treatment of 28
Selective serotonin reuptake inhibitors 2
Semantic memory 38
Sensitization, central 125
Sensory
 disturbances 2f
 hypersensitivity 83
 motor aura 83
Sentinel headaches 65
Septic cerebral venous sinus thrombosis 31
Septic sinus thrombosis 31
Serotonin reuptake inhibitors 2
Sexual activity 22
Short-lasting unilateral neuralgiform headache 119, 121
Short-lasting unilateral neuralgiform headache attacks 118, 119, 121
 with cranial autonomic symptoms 117
  classification of 120
  secondary 120
Short-lasting unilateral neuralgiform headache with conjunctival injection and tearing 118, 177, 149
 classification of 120
 secondary 120
Sigmoid sinus 56
Silver-beaten appearance 56
Single-gene testing 41
Sinonasal cerebrospinal fluid 162
Sinus
 stenosis of 155
 straight 31f
 thrombosis 164
  prevent 61
Sinusitis, complicated 21
Sjögren's syndrome 11, 155
Skin biopsy 42
Skull radiograph 56
Sleep
 disruptions 86
 regulation of 130
Sneezing 17
Sodium valproate 109
Speech 83
Sphenopalatine block 96

Sphenopalatine ganglion 94-96, 112, 134, 175
 blockade 119, 120
 neuromodulation 111
 stimulation 111, 177
Spinal cord 177
 stimulation 177
Spinal imaging 165
Spinal longitudinal extradural collection 165
Spinal pachymeningeal enhancement 166f
Spine
 computed tomography scan of 165
 disorders 163
 magnetic resonance imaging of 165
 surgery 163
Splenius semicapitis muscle 95
Spontaneous intracranial hypotension 162-164
 differential diagnosis of 164b
Sports-related injuries 17
Status migrainosus 135
Stenosis 59
Stenting 19
Steroids 105, 108, 119, 123, 142t
Strenuous physical activity 22
Stria terminals, bed nucleus of 134
Stroke 10, 16, 21, 34, 42, 65, 172
 care, acute 16
 ischemic 67-69
 location, influence of 68
 prevention 19t
 symptoms 18
 syndromes, familial 34
 treatment, acute 18
 types of 66t
 with migraine 34
Stroke-like episodes 10, 37
 syndrome 10
Subadventitial hematoma growth, formation of 17
Subarachnoid hemorrhage 2, 18, 21, 46, 47, 49, 65, 66, 66b
Subarcuate artery 55
Subcortical infarcts 36, 37, 43, 68
Subcortical lacunar lesions 40
Subcutaneous sumatriptan 107
Subdural collections, unilateral 164
Subdural fluid collections 164
Subdural hematoma 21, 164
 left-sided 165f
Subdural hemorrhage 164, 168
Sudden neck movements 17
Suicide headache 103
Sulfonamides 155
Sumatriptan 79
 injection 105
 intranasal 107
 nasal spray 105

Superior sagittal sinus 27f, 30f, 56, 58, 59
  pressure 154
Superior vena cava syndrome 155
Supraorbital nerve 94
Supratrochlear nerve 143
Surgery 63, 163
Surgical management 167
Sympatholytic therapy 50
Syncopal attacks 144
Syndrome of inappropriate antidiuretic hormone 23
Syphilis 11
Systemic angiopathy 36
Systemic infection 31
Systemic lupus erythematosus 11, 155
Systemic sclerosis 11
Systemic vasculitis 11

T

Tachyarrhythmias 50
Takayasu arteritis 11
Tamoxifen 155
Temporal lobe 40
  anterior 35, 41f
Tension-type headache 125, 126, 128, 131, 140, 148, 153
  chronic 127, 128fc, 129
  economic burden of 126
  pure chronic 127
Tentorium cerebelli 56
Testosterone 154
Tetracycline 155
Thalamus 175, 177
Therapeutic plasma exchange 32
Thunderclap headache 1, 21, 22, 22fc, 23, 24
  causes of 21t
Thyroxine 155
Tinnitus 172
Topiramate 89, 91, 91t, 106, 108, 109, 119, 120, 150, 159
Torticollis, benign paroxysmal 82, 86
Toxoplasma 11
Trans medullary vein 57f
Transarterial approach 60
Transarterial route, complications of 61
Transcortical neuromodulation 178
  method 178
Transcranial direct current stimulation 176, 179
Transcranial Doppler 48, 51
  ultrasonography 48
Transcranial magnetic stimulation 98, 176, 178, 179
Transient ischemic
  attack 19, 34, 36, 37, 40, 65, 66, 69, 106, 107
  episodes 38
  stroke 36
Transient visual obscuration 153, 164
Transluminal balloon angioplasty 50
Transverse sinus 58f
  right 57f
  stenosis 155
Trapezius muscles 94
Trauma 163
  mild 163
Triamcinolone 142
Trigeminal autonomic cephalalgias 103, 116, 118f, 139, 147, 148, 175
  classification of 117b
Trigeminal ganglion 134
Trigeminal innervation 133
Trigeminal nerve 134
  intracisternal portion of 111
  microvascular decompression of 119
  stimulation, external 178, 178t
  supraorbital branches of 178
  supratrochlear branches of 178
Trigeminal neuralgia 120, 121
  ablation of 119
Trigeminal nucleus caudalis 108
Trigeminocervical complex 84, 133, 134, 175
Trigeminovascular system 73, 133
Trigger point injections 130, 138
Triptans 72, 107, 135, 150
Tuberculosis 11, 164
Tumor necrosis factor alpha 47
Turner syndrome 17, 155

U

Ubrogepant 75, 78
Ultrasonography-guided approach 94
Uncal herniation 164
Underlying cause, treatment of 156, 157
Upper limb symptoms 2f
Upper respiratory tract infection 78
Urinary tract infection 78
Urokinase 49

V

Vaccine stimulates neoantigen formation 32
Vagal nerve stimulation 112, 119, 178
Valproic acid 91, 92
Valsalva maneuver 153
Vascular diseases 17
Vascular Ehlers–Danlos syndrome 17
Vascular flap, presence of 16
Vasculitic pattern 12
Vasoactive intestinal peptide 84
Vasoactive medications 2
Vasoconstriction, treatment of 6
Vasogenic edema 31f
Vasograde score 47t
Vasopressors 49
Vasospasm 46, 52
  predictors of 47
  risk of 47
Vasovagal attacks 144
Venous flow, restoration of 27
Venous hypertension 61, 155
Venous infarcts 29
Venous outflow angioarchitecture 55
Venous sinus stenting 159
Venous stroke 69, 69b
Venous thrombosis 61
Verapamil 50, 106, 108, 109, 119, 123, 139, 150
Vertebral artery 55
Vertigo 164
  benign paroxysmal 82, 86, 172
  episodes of 172
  medication-induced 172
Vessel perforation 61
Vestibular migraine 170, 172, 172b, 173
  diagnostic index 171
  probable 172b
Vestibular paroxysmia 172
Vestibular rehabilitation 173
Vestibular schwannoma 172
Vestibular symptoms 83
Visual analog scale 118, 138
Visual aura 83
Visual impairment, prevention of 156, 158
Visual obscuration 153
Visual snow 85
Vitamin A 155
Vomiting 153
Voxel-based morphometry 128

W

Whiplash injury 17, 163
White matter edema 57f
William syndrome 17

X

X-linked recessive 37

Y

Yawning 83

Z

Zavegepant 75, 77, 78
Zolmitriptan 173
  intranasal 105, 107